Emotions and Health, 1200–1700

Studies in Medieval and Reformation Traditions

VOLUME 168

The titles published in this series are listed at brill.com/smrt

Emotions and Health, 1200–1700

Edited by

Elena Carrera

BRILL

LEIDEN • BOSTON
2013

Cover illustration: "Ira." *Theatrum sanitatis*, facsimile of Ms. 4182 of the Biblioteca Casanatense in Rome, ed. Manuel Moleiro Rodríguez (Barcelona, 1998), cxc. Courtesy: Wellcome Library, London.

Library of Congress Cataloging-in-Publication Data

Emotions and health, 1200–1700 / edited by Elena Carrera.
pages cm. — (Studies in medieval and Reformation traditions)
Includes bibliographical references and index.
ISBN 978-90-04-25082-6 (hardback : alk. paper) — ISBN 978-90-04-25293-6 (e-book)
1. Emotions—Health aspects—History. 2. Emotions—Early works to 1850. 3. Emotions in literature. 4. Medicine and psychology—History. I. Carrera, Elena, editor of compilation.

RC455.4.E46E465 2013
362.19689—dc23

2013014421

This publication has been typeset in the multilingual "Brill" typeface. With over 5,100 characters covering Latin, IPA, Greek, and Cyrillic, this typeface is especially suitable for use in the humanities. For more information, please see www.brill.com/brill-typeface.

ISSN 1573-4188
ISBN 978-90-04-25082-6 (hardback)
ISBN 978-90-04-25293-6 (e-book)

This book is printed on acid-free paper.

MIX
Paper from responsible sources
FSC® C109576
FSC
www.fsc.org

Printed by Printforce, the Netherlands

CONTENTS

ACKNOWLEDGEMENTS

First and foremost, I wish to express my gratitude to the contributors for their expertise and their commitment to this edited volume, which began life as a symposium on this theme held at the Queen Mary Centre for the History of the Emotions in 2010. I would like to thank the Wellcome Trust for its generous support of our Centre's activities and for funding a sabbatical leave during 2010–2011, which allowed me to carry out the research I present here. I thank Thomas Dixon, Rhodri Hayward, Colin Jones and many other colleagues at Queen Mary for providing a most stimulating, supportive and convivial research environment. Thanks also to CUA press for granting permission to reproduce, in Nicholas Lombardo's chapter, material from various parts of his *The Logic of Desire: Aquinas on Emotion* (Washington, D.C.: The Catholic University of America Press, 2011), with some adaptations and additions. Finally, I thank Andrew Gow and Ivo Romein at Brill for their enthusiastic support, and the anonymous reviewers for their helpful and encouraging comments.

London
September 2012

LIST OF FIGURES AND TABLE

NOTES ON CONTRIBUTORS

NICOLE ARCHAMBEAU is Lecturer in History and Religious Studies at the University of California, Santa Barbara. She has published on experiences of war and plague, and on anxiety and confession in the fourteenth century, and is currently completing *Body and Soul under Siege: Surviving Plague, War, and Anxiety in Southern France.*

ELENA CARRERA is Senior Lecturer in Spanish Golden Age Culture at Queen Mary University of London, and has published on the history of emotions, the history of madness, and mysticism. She is the author of *Teresa of Avila: Authority, Power and the Self in Mid-Sixteenth Century Spain* (Legenda, 2005).

PENELOPE GOUK is Honorary Research Fellow at the University of Manchester. She has published extensively on early modern conceptions of music, including *Music, Science and Natural Magic in Seventeenth-Century England* (Yale University Press, 1999), and on music and emotion, in *Representing Emotions: New Connections in the Histories of Art, Music and Medicine* (Ashgate, 2005), jointly edited with Helen Hills.

ANGUS GOWLAND is Reader in Intellectual History at University College London. His research focuses on early-modern ideas about melancholy and dreams, and the interaction in this area between medicine, ethics, theology and politics. He is the author of *The Worlds of Renaissance Melancholy: Robert Burton in Context* (Cambridge University Press, 2006).

NICHOLAS E. LOMBARDO, O.P., is Assistant Professor of Theology at The Catholic University of America in Washington, D.C., and author of *The Logic of Desire: Aquinas on Emotion* (CUA Press, 2011).

WILLIAM F. MACLEHOSE is Lecturer in History of Medieval Science and Medicine at University College London. His research focuses on the connections between medical, natural philosophical, and religious thought in western Europe during the twelfth and thirteenth centuries. He is the author of *A Tender Age: Cultural Anxieties over the Child in the Twelfth and Thirteenth Centuries* (Columbia University Press, 2008).

MICHAEL R. SOLOMON is Professor of Romance Languages at the University of Pennsylvania. He is the author of *The Literature of Misogyny in Medieval Spain* (Cambridge UP 1996) and *Fictions of Well-Being: Sickly Readers and Vernacular Medical Writing in Late Medieval and Early Modern Spain* (University of Pennsylvania Press, 2010).

ERIN SULLIVAN is Lecturer and Fellow at the Shakespeare Institute, University of Birmingham, where she works on the relationship between medical, religious and literary culture in Renaissance England. She has published work in *Cultural History* and *Studies in Philology,* and is currently completing *Beyond Melancholy: Sadness and Selfhood in Renaissance England.*

INTRODUCTION

The history of emotions has become a complex field of research since Carol Stearns and Peter Stearns compellingly argued in 1985 that the study of emotional experience in the past needed to distinguish between the prescriptive guidelines provided in advice handbooks and actual experiences and expressions of emotion.[1] William Reddy's emphasis since 1997 on the performative value of emotional words and gestures (his notion of 'emotives') and his historical approach to emotional styles, together with Barbara Rosenwein's introduction of the concept of co-existing 'emotional communities' which change over time, have helped to establish new paradigms for looking at a wide range of sources, beyond advice manuals and books of manners, to find evidence of prevailing sets of emotional norms in different social and cultural contexts from the past.[2] As Reddy noted in a recent interview, the history of emotions has opened up new approaches to social, cultural and political history, rather than producing a specialized field of research.[3] This collection of essays takes a new look at prescriptive and descriptive discussions of emotions in the context of medical advice circulating in Europe between 1200 and 1700 (the gap between the periods studied by Rosenwein and Reddy), also considering some of the co-existing theological, religious and philosophical discursive representations of emotional experience, related to alternative explanatory models of health and well-being.

The proposal made by Peter and Carol Stearns to separate between cultural paradigms and actual experience of emotion was at odds with

1 Peter N. Stearns and Carol Z. Stearns, "Emotionology: Clarifying the History of Emotions and Emotional Standards," *American Historical Review* 90 (1985): 813–36; *Anger: The Struggle for Emotional Control in America's History* (Chicago, IL: University of Chicago Press, 1986). See also Peter Stearns, *Jealousy: The Evolution of an Emotion in American History* (New York: New York University Press, 1989); *American Cool: Constructing a Twentieth-Century Emotional Style* (New York: New York University Press, 1994).

2 William Reddy, *The Invisible Code: Honor and Sentiment in Postrevolutionary France, 1815–1848* (Berkeley, CA: University of California Press, 1997); *The Navigation of Feeling: A Framework for the History of Emotions* (Cambridge: Cambridge University Press, 2001); *The Making of Romantic Love: Longing and Sexuality in Europe, South Asia, and Japan, 900–1200 CE* (Chicago: Chicago University Press, 2012); Barbara Rosenwein, *Emotional Communities in the Early Middle Ages* (New York: Cornell University Press, 2006).

3 See Jan Plamper, "The History of Emotions: An Interview with William Reddy, Barbara Rosenwein, and Peter Stearns," *History and Theory* 49 (2010): 237–65.

the Foucauldian emphasis on the self as a discursive construct, and the increasingly audible voices in the 1980s of cultural anthropologists claiming that there is no experience of emotion outside of culture. Among the latter, Catherine Lutz raised serious concerns about the fact that emotions had been primarily conceived of "as pre-cultural facts, as features of our biological heritage that can be identified independently of our cultural heritage," and urged scholars to expand the domains in which emotions should be studied, shifting away from "the supposedly more permanent structures of human existence—in spleens, souls, genes, human nature, and individual psychology" and looking instead at history, culture, ideology, and transient human goals.[4] In assuming that the existing conceptualizations of emotion had emphasized their status as pre-cultural facts, Lutz did take a presentist approach. She did not take into consideration, for instance, the acute awareness of inherited explanatory paradigms of health and well-being shown in medieval and early modern Aristotelian and Galenic discussions of states such as anger, fear, joy, sadness or shame as being related both to transient goals (their cognitive component) and to changing bodily qualities (their physiological manifestation). As this volume will show, medieval and early modern Galenic authors saw physical, emotional and spiritual health and well-being as being based less on innate physiological factors than on a balanced lifestyle. They consciously drew on authoritative texts to account for the ways in which people's particular experiences of moderate and immoderate passions could both alter and be altered by their fluctuating physiological states.

Since Lutz made her influential claims, a rapidly growing number of historical and cultural studies have recognized the historicity of emotion and have explored a wide range of historical sources in search of clues about the changing ways in which societies (or social groups) have shaped the experience, interpretation and expression of emotions, and about the kinds of emotional regimes they have promoted.[5] It is perhaps time to

---

[4] Catherine Lutz, "Emotion, Thought, and Estrangement: Emotion as a Cultural Category," *Cultural Anthropology* 1 (1986): 287–309 (287, 297–98). See also the seminal collection of essays, Rom Harré, ed., *The Social Construction of Emotions* (Oxford: Basil Blackwell, 1986).

[5] Among the most notable studies, see Reddy, *The Navigation of Feeling*; Penelope Gouk and Helen Hills, eds. *Representing Emotions: New Connections in the Histories of Art, Music and Medicine* (Aldershot: Ashgate, 2005); Rosenwein, *Emotional Communities*; Thomas Dixon, *From Passions to Emotions: the Creation of a Secular Psychological Category* (Cambridge: Cambridge University Press, 2006); Fay Bound Alberti, ed., *Medicine, Emotion and Disease, 1700–1950* (Basingstoke: Palgrave Macmillan, 2006); Susan Broomhall, ed., *Emotions in the Household, 1200–1900* (Basingstoke: Palgrave Macmillan, 2008); Piroska Nagy

reconsider the changing historical relationship between categories such as 'emotion' and 'health' and explore how they have been associated with highly durable (though now obsolete) categories such as the humours, the spirits and the sensitive soul.

This collection of essays examines some of the significant roles attributed to the emotions in pre-modern Europe. For instance, while Aquinas saw the emotions as signs of virtue, the Neostoic approaches revived in the late Renaissance saw them as signs of moral impairment. In the Galenic medical approaches prevailing well into the seventeenth century they were considered as lifestyle factors which could be beneficial or harmful to health, depending on their intensity. The essays thus seek to revisit some of the most longstanding conceptual structures within which the medieval and early modern notions of emotion were inscribed. In using the label 'emotions' in the title of the volume, the contributors do not assume that it refers to a universal and ahistorical set of categories or a universally recognizable set of states. The label, however, provides a practical means of examining pre-modern discussions of the prevailing medical and philosophical categories of 'passions,' 'accidents of the soul,' 'passions of the heart,' 'movements of the soul,' 'affections of the mind,' 'affects' and 'perturbations,' as well as descriptions, formulations and evaluations of states conventionally referred to in terms such as grief, sorrow, sadness, despair, anxiety, fear, terror, anger, wrath, pleasure and joy in Latin or in other medieval and early modern European languages. In this introduction, I aim to show how this collection of essays contributes to furthering the vibrant field of the history of medieval and early modern 'emotions.' After mapping out the most significant recent publications in the field, I will provide an outline of each of the essays, and then go on to draw out the key themes and arguments with which the volume as a whole engages.

Reddy's approach to the history of emotions since the Enlightenment fruitfully crosses traditional disciplinary boundaries between history, anthropology, cognitive psychology and neuroscience.[6] The essays edited by Penelope Gouk and Helen Hills establish insightful links between the

---

and Damien Boquet, eds, *Le sujet des émotions au Moyen Âge* (Paris: Éditions Beauchesne, 2009); Ute Frevert, *Emotionss in History—Lost and Found* (Budapest/New York: Central European University Press, 2011); Frevert *et al.*, eds, *Gefühlswissen: Eine lexikalische Spurensuche in der Moderne* (Frankfurt am Main: Campus, 2011); Jonas Liliequist, ed., *A History of Emotions, 1200–1800* (London: Pickering and Chatto, 2012).

[6] Reddy, *The Navigation of Feeling.*

ways in which emotions have been represented in art, music and medicine from the fourteenth to the twentieth century. The collection edited by Susan Broomhall explores the affective ties and displays of emotion within extended domestic communities in central and northern Europe between the thirteenth and the eighteenth centuries.[7] Looking at the early modern contexts of politics, art, literature, medicine, religion, philosophy and education, the volume edited by van Jan Frans Dijkhuizen and Karl Enenkel shows how, in this period, emotional suffering was inextricably linked to physical pain.[8] The collection edited by Jonas Liliequist examines medieval and early modern repertoires and representations of emotion, primarily in French and English literature, though it also offers some insights into art and music theory, and covers the less studied geographical areas of Greenland, Sweden and the Ottoman Empire.[9] Reddy's most recent contribution to the history of emotions focuses on the courtly love phenomenon in twelfth-century Europe, contrasting it to the representation of sexual practices in twelfth-century South-East Asia and in Heian Japan.[10] The present collection of essays seeks further to contribute to the opening up of the fields of medieval and early modern history of the emotions and medical history by exploring their intersections with theology, religion, history of beliefs, drama, music, and moral and natural philosophy. It focuses on views and practices in western Europe, though it also seeks to acknowledge the huge influence of Islamic medical authors like Avicenna.

In discussing the pre-modern understanding of the emotions as movements of the sensitive soul within the body, this collection of essays builds on the existing scholarly explorations of the link between emotions and the body, such as Gouk and Hills's, Dijkhuizen and Enenkel's, and Bound Alberti's.[11] In seeking to provide a greater understanding of the medieval and early modern perceptions of the interaction of body and soul than is currently available, it takes into consideration the most influential

---

[7] Broomhall, ed., *Emotions in the Household, 1200–1900.*

[8] Jan Frans van Dijkhuizen and Karl A. E. Enenkel, eds, *The Sense of Suffering: Constructions of Physical Pain in Early Modern Culture* (Leiden and Boston: Brill, 2009).

[9] Liliequist, ed., *A History of Emotions, 1200–1800.*

[10] Reddy, *The Making of Romantic Love.*

[11] Gouk and Hills, eds., *Representing Emotions;* van Dijkhuizen and Enenkel, eds, *The Sense of Suffering*; Bound Alberti, ed., *Medicine, Emotion and Disease.* See also her more recent monograph, Bound, *Matters of the Heart: History, Medicine and Emotion* (Oxford: OUP, 2010).

monographs on emotion in the pre-modern period.[12] In covering both the late medieval and early modern periods, it aims to show the continuity of ideas on the interaction of body and mind, and on the embodied soul as a purposeful composite, across a wide range of cultural discourses: scholasticism, Galenic medical texts, popular accounts of visions and experiences involving the imagination, religious narratives related to canonization inquests, moral and philosophical texts drawing on Aristotelian, Neoplatonic and Neostoic traditions, discussions on music, and ephemeral publications such as the London Bills of Mortality.

In the first essay in the collection, Nicholas Lombardo offers an overview of the key concepts of passion and affection in Aquinas in their historical context, and analyses how they relate to Aquinas's larger theological project and his understanding of psychological health and virtue. He shows how Aquinas defined the passions as involving both the soul and the body (producing bodily alterations) in prompting action in response to a perceived good or evil, and distinguished them from intellectual affections, which only involved the soul (the will), though he also stressed the interaction between affections and passions in experiences like wilful joy. He demonstrates that, while endorsing the Aristotelian notion of passion as receptiveness to being acted upon by a perceived stimulus, Aquinas emphasized that the passions are also active expressions of the sense appetite's inclinations and movements oriented towards a *telos*. In response to the existing evaluations of Aquinas's views on the passions as negative, Lombardo furthermore argues that Aquinas understood imperfection and deficiency in Aristotelian terms as potentiality, allowing for movement and dynamism, and notes how he even claimed that, when oriented towards human flourishing, pleasure can strengthen the use of reason, while moderate fear can focus the mind, and that sorrow and anger, if moderate and appropriate, can be marks of virtue.

The social dimension of emotional experience, its expression and its amenability to change is the focus of Nicole Archambeau's essay, which looks at first- and third-person accounts of the inconsolable sorrow

[12] Among them, Gowland's *The Worlds of Renaissance Melancholy* (Cambridge: Cambridge University Press, 2006) and Schmidt's *Melancholy and the Care of the Soul* (Aldershot: Ashgate, 2007) established with great clarity the medical, religious and political contexts which shaped the early modern fascination with melancholy. For studies which relate medical theory to cultural practices, see Gail Kern Paster, *Humoring the Body: Emotions and the Shakespearean Stage* (Chicago: University of Chicago Press, 2004); Gail Kern Paster, Katherine Rowe and Mary Floyd-Wilson, *Reading the Early Modern Passions: Essays in the Cultural History of Emotion* (Philadelphia: University of Pennsylvania Press, 2004).

and inner struggle of Lady Mathildis de Sault (a noblewoman in mid-fourteenth-century Provence who lost her baby daughter) in the context of the canonization inquest which shaped the narratives. Archambeau discusses the inquest descriptions of this noblewoman's extreme sadness, and her avowed desire to kill the wet nurse, against the background of references to sorrow and despair as causes and symptoms of insanity produced in Montpellier in the early fourteenth century. She also refers to prevailing aristocratic social codes and practices related to revenge, and to spiritual discourses of sin and forgiveness which might have shaped Lady Mathildis' interpretation of the desire to kill as a sinful temptation, helping her to transform her sorrow into a healthier, more acceptable mental state.

Taking a close look at the history of medical ideas on fear, William MacLehose examines the discussion in medical texts written between the first and the fourteenth centuries of the relation between body, mind and accidents of the soul in the disease known as 'incubus.' He shows how the medieval medical approach to the 'incubus' saw it as a nosological category which included both bodily sensations (suffocation, paralysis, inability to speak) and mental and emotional responses (particularly fear), and how medieval medical authors sought to explain the somatic and emotional aspects of the condition through the role of the brain and fantasy or imagination. While the literary and folkloric traditions of a demon known as an incubus who attacks people in their sleep are well-known, MacLehose's analysis focuses on the connections made in scholastic medicine between sleep and emotions, and between the humoral composition of the body and the functionings of the mind and soul.

In view of recent scholarly debates about emotions as either biological phenomena requiring interpretation or as mental processes based on cognitive evaluations, Elena Carrera argues that medieval and early modern medical writers tended to stress the two-way interaction between cognitive processes and physiological alterations in the events they referred to as 'accidents of the soul,' 'passions of the heart' or 'affections of the mind.' Departing from the existing critical emphasis on explaining the early modern passions as the effect of humoral imbalances and temperament, she discusses medieval and early modern medical accounts of the passions as movements of spirit (a subtle bodily substance distilled from the blood), which could cause significant temperamental and bodily changes. She examines in particular the views on anger, its dependence on physiological disposition, and its effects on bodily and mental health discussed in handbooks for physicians, manuals for surgeons, regimens of health and plague tracts, circulating in Latin, English, Spanish, French, German, Catalan and Portuguese between 1250 and 1700. Analyzing the nuanced distinctions made in some medical texts between different types of anger, their qualities, intensity and external manifestations, she demonstrates that, despite the general view that excessive anger was detrimental to health, the therapeutic value of moderate anger was also acknowledged.

Focusing on the vernacular dissemination in late medieval and early modern Spain of medical ideas on the seemingly related concepts of coitus and love, Michael Solomon points out that traditional medical advice on coitus did not usually refer to love or desire, but simply stressed the need for regular and moderate evacuation of bodily fluids as part of a healthy lifestyle or regimen. By contrast, plague treatises tended to emphasize the detrimental effect of excessive coitus, either arguing that it made people more susceptible to contagion, or simply recommending complete sexual abstinence without any further explanation. Regimens of health typically referred to happiness, sadness, anger and fear as the movements of the soul which should be regulated as part of a healthy lifestyle, and very few medical texts mentioned love among those movements of the soul. When medical authors discussed love, they presented it primarily as a disease or ailment, characterized by an obsessive fixation on the beloved, which could be treated through a number of distracting techniques such as travelling and spending time with friends. Solomon suggests that the rise of vernacular medical treatises in the late medieval and early modern period tended to conflate the medical distinction between love and coitus, providing new health-preserving imperatives that allowed lay readers to cast their affective desires in the form of widely accepted concepts of health and hygiene.

Moving on to late sixteenth- and early seventeenth-century England, Erin Sullivan examines the notion of death from sorrow in medico-philosophical treatises, mortality records and popular drama, and argues convincingly that the idea of dying of a broken heart was not simply accepted as a dramatic convention, but was believed to be a real physiological danger. Showing how medical texts described sadness as taking place in the soul and the body simultaneously, involving first the brain and then the heart, placing a strain on it by drying, contracting, dulling and sometimes extinguishing the vital spirits, Sullivan also looks at social historical evidence of the perceived effects of sadness on the body and mind. She provides a detailed analysis of the significant presence of the category 'grief' (meaning both physical pain and emotional distress) among all the causes of death entered in the extant weekly and yearly London Bills of Mortality from the years 1629–1660, relating it to the scant available information about the social contexts of deaths from grief. She also takes into account the wider background of philosophical views on the impact of friendship on health in discussing how stage representations tended to underline the inefficacy of stoic moral counsel, and stress the therapeutic value of expressing sadness to a sympathetic listener and the detrimental effects of the lack of sympathy.

Offering a broad intellectual historical perspective on emotion in early modern Europe, Angus Gowland examines medical, moral philosophical and spiritual notions of the human self and subjectivity. Drawing on a Foucauldian conception of the subject as being discursively constituted within a network of relations of power and knowledge, he differentiates between 'selfhood' as what is idiosyncratic to an individual (e.g., his or her temperament or unique mixture of humours) and 'subjectivity' as a non-individuated, generic set of characteristics, potentialities, operations and actions (i.e. the functionalist Galenic notion of natural capacities versus diseased states, or the Aristotelian conception of the ensouled body engaging in sequences of activities). In exploring the relationship between theories of body and soul within the dominant orthodox Galenic medicine and Aristotelian faculty psychology, he shows how these were negotiated and reshaped in the Renaissance, when Platonic, Neoplatonic, Aristotelian and Neostoic identifications of the rational self (or intellect) as an inner locus of authenticity co-existed with the Aristotelian notion of the human subject as an embodied social being, with Ciceronian and Senecan moral conceptions of the self, and with Christian ideas about the will and the conscience. He then examines how the Renaissance melancholic subject was constructed by such disparate discourses as a morally impaired rational animal with imperfectly actualized potentialities, intense desires and a depraved will, and how melancholy was seen as a condition of corruption and dysfunction, characterized by a deranged imagination and extreme emotional perturbations, though it was sometimes associated with inspired states of self-alienation.

Revisiting the medical notions of spirit and the passions, Penelope Gouk establishes significant connections between a number of crucial Renaissance and early modern approaches to the effects of music on the body and soul via the spirit. While the philosopher Francis Bacon (d. 1626) and the physician Richard Brocklesby (d. 1797) saw the power of music as an object of experimental research aimed to improve medical practice, Thomas Wright (d. 1620) considered it as a means of redirecting the passions to good ends and the Neoplatonist philosopher and physician

Marsilio Ficino (d. 1499) conceptualized it as a spiritual medicine appropriate only to a minority of scholars. Nonetheless, as Gouk shows, they all stressed that music has a stronger effect than anything else transmitted through the senses, and that the motion of music can alter the passions by replenishing the spirits or by composing their disordered movements. Brocklesby and Ficino stressed the value of music as a therapeutic tool and a means of prolonging life, and Bacon explained how musical sounds, through sympathetic vibration, could both arouse and moderate passions. Noting how the four authors endorsed the medical belief that moderate passions are beneficial to health (in strengthening the spirits, condensing them and maintaining their gentle heat), Gouk also discusses the links between the medical notion of the spirits, religious views on divine inspiration, and Stoic, Neoplatonic and Newtonian notions of the *spiritus mundi*.

These eight essays offer complementary evidence and interpret it from different angles, shedding nuanced light on a number of themes, which are still hotly debated among historians of emotion, and which are of particular relevance in understanding medieval and early modern views on the passions and accidents of the soul: 1) emotions and emotion terms as objects of historical study; 2) the question whether historical representations and discussions of emotion might have been influenced by a combination of culturally specific and cross-cultural goals and values; 3) the extent to which 'emotional communities' can be seen as social groups belonging to well-defined historical contexts or as trans-historical ideological groups; 4) the impact of language in defining context-bound emotion categories and constructing subject positions in relation to them; 5) the emotions as interactions of mind and body.

Emotions as Categories of Study

A recent dominant trend within psychology has followed Paul Ekman in focusing on a basic set of six emotions (anger, fear, disgust, surprise, happiness and sadness) which can be understood as genetic (rather than learnt) physiological states, manifesting in universally recognizable facial expressions and bodily gestures. One of the two main questions posed by such an approach is whether taxonomies (or classifications of different types of emotion) can travel across cultures. The other question, discussed in greater detail in the last section of this introduction, is whether emotions can be understood as physiological states only.

Within the discipline of psychology, Ekman's assumption that facial expressions can be innately recognized as being associated with particular emotions has not gone unchallenged.[13] In the wider community of scholars of emotion, Ekman's views have been criticized as 'universalist,' and seen to be diametrically opposed to the claims made by social constructionists since the 1980s about the importance of ritual practices and collective performance in shaping emotions as learnt processes.[14] The gap between these two dominant trends has been filled in by cultural historians like Gail Kern Paster, Katherine Rowe and Mary Floyd-Wilson, who emphasize the importance of studying culture-specific variation in the expression of emotion, arguing that the scientific approach to objectively measurable emotional output propounded by behavioural and evolutionary psychologists like Ekman is too reductive.[15] It has also been bridged by social scientists who have advocated a non-reductive social constructionist perspective, acknowledging that some emotions involve raw organic processes and that some of their physical expressions can be seen as universal, though arguing that they can only be known or discussed through language. Among them, Graham Richards has suggested that emotions are not 'natural phenomena' which can be seen or experienced as they really are, and that therefore the most compelling scholarly task is to examine how emotions, as "fundamentally incoherent biological states," are given meaning and a structure by reference to observable 'public-world phenomena' and to the verbal categories available.[16]

In historical studies of emotion, one cannot rely on directly observable 'public' (or external) references, though one can pay attention to the structuring role of significant events and prevailing ideas. It can be challenging

---

[13] Paul Ekman, "Basic Emotions" and "Facial Expressions," in *Handbook of Cognition and Emotion*, ed. T. Daglesih and M. J. Power (New York: John Wiley & Sons Ltd., 1999), 45–60, 301–20; see also his earlier review: "Cross-Cultural Studies of Facial Expression," in *Darwin and Facial Expression: A Century of Research in Review*, ed. Paul Ekman (New York: Academic Press, 1973), 169–222. One of the most prominent critics of Ekman within psychology is James A. Russell, who argues that similar facial movements found in comparable situations in different cultures are best described as social behaviours, rather than emotions; "Is There Universal Recognition of Emotion from facial Expression? A Review of the Cross-Cultural Studies," *Psychological Bulletin* 115 (1994): 102–41.

[14] See, for instance, Rosenwein's criticisms of the approaches promoted by Ekman's followers and by life scientists as universalist and 'presentist,' in Plamper, "The History of Emotions," 253.

[15] *Reading the Early Modern Passions*, 3–4.

[16] Graham Richards, "Emotions into Words—Or Words into Emotions?," in *Representing Emotions*, ed. Gouk and Hills, 49–68 (49, 52); see also Dixon, " 'Emotion': The History of a Keyword in Crisis," *Emotion Review* 4:4 (2012): 338–44.

to ascertain how words and categories might have been used in particular social and cultural contexts, even though it is possible to reconstruct the immediate lexical contexts of a number of significant textual documents. In using textual evidence, one option is to focus on 'emotion words,' as Rosenwein has shown, looking at the prevalence of certain emotion terms in early medieval texts like moral treatises and funerary inscriptions in connection with the values of the social groups in which those texts were produced.[17] It is also possible to focus on explaining differences between pre-modern categories and our own, as the recent volume edited by Paster, Rowe and Floyd-Wilson has done, seeking to demonstrate that "taxonomies of emotions do not track or translate across cultures or historical periods."[18] However, while placing the emphasis on difference, this collection of essays also seeks to acknowledge how certain categories such as the 'accidents of the soul' and the 'spirits,' which have become obsolete or reinterpreted in our scientific era, had been successfully tracked and successfully translated across cultures and historical periods in the past.

Cross-Cultural Goals and Values

Despite the existing scholarly emphasis on the culturally specific ways in which emotions are experienced, expressed, interpreted and represented, and despite the short-terms goals to which individual and collective experiences of emotion might be related, it is still possible to conceptualize the function of emotion as being attachable simultaneously to short- and long-term goals, and to culture-bound and cross-cultural values. For instance, looking at the evidence presented by Archambeau, we can see how short-term goals (like Mathildis' desire to kill the wet-nurse in response to the death of her baby) may be situational, while long-term goals such as attaining acceptance or long-lasting well-being, might be shared by a wider emotional community across geographical and chronological boundaries. This, however, does not mean that long-lasting goals or values can be seen as universal, or can be universally recognized. For example, the modern concept of 'acceptance' may have a similar structure to what a noblewoman from fourteenth-century Provence may call

[17] See Rosenwein's account of her methodological approach in Plamper, "The History of Emotions," 250–54; see also Rosenwein, "Emotion Words," in *Le sujet des émotions*, ed. Nagy and Boquet, 93–106.

[18] *Reading the Early Modern Passions*, 4.

'mercy,' though the two concepts are embedded within different sets of culturally specific values: the modern notion of 'acceptance' comes with a post-psychoanalytic cultural baggage, while Methildis' concept of mercy, as Archambeau shows in her essay, can be seen as part of a Christian 'cultural script.'

Furthermore, it is possible to see how emotions do not simply have culturally specific manifestations, but are also interpreted in terms of personal goals and evaluations, which are embedded within social values. For instance, in the medieval and early modern medical texts discussed by Carrera in this volume, a man's desire for revenge was usually associated with anger, while in the canonization inquest examined by Archambeau, Mathildis' vengeful desire to kill was associated with sorrow, rather than anger. One of the competing explanations for why this might have been so is the prevalence in medieval culture of the Aristotelian assumption that women lacked the necessary physiological heat to be able to experience proper anger. Another explanation was the general belief that excessive anger was sinful, a recurrent theme in medieval and early modern theology.

Together, the essays show that, among the numerous competing goals and values which might have shaped how medieval and early modern people experienced their passions, the most enduring value and goal across cultures and time boundaries was health, or well-being. However, they also show that there were significant differences between co-existing medical views on how the passions might be understood as symptoms or causes of disease, and how they might also contribute to curing diseases of contrary qualities. While most of the medical treatises examined by MacLehose, Solomon, Sullivan and Gowland emphasize more the negative impact of excessive passions, some of the medical authors examined by Carrera promoted the positive value of moderate passions. Moderation also appears to be crucial in the four different cultural contexts examined in Gouk's essay, in which music was seen as an effective way of moderating the passions, as a means to prevent disease and premature death.

Emotional Communities

In explaining her notion of 'emotional community' as applicable to any social group with common interests and goals, and shared emotional styles and valuations, Rosenwein suggests that the terms used by Aquinas in his discussion on the passions in the *Summa theologiae* can be assumed to have been valid not only to the community of his immediate disciples, but also more generally "across the entire thirteenth and fourteenth centuries in Western Europe."[19] However, in a more recent essay (2012), she offers an alternative reading of Aquinas, arguing that his views on love were grounded on the systematizing approaches to its theological function by earlier scholastics, and that his theory of emotions did not constitute a turning point because "he did not catalyse an emotional transformation."[20] The fact that Aquinas' views on the passions do not seem to have had a direct impact on thirteenth-century society does seem to question the universal validity of the phrase 'emotional communities' as an analytical tool in writing the history of the emotions. As Rosenwein notes, the existing attempts to write larger narratives based on turning points is "unsatisfactory or incomplete."[21]

Part of the problem is that theories of emotions are not really amenable to socio-historical analysis. Nonetheless, in the light of Lombardo's discussion in this volume, we can see Aquinas' systematic account of the passions as a significant landmark in the history of ideas, while acknowledging that his views co-existed with other relevant (theological, philosophical, medical and popular) interpretations. Writing from a theological perspective, Lombardo shows how, despite using terms of emotion similar to those of his contemporaries, Aquinas gave them a different value. For instance, his interpretation of sexual pleasure was at variance with that of other influential theologians, like Bonaventure. Yet his attempts to give all moderate passions a positive value were not appreciated by the Dominicans in his immediate context.

Looking at Aquinas' arguments in the wider framework of medieval ideas presented in this volume, we can see how his emphasis on moderation was shared by influential medical authors such as Arnald of Villanova, who, like him, were trained in scholasticism. Aquinas' recommendations on how taking a nap or having a bath might help when one is too sad might seem at odds with modern readings of his theology. Yet, they show his awareness of prevailing therapeutic practices and beliefs (i.e., that the dry and cold qualities of sadness could be counteracted by the moisture and warmth gained from having a bath) which were both embedded in his historical context and also connected with older, enduring interpretative frameworks: Hippocratic and Galenic regimens of health.

---

19 Plamper, "The History of Emotions," 253.

20 Rosenwein, "Theories of Change in the History of the Emotions," *A History of Emotions*, ed. Liliequist, 7–20 (18).

21 "Theories of Change," 7.

While Aquinas' views on the positive value of the passions might not have been much appreciated in the thirteenth century, they had a marked impact among philosophers and spiritual writers in the Renaissance, who drew directly on his treatise on the passions of the soul. In establishing relationships between ideas propounded by authors belonging to different social contexts, the notion of 'emotional community' can still be useful beyond the framework of historical analysis of social and political change in which Rosenwein first used this phrase. One can perhaps evoke here her image of "smaller circles" representing subordinate emotional communities, partaking in a larger emotional community, a larger circle intersecting with other circles.[22] Even though some of the texts discussed in this volume were produced within fairly defined social and ideological communities (like the thirteenth-century Provençale social elite in Archambeau's essay), their ideas can also be considered in relation to wider intersecting cultural traditions, such as Galenism, folk medicine or Christianity, which had a common long-term goal: promoting well-being.

Language, Emotion and Subjectivity

The idea that emotions can only be known or discussed through language has encouraged historians of emotion to look for the terms which were available and had a particular explanatory value in referring to emotional states. In doing this, the contributors to this volume also recognize the importance of context in defining how the terms were used. For instance, Archambeau draws attention to how the emotion terms she examines (e.g., *tristicia, dolore* and *consolacio*) were shaped by the requirements of the canonization inquest in which they were recorded. MacLehose shows how the popular use of the term 'incubus' to refer to the experience of being attacked at night by a supernatural creature contrasts with the medical interpretation of the phenomenon as being caused in the sufferer's body and mind. Carrera shows how terms like anger and wrath derived distinct meanings from the available translations of authoritative texts by Galen. Sullivan argues that, despite the different contextual meanings of the terms 'grief,' 'sorrow' and 'sadness' in modern English, they are used interchangeably in the medical texts and the plays she examines. Gouk distinguishes between the different contextual meanings of the term

22 Rosenwein, *Emotional Communities*, 24.

'spirit' in early modern medicine, religion and natural philosophy, while showing that those meanings were not completely separate.

Some of the essays also explore the ways in which the terms available offered positions from which people might be able to interpret their own subjectivity. Solomon suggests that the popularization of medical texts on lovesickness encouraged people to experience unrequited love and unfulfilled sexual desire as a malady, and to see sex as its main cure. Looking at discursive constructions of melancholic subjectivity, Gowland examines how the term 'melancholy' was used in medicine, moral philosophy, political thought, natural philosophy and theology to refer to the sub-human condition of being subject to irrational impulses and disturbing emotions, being thus unable to form adequate relationships with other individuals, with the community, with nature and with God.

Emotion, Soul and Body: The Mind

In looking at the impact of verbal categories across medieval and early modern cultures, this collection of essays attempts to show the endurance of the Aristotelian and Galenic understanding of passions such as anger, fear, sadness and joy as cognitive and physiological events, located in the soul (or the mind) and the body simultaneously. The Latin phrase *accidentia animae* (literally, 'the things that happen to the soul') referred to the functions of the soul related to embodied human life, rather than to the theological concept of the immortal soul. It was translated into English first as 'accidents of the soule,' and later as 'accidents of the mind,' 'affections of the mind' and 'passions of the mind.'

The various notions of soul discussed in the essays in this collection relate primarily to either a Platonic or an Aristotelian tradition. In the Platonic tradition represented by the metaphysical works of Ficino, the human soul was considered to be the knot binding the higher realm of God and mind with the lower realm of quality and matter (the body). In the Aristotelian tradition endorsed by Galenic medical writers the human being was thought of as a body-soul composite. Some very influential authors, like Avicenna and Aquinas, straddled both traditions. Aquinas drew on Christian revisions of Aristotle to explain the 'passions of the soul' (*animales passiones*) as involving the soul's functions related to embodied life (sensation, perception, imagination and movement towards a goal), and thereby producing bodily change (*transmutatio corporalis*). He also explained that the kind of joy or love which can be attributed to the human intellect (*appetitum intellectivum*), and to disembodied beings like God and the angels, are simply acts of will (*actum voluntatis*); they are not passions because they do not involve bodily change.[23] While theologians like Aquinas wrote both about the soul as an immortal immaterial entity and about the soul's capacities related to embodied life, Galenic physicians focused on the latter.

The Latin term *mens* was used in medieval and Renaissance philosophy and theology to refer to the human immaterial intellective power; namely, the capacity to go beyond the body's potentialities and dispositions to connect with celestial beings (God and the angels) through contemplation. By contrast, the term 'mynde' was used in medieval and Renaissance medical texts in English (as equivalent to the Latin terms *animus* and *anima*) to denote the types of experiences which we categorize today as either 'cognitive' or 'emotional.' Thus, the late fifteenth-century English edition of the health guide attributed to Joannes de Burgundia, *Gouernayle of Helthe,* refers to "mynde" in connection with the understanding and with affective states such as 'gladness.'[24] Thomas Elyot includes fear, anger, sorrow, hope, pleasure and displeasure among the "affections of the mynde," and also warns about the negative impact of excessive thinking and worrying ("busynesse of mynde") on the body's vital functions.[25] Well into the seventeenth century, health was characterized both by a lively body and a cheerful mind.

This enduring, though largely understudied, conceptualization of health as involving a cheerful 'mind' seems particularly relevant at a time when the categories of 'emotion' and 'cognition' are increasingly recognized as being inextricably linked. The essays in this collection thus aim to bring to the fore medieval and early modern Aristotelian and Galenic ideas which have not been taken into account in recent studies of emotion, such as that of the theorist Jon Elster. In his classification of emotions in terms of their amenability to scientific study, Elster claims that Aristotle "anticipated the key elements of the modern theories and, moreover, had important insights that have not been rediscovered."[26] His study, however, only goes back to Darwin and William James.

---

23 *Summa Theologiae*, 1a.2ae. 22.3.

24 Joannes de Burgundia, *Gouernayle of Helthe* (London: Caxton, 1490).

25 *Castel of Helth* (London: Thomas Bertheleti, 1539), 69v.

26 Jon Elster, *Alchemies of the Mind: Rationality and the Emotions* (Cambridge: Cambridge University Press, 1998), 48.

Some of the research conducted in 'affective neuroscience' in the last two decades has become closer to the Aristotelian and Galenic approaches by questioning traditional views of cognition and affect as separable (and often opposing) forces or processes within the mind, suggesting that they are interrelated processes, and that their distinction is phenomenological, not ontological.[27] Emphasizing the physiological basis of cognition, affective neuroscientists have located different emotions in different regions of the brain.[28] By contrast, medieval and early modern medical authors saw the interaction between emotion, cognition and action as having a wider physiological basis, and thus explained the passions as movements of subtle bodily spirit between the brain, the heart and the outer surface of the body. Even though research in neuroscience is still focused primarily on locating cognitive and affective functions in particular brain areas (due in part to the methodological restrictions imposed by the use of the existing neuroimaging technology), the paradigms of much of this new type of research have contributed to moving the discussion of emotion beyond the mind-body dualism. It is therefore to be hoped that the new evidence and the thought-provoking arguments presented by the contributors to this volume will move readers across the disciplines of history of medicine, history of ideas, cultural history, sociology, anthropology, psychology and neuroscience to take a fresh look at these old ways of conceptualizing the interaction of mind and body.

Elena Carrera

---

[27] Seth Duncan and Lisa Feldman Barrett, "Affect is a Form of Cognition: A Neurobiological Analysis," *Cognition and Emotion* 21 (2007): 1184–211.

[28] See, for instance, Bruno Wicker, Christian Keysers, Jane Plailly, Jean-Pierre Royet, Vittorio Gallese and Giacomo Rizzolatti, "Both of Us Disgusted in My Insula: The Common Neural Basis of Seeing and Feeling Disgust," *Neuron* 40 (2003): 655–64.

EMOTIONS AND PSYCHOLOGICAL HEALTH IN AQUINAS[1]

Nicholas E. Lombardo

This essay aims to reconstruct the views of Thomas Aquinas on the emotions and psychological health. First, Aquinas's account of the emotions will be presented in its historical context, with special attention to the passions and their relationship to virtue and human flourishing. It will then reconstruct Aquinas's views on the emotions and psychological health, focusing especially on sadness. For Aquinas, our emotions (even seemingly negative ones such as sadness, fear, and anger) are healthy when they operate according to their inner structure and unhealthy when they do not.

The Emotions in Aquinas

When Aquinas finished the *Prima secundae* of the *Summa theologiae* in 1271,[2] questions 22–48 probably constituted the longest sustained discussion of the passions ever written.[3] This *Treatise on the Passions*, as questions

[1] This essay reproduces, with some adaptations and additions, material from various parts of Nicholas E. Lombardo, *The Logic of Desire: Aquinas on Emotion* (Washington, D.C.: The Catholic University of America Press, 2011), xi–xii, 1–20, 34–43, 94–117, 190–198, 201–223, 272. Used with permission.

[2] For a discussion of the historical origins and precise chronology of the *Summa theologiae* and Aquinas's other works, see Jean-Pierre Torrell, *Saint Thomas Aquinas*, vol. 1, *The Person and His Work*, trans. Robert Royal (Washington, D.C.: The Catholic University of America Press, 1996), esp. 146–47, 330–61. On the origins of the *Summa*, see also Leonard E. Boyle, "The Setting of the *Summa theologiae* of Saint Thomas," in *Facing History: A Different Thomas Aquinas* (Louvain-La-Neuve: Fédération Internationale des Instituts d'Études Médiévales, 2000), 65–91, and M. Michèle Mulchahey, *"First the Bow Is Bent in Study": Dominican Education before 1350* (Toronto: Pontifical Institute of Mediaeval Studies, 1998), 278–306. For an accessible introduction to the *Summa* and the history of its reception, see Jean-Pierre Torrell, *Aquinas's* Summa: *Background, Structure, and Reception* (Washington, D.C.: The Catholic University of America Press, 2005).

[3] To my knowledge, the longest sustained discussion of the passions before Aquinas is found in Aristotle's *Rhetoric*, and Aristotle's treatment is neither as long nor as systematic as Aquinas's. Paul Gondreau states that the *Treatise on the Passions* "dwarfs the only known historical precedents [for a systematic treatment of the passions], both of which Aquinas draws upon: Nemesius of Emesa's short treatise on the passions in his *De natura hominis* and, following this, John Damascene's treatise on the same in his *De fide orthodoxa* (Aristotle left us no systematic treatment of the passions)." See "The Passions and the

22–48 of the *Prima secundae* have come to be known, is the culmination of a lifetime of reflection and the centerpiece of a much larger project. Aquinas's attention to the passions spans his entire literary output, beginning with his commentary on the *Sentences* of Peter Lombard, and permeates each part of the *Summa theologiae*.[4] In the *Summa*, he thoroughly integrates his discussion of the passions with his metaphysics and his account of human nature, the desire for happiness, virtue, vice, sin, and grace. Yet most studies of Aquinas on the passions focus almost exclusively on the *Treatise on the Passions* and Questions 80–82 of the *Prima pars*, and do not consider his treatment of the passions vis-à-vis original sin, grace, and specific virtues and vices. In its integration within such an expansive project, the *Treatise on the Passions* is without historical precedent, as is the *Prima secundae*, the section of the *Summa* in which it is found.

Historical evidence suggests that Aquinas began writing the *Summa theologiae* to correct the casuistry prevalent in manuals for confessors and other works of moral theology. He was concerned that the moral theology taught to Dominican students and others had a skewed emphasis on vice and sin and lacked sufficient theological and anthropological context. Consequently, one of Aquinas's principal objectives in writing the *Summa* was to give a balanced foundation for the study of Christian ethics. For this reason, Leonard Boyle suggests that the *Prima secundae*, Aquinas's analysis of human actions and passions *par excellence*, is the heart of the *Summa theologiae*. In any case, nothing comparable to the *Prima secundae*

Moral Life: Appreciating the Originality of Aquinas," *The Thomist* 71 (2007): 419–50, at 426; *The Passions of Christ's Soul in the Theology of St. Thomas Aquinas* (Münster: Aschendorff Verlag, 2003), 106. Servais Pinckaers notes that "to our knowledge, there does not exist in the Fathers nor in the Middle Ages a study of the human passions comparable for its length and its quality. It is a unique, classic work—and is too neglected." See Pinckaer, "Les passions et la morale," *Revue des sciences philosophiques et théologiques* 74 (1990): 379–91, at 379. Simo Knuuttila refers to it as "the most extensive medieval treatise" on the passions; *Emotions in Ancient and Medieval Philosophy* (Oxford: Oxford University Press, 2004), 239. Mark Jordan argues that Aquinas's extended discussion of the passions in the *Prima secundae* constitutes a structural innovation vis-à-vis the work of his predecessors. See Jordan, "Ideals of *Scientia moralis* and the Invention of the *Summa theologiae*," in *Aquinas' Moral Theory: Essays in Honor of Norman Kreztmann*, ed. S. MacDonald and E. Stump (Ithaca: Cornell University Press, 1999), 79–97, at 84–90.

[4] Besides the *Summa*, the most significant places where Aquinas discusses the passions include (listed in approximate chronological order): *Scriptum super libros Sententiarum* II.36, III.15–16, III.26–27, III.34, IV.49; *De veritate* 22.3–4, 25–26; *Summa contra gentiles* I.89–91; *Sententia libri De anima, passim*, esp. III.14; *De malo, passim*; *De virtutibus* 1.4–5, 4.1–2; *Sententia libri Ethicorum, passim*, esp. II.5. Of these, Aquinas's discussion of the passions in the *Scriptum super libros Sententiarum* and *De veritate* 25–26 are probably the most important.

in scope or content existed before Aquinas or during his lifetime. There are contemporary parallels to the *Secunda secundae* and its discussion of particular virtues and vices, such as the *Summa de vitiis et virtutibus* of William Peraldus, and there are parallels to the *Summa theologiae* considered as a whole, notably the *Summa theologiae* of Alexander of Hales, one of the principal models for Aquinas's work, but there are no parallels to the *Prima secundae*.[5] Aquinas's account of the passions also represents an original synthesis of every major thinker available to him, particularly Aristotle, Augustine, Nemesius of Emesa, John Damascene, and his teacher, Albert the Great.[6] When his writings are considered under the rubric of emotion—a modern concept considerably broader than the ancient and medieval concept of passion—the scope of his achievement becomes even more impressive.

Nonetheless, despite renewed interest in emotion among contemporary philosophers and theologians, Aquinas's account of emotion remains neglected. Robert Solomon's anthology of classic texts on emotion, a standard philosophy textbook, does not include anything from Aquinas.[7] Martha Nussbaum gives him only cursory mention in her massive work on emotion.[8] In his book *Aquinas on Mind*, Anthony Kenny criticizes Aquinas's

---

[5] See Boyle, "Setting of the *Summa*," Torrell, *The Person and his Work*, 142–59; and Gondreau, *Passions of Christ's Soul*, 22, 45–46, 107–10. Jordan provides an extended discussion of the originality and historical context of the *Secunda pars* and the relationship between the *Prima secundae* and the *Secunda secundae*, and comes to a conclusion similar to Boyle's about the centrality of the *Secunda pars* to Aquinas's project, suggesting that "any account of the *Summa*'s purposes that fails to explain the unprecedented size and scope of the moral teaching in the work will be an inadequate account." See Jordan, "Ideals of *Scientia moralis* and the Invention of the *Summa theologiae*," 79–97, at 97.

[6] For discussions of Aquinas's sources, and those he deliberately excludes, see Gondreau, *Passions of Christ's Soul*, 101–35; Jordan, "Aquinas's Construction of a Moral Account of the Passions," *Freiburger Zeitschrift für Philosophie und Theologie* 33 (1986): 71–97; and John Patrick Reid, Introduction, notes and appendices to *Summa theologiae*, vol. 21: *Fear and Anger* (London: Blackfriars, 1965), 146–50.

[7] Robert C. Solomon, *What Is an Emotion? Classic and Contemporary Readings*, 2nd edn (New York: Oxford University Press, 2003).

[8] Martha C. Nussbaum, *Upheavals of Thought: The Intelligence of Emotions* (Cambridge: Cambridge University Press, 2003). Although sympathetic to her account of emotion, Carlo Leget expresses surprise at Nussbaum's neglect of Aquinas: "Given, however, Nussbaum's historical interest and the Aristotelian and Stoic traditions she draws upon, it is surprising that in her study hardly any attention is paid to the work of Thomas Aquinas. Aquinas's account not only belonged to the very same intellectual tradition upon which Nussbaum builds; he also composed the most extensive treatise on emotions in his day, one that has had a considerable influence on later Western thought." See "Martha Nussbaum and Thomas Aquinas on the Emotions," *Theological Studies* 64 (2003): 558–81.

account of the passions as forced, derivative, and not entirely coherent, despite his great sympathy for many aspects of his thought.[9]

Interest in Aquinas's account of emotion, however, is growing. Recent studies have made extraordinary statements about Aquinas's influence on subsequent medieval and early modern thinkers. Peter King states that Aquinas "set the agenda for later medieval discussions of the passions" such that "later thinkers could do no better than to begin with his account, even when they disagreed with it."[10] In her book, *Passion and Action: The Emotions in Seventeenth-Century Philosophy*, Susan James devotes a chapter to Aquinas. Of all the medievals, she claims, he exerted the greatest influence on early modern theorists of the passions, and perhaps even eclipsed Aristotle.[11] Eileen Sweeney suggests that Descartes and Hobbes should be understood "as reacting to and constructing alternatives to Aquinas's arrangement of the passions."[12] Thomas Dixon's historical study of the categories of passion and emotion singles out Augustine and

---

[9] Anthony Kenny, *Aquinas on Mind* (New York: Routledge, 1993), 63: "Aquinas divides the sensory appetite into two sub-faculties: one which is the locus of affective drives, and another which is the locus of aggressive drives. It would be unprofitable to follow in detail his justification for this anatomizing; it consists largely of forced assimilation of diverse classifications made by previous philosophers and theologians. Altogether, it cannot be said that Aquinas' treatment of sensory desire is quite coherent." Kenny does, however, express admiration for many aspects of Aquinas's thought, especially his philosophy of mind; see preface, 1–14. Moreover, his earlier influential book on the philosophy of emotion is informed by his engagement with Aquinas; Kenny, *Action, Emotion, and Will* (London: Routledge and Kegan Paul, 1963). Consequently, Kenny's criticism should not be interpreted as a categorical dismissal of Aquinas's account of emotion. While he seems to consider many of its significant features unworthy of much consideration, he does not deny the enduring relevance of Aquinas's philosophical anthropology to contemporary philosophy of emotion.

[10] Peter King, "Late Scholastic Theories of the Passions: Controversies in the Thomist Tradition," in *Emotions and Choice from Boethius to Descartes*, Studies in the History of the Philosophy of Mind, 1, ed. Henrik Lagerlund and Mikko Yrjönsuuri (Dordrecht: Kluwer, 2002), 229.

[11] Susan James, *Passion and Action: The Emotions in Seventeenth-Century Philosophy* (Oxford: Clarendon Press, 1997), 30: "However, the Scholastic interpreter [of Aristotle] who exerted the greatest influence on early-modern theorists of the passions was undoubtedly Thomas Aquinas. His analyses of the differences between activity and passivity, alongside his description and classification of the passions of the soul, were reiterated and discussed throughout the seventeenth century, and may well have been more widely read than Aristotle's own texts."

[12] Eileen Sweeney, "Restructuring Desire: Aquinas, Hobbes, and Descartes on the Passions," in *Meeting of the Minds: The Relations between Medieval and Classical Modern European Philosophy*, ed. Stephen F. Brown (Turnhout: Brepols, 1998), 215.

Aquinas as the two principal representatives of the Christian tradition prior to the early modern period.[13]

Furthermore, a number of analytic philosophers have offered sympathetic reconstructions and appraisals of Aquinas's understanding of the passions.[14] The revival of virtue ethics inspired by Alasdair MacIntyre's *After Virtue* seems partly responsible for much of this interest, since Aquinas is one of the primary representatives of the virtue ethics tradition, and his account of the passions is closely connected to his account of virtue.[15]

There has been a similar renewal of interest in Thomist scholarship.[16] Thomist scholars have always looked to Aquinas as a primary point of

---

[13] Thomas Dixon, *From Passions to Emotions: The Creation of a Secular Psychological Category* (Cambridge: Cambridge University Press, 2003), 26–61.

[14] See Mark P. Drost, "Intentionality in Aquinas' Theory of the Emotions," *International Philosophical Quarterly* 31 (1991): 449–60; Robert C. Roberts, "Thomas Aquinas on the Morality of Emotions," *History of Philosophy Quarterly* 9 (1992): 287–305; Norman Kretzmann, "Philosophy of Mind," in *The Cambridge Companion to Aquinas*, ed. Norman Kretzmann and Eleonore Stump (Cambridge: Cambridge University Press, 1993), 128–59, esp. 144–46; Mark Stephen Pestana, "Second Order Desires and Strength of Will," *Modern Schoolman* 72 (1996): 173–82; Peter King, "Aquinas on the Passions," in *Thomas Aquinas: Contemporary Philosophical Perspectives*, ed. Brian Davies (New York: Oxford University Press, 2002), 353–84; Claudia Eisen Murphy, "Aquinas on Our Responsibility for Our Emotions," *Medieval Philosophy and Theology* 8 (1999): 163–205; Pasnau, *Thomas Aquinas on Human Nature*, 200–64.

[15] Alasdair MacIntyre, *After Virtue*, 2nd edn (Notre Dame, Ind.: University of Notre Dame Press, 1984).

[16] Among the most significant studies in English, see Gondreau, *The Passions of Christ's Soul*, which also offers a survey of Thomist scholarship on Aquinas and human affectivity; Craig Titus, *Resilience and the Virtue of Fortitude: Aquinas in Dialogue with the Psychosocial Sciences* (Washington, D.C.: The Catholic University of America Press, 2006), a pioneering attempt to integrate contemporary psychology with Aquinas's anthropology and ethics.; Kevin White, "The Passions of the Soul (Ia IIae, qq. 22–48)," in *The Ethics of Aquinas*, ed. Stephen J. Pope (Washington, D.C.: Georgetown University Press, 2002), 103–15; Diana Fritz Cates, *Aquinas on the Emotions: A Religious-Ethical Inquiry* (Washington, D.C.: Georgetown University Press, 2009); Robert Miner, *Thomas Aquinas on the Passions: A Study of* Summa Theologiae, *1a2ae 22–48* (Cambridge: Cambridge University Press, 2009). In French, see Pinckaers, "Les passions et la morale," and Jean-Pierre Torrell, *Saint Thomas Aquinas*, vol. 2, *Spiritual Master*, trans. Robert Royal (Washington, D.C.: The Catholic University of America Press, 2003), esp. 244–65; Servais Pinckaers, *Passions et Vertu* (Paris: Editiòns Parole et Silence, 2009). In Spanish, Marcos Manzanedo has written an excellent series of articles in *Studium*, offering a close textual analysis of Aquinas's work on the passions, and giving special attention to the development of his thought over the course of his lifetime. In Italian, Matteo Laghi, "Passio et 'passione' nella letteratura tomista: Riflessioni in merito allo Status Quaestionis," *Divus Thomas* (Piacenza) 103 (2000): 59–92; Constantino Marmo, "Hoc autem etsi potest tollerari: Egidio Romano e Tommaso d'Aquino sulle passioni dell'anima," in *Documenti e studi sulla tradizione filosofica medievale*, vol. 2 (Spoleto, Italy: Centro italiano di studi sull'alto Medioevo, 1991), 281–315; Italo Sciuto, "Le passioni dell'anima nel pensiero di Tommaso d'Aquino," in *Anima e corpo nella cultura medievale*,

reference regarding the passions; nonetheless, until the twentieth century, his treatment of them was neglected, because the centrality of the passions to his anthropology and ethics was insufficiently appreciated.[17] The neglect of Aquinas's treatment of the passions began with Aquinas's contemporaries and immediate successors, who were more interested in his discussion of specific virtues and vices in the *Secunda secundae* than the more abstract anthropological principles found in the *Prima secundae*.[18] It was perhaps its originality that caused it to be overlooked.[19] One of the most popular and influential guides for confessors in the Middle Ages, which was written by a Dominican and sought to popularize the moral teaching of Aquinas, quotes the *Secunda secundae* frequently but only refers to the *Prima secundae* occasionally. While this focus on the *Secunda secundae* is not surprising, considering the work's orientation toward concrete pastoral advice rather than theory, it is consistent with the supposition that even Aquinas's fellow Dominicans did not fully appreciate the relevance of the *Prima secundae*, let alone the *Treatise on the Passions*, to his overall project.[20] Since then, there has been sustained interest in the passions among Thomist scholars and an unbroken chain of scholarship, with varying degrees of attentiveness to non-Thomist philosophy and scientific psychology.[21] During the early and mid-twentieth century, the passions received relatively intense attention before passing into a period of mild neglect. They are now receiving more attention within Thomist

---

ed. C. Casagrande and S. Vecchio (Florence: Edizioni del Galluzzo, 1999), 73–93; and Antonio Stagnitta, *L'anthropologia in Tommaso d'Aquino: saggio di ricerca comparata sulle passioni e abitudini dell'uomo* (Naples: E.D.I. Editrice, 1979). In German, Alexander Brungs, *Metaphysik der Sinnlichkeit: Das System der Passiones Animae bei Thomas von Aquin* (Halle/Saale: Hallescher Verlag, 2002).

[17] Gondreau, *The Passions of Christ's Soul*, 23.

[18] The breakdown of extant manuscript copies of the *Summa* reflects their interests: the *Tertia pars* accounts for 18%, the *Prima secundae* for 20%, the *Prima pars* for 25%, and the *Secunda secundae* for 37%. See Boyle, *Setting of the Summa*, 85–86.

[19] Boyle, *Setting of the Summa*, 85–86.

[20] See Boyle, "The 'Summa confessorum' of John of Freiburg and the Popularization of the Moral Teaching of St. Thomas and Some of His Contemporaries," in *Facing History: A Different Thomas Aquinas* (Louvain-La-Neuve: Fédération Internationale des Instituts d'Études Médiévales, 2000), 50.

[21] Of special note is the work of two Dutch psychiatrists, Anna Terruwe and Conrad Baars, who pioneered the integration of Thomistic psychology with clinical practice. Each published numerous books. A synthesis of their mature thought can be found in Anna A. Terruwe and Conrad W. Baars, *Loving and Curing the Neurotic: A New Look at Emotional Illness* (New Rochelle, N.Y.: Arlington House, 1972). A revised version was republished in two separate volumes: *Healing the Unaffirmed* (Staten Island, N.Y.: Alba House, 1976) and *Psychic Wholeness and Healing* (Staten Island, N.Y.: Alba House, 1981).

circles, in large part due to the scholarship of Servais Pinckaers and Jean-Pierre Torrell, as well as the growing interest of analytic philosophers in both Aquinas and emotion. Nonetheless, as Torrell notes, the *Treatise on the Passions* "has scarcely attracted the attention of moralists," and, as Mansfielld has suggested, "perhaps no aspect of Aquinas's moral theory has been more neglected than his treatment of the *passiones animae*."[22]

The Place of Emotion in Aquinas's Theological Project

Despite the neglect of Aquinas's account of emotion, it is not an exaggeration to say that emotion is central to his theological project. Aquinas's account of emotion centers on his account of desire. In turn, it is desire that gives the *Summa theologiae* its *exitus-reditus* structure: Aquinas begins with God and then traces how creation flows from God's desire and returns to him through ours. Consequently, to follow the theme of emotion through the *Summa* is to follow the guiding principle around which Aquinas organized his most mature thought. The *Summa* is often compared to the great cathedrals of the Middle Ages for its vast structure and its comprehensive synthesis of so many component parts. Looking at the theme of desire and emotion is like stepping away from the many side chapels of the *Summa* and looking down the nave.

Desire and emotion are not just central to the structure of the *Summa*: they are central to Aquinas's project and especially his ethics. For Aquinas, ethics is nothing other than the study of human psychology insofar as it flourishes or fails to flourish. Unlike approaches that regard psychology and ethics as two distinct categories that are only occasionally concerned with each other, or perhaps extrinsically related in a calculus where psychological well-being is weighed against doing what is right, Aquinas's approach offers a refreshing synthesis of psychology and ethics. In many popular understandings, there is something paradoxical about divine commandments: God gives us desires and then commands us not to act on them. For Aquinas, there is no paradox, because God commands us *through* the desires he gives us. The commandments of divine revelation are ancillary to our natural inclinations; they are signposts to the fulfilment of desire, shorthand conclusions following from the logic of human nature.

[22] Torrell, *Spiritual Master*, 259; Richard K. Mansfield, "Antecedent Passion and the Moral Quality of Human Acts According to St. Thomas," in *Virtues and Virtue Theory: Proceedings of the American Catholic Philosophical Association* 71 (1997): 221–31, at 221.

The positive role of emotion in Aquinas's theology derives in no small part from the cultural milieu of the Dominican Order to which Aquinas belonged, even apart from the influence of individual Dominicans such as his teacher Albert the Great, who had pioneered the study of Aristotle and the integration of theology with natural science. The order had grown out of an informal band of itinerant preachers devoted to defending the goodness of the material world against the dualistic beliefs of the Cathars of southern France. These origins gave Dominic and his companions an especially acute attentiveness to the goodness of creation. Insofar as they established the government and basic structure of the order, and consciously and unconsciously shaped the distinctive traits of Dominican culture, their legacy undoubtedly influenced Aquinas toward a more pronounced appreciation of creation—and therefore of emotion. His account of emotion, then, in part reflects the cultural dispositions of the early Dominicans. This genealogy underscores its rootedness in practical concerns and the analysis of ordinary human experience, and also helps to explain its balance and humaneness.

Categories of Emotion in Aquinas's Writings

The word "emotion" has no direct parallel in the Latin vocabulary of the thirteenth century.[23] Since the mid-twentieth century, scholars of Aquinas writing in English frequently identify what he calls the passions of the soul (*passiones animae*) with the emotions, translating *passio* as "emotion," rather than the more literal "passion."[24] This translation is seriously misleading. While it is accurate to regard many of the passions as emotions, Aquinas also speaks of affections (*affectiones* or *affectus*) that are not passions and yet clearly correspond to the category of emotion. For example, he speaks about certain kinds of joy or love that he explicitly says are not passions, but clearly should be considered emotions. Moreover, Aquinas also writes about a category called the passions of the body (*passiones*

[23] The closest etymological parallel to emotion in Latin is *motus*, or movement, which is occasionally used in a psychological context (sometimes as *motus animae*) to refer to a movement of the soul; see Dixon, *From Passions to Emotions*, 39–40. It will be argued that the closest parallel in meaning is *affectus* or *affectio*, that is, affection.

[24] Many of the volumes of the Blackfriars *Summa* edited by Thomas Gilby adopt this practice. Eric D'Arcy prefaces his translation of Questions 22–39 of the *Treatise on the Passions* with a detailed explanation for his choice of emotion for *passio*. Sse Introduction and notes to *Summa theologiae*, vol. 19: *The Emotions* and vol. 20: *Pleasure* (New York: McGraw-Hill; London: Eyre and Spottiswoode, 1967, 1975).

corporalis) that encompasses phenomena that we would hesitate to describe as emotions, such as itches, pangs, hunger, and thirst.

For reasons that cannot be discussed here, Aquinas's category of affection (in Latin, *affectus* and its synonym *affectio*) should be seen as corresponding to the contemporary category of emotion.[25] Within his category of affection there are two subgroups. First, there are *passions of the soul*, which are movements of the sense appetite, and therefore involve both the body and the soul. We share these in common with animals. Second, there are *intellectual affections*, which are movements of the will, and therefore only involve the soul. We share these in common with angels and God. According to Aquinas, in ordinary experience, passions of the soul and intellectual affections are tightly interwoven: for example, joy in the will overflows to the sense appetite.

The Passions: Movements of the Sense Appetite

Aquinas writes far more about the passions than about intellectual affections, and his thought about the passions is far more developed and systematic. Moreover, as one would expect, scholarship has focused on his views on the passions. Consequently, the discussion here will focus on Aquinas's treatment of the passions. This section will give an overview of the passions and their relationship to human flourishing, as a prelude to reconstructing the relationship between the emotions and psychological health.

"Passion," writes Aquinas, "is a movement of the sense appetite caused by imagining good or evil."[26] This pithy definition, borrowed from John Damascene and replete with Aristotelian terminology, summarizes Aquinas's understanding of the passions of the soul. A passion is a physiological and psychological response to the apprehension of a sensible good or a sensible evil, that is, an object that is known through the senses, and judged to be either good or evil.[27] It is nothing other than the movement

---

[25] For a discussion of the category of affection in Aquinas and its correspondence with the modern category of emotion, see Lombardo, *The Logic of Desire*, 75–93, 224–29. See also Dixon, *From Passions to Emotions*, 26–61, esp. 40. Dixon's work first drew my attention to the significance of affection in Aquinas vis-à-vis the contemporary category of emotion.

[26] "Passio est motus appetitivae virtutis sensibilis in imaginatione boni vel mali." *ST* I–II 22.3. See also John Damascene, *De fide orthodoxa* 2.22. The translations from the *Summa theologiae* are my own, working in consultation with the English Dominican and Blackfriars translations.

[27] When he discusses the passions, Aquinas often refers to the object of a passion without any qualifier such as "sensible." It is simply an object, or a good, or an evil. However,

of the sense appetite, a passive power, from dormancy to act, in response to the apprehension of an object to which the sense appetite is inclined.[28] There are thus two aspects of a passion: receptivity to a sensible object's stimulation—apprehension of an intention being a necessary precondition for a passion[29]—and movement toward some *telos*. The perceptive and cognitive faculties "present" the finished product of an intention to the sense appetite, and if the intention corresponds to its capacities and inclinations, the sense appetite is triggered and a passion results.

Passion as Receptivity

Passion (*passio*) has a wide range of equivocal meanings in ancient and medieval philosophy and theology, as does its Greek cognate, *pathos*. The word is most commonly used to refer to the passions of the soul, but the passions of the soul constitute only one species of passion. More generally, passion signifies passivity and the "act" of being acted upon. It refers especially to suffering, that is, to ways of being acted upon that are unpleasant because they somehow rub against natural tendencies and inclinations. Cognizant of the ambiguities surrounding the word, Aquinas attempts to clarify matters by rehearsing its various meanings in multiple places in the *Summa theologiae*.[30] The most relevant and thorough discussion is at the beginning of the *Treatise on the Passions*, where Aquinas analyzes three uses of the Latin word *pati* (to suffer or undergo), the verb form of *passio*:

---

it is evident that, for Aquinas, the proper object of the sense appetite is a sensible object. First, in his view that sense appetite responds to sense cognition (see especially *ST* I 81.1), Aquinas makes plain that the objects of sense appetite are known through sense cognition, and thus must be sensible. Second, Aquinas specifies the object of concupiscible passions as "a straightforward sensible good or evil," and the object of irascible passions as "a good or evil that is arduous or difficult" ("bonum vel malum secundum quod habet rationem ardui vel difficilis," *ST* I–II 23.1). See also *ST* I–II 46.3. While Aquinas does not explicitly describe the object of irascible passion as sensible here, it is evident from the context that it is not just an arduous good or evil, but an arduous sensible good or evil. Hence both sorts of passions have sensible objects, according to Aquinas. Nonetheless, it is important to note that concepts and abstract ideals can elicit a response from the sense appetite, insofar as they involve sensible characteristics in the subject's apprehension of them. See Lombardo, *The Logic of Desire*, 90–91.

[28] See *ST* I–II 22.2–3, 41.1, 45.2.

[29] For passion's dependence on apprehension, see *ST* I–II 17.7, 45.4, 62.4, 75.2, 77.1, and for its specific dependence on the apprehension of intentions, see *ST* I 78.4, 81.2–3; and esp. *ST* I–II 22.2.

[30] *ST* I 79.2, 97.2; *ST* I–II 22.1, 41.1.

> First, in a general way, all receiving is passion [*pati*], even when nothing is lost, and so it could be said that the air "undergoes" when it is illuminated. However, this kind of passion is more about *being perfected* than *undergoing*. Second, passion properly means that something is received while something else is lost. This happens in two ways. When something is lost that is not suitable to a thing, just as when the body of an animal is made healthy, it is called "passion" because the animal's body receives health and sickness is removed. In another way, sometimes the opposite happens: getting sick is called "passion" because weakness is received and health is lost. This last case is what is most properly called passion.[31]

Passion, then, is the "act" of being acted upon. It implies the potential to be actualized and thus perfected. Insofar as this potential is bound up in the tendency toward something not yet attained, it also implies a metaphysical deficiency.[32] Just as the term "appetite" encompasses many kinds of inclination, and not just the sense appetite, the term "passion" encompasses many kinds of receptivity. Others had distinguished passion's various meanings before,[33] but Aquinas synthesizes these various meanings into a coherent unity. He also organizes them into a hierarchy of ascending specificity: passion as reception of a quality, passion as reception of a quality in place of another, and passion as reception of an inferior quality in place of another. By doing so, he puts the more negative connotations of passion in a context that lessens their significance.

Then Aquinas applies the three senses of passion outlined above to the powers of the soul:

> Passion can be in the soul in each of these three ways. Regarding the first sort of passion, which involves only reception, Aristotle says that sensing and understanding are a kind of passion. The sort of passion that involves loss always involves bodily change. Passion in this stricter sense is not in the soul except insofar as the composite of body and soul undergoes it. But here again there is a distinction: when the bodily change is for the worse, it

31 "Uno modo communiter, secundum quod omne recipere est pati, etiamsi nihil abjiciatur a re: sicut si dicatur aerem pati quando illuminatur. Hoc autem magis est perfici quam pati. Alio modo dicitur proprie pati, quando aliquid recipitur cum alterius abjectione; sed hoc contingit dupliciter. Qandoque enim abjicitur id quod no est conveniens rei: sicut cum corpus animalis santur dicitur pati, quia recipit sanitatem, aegritudine abjecta. Alio modo quando e converso contingit: sicut aegrotare dicitur pati, quia recipitur infirmitas, sanitate abjecta. Et hic est propriisimus modus passionis." *ST* I–II 22.1.

32 *ST* I–II 22.2 ad 1.

33 In his discussion of the passions, John Damascene also writes about the equivocal meanings of *pathos*. See *De fide orthodoxa* 2.22.

> is even more strictly passion than when the bodily change is for the better. Hence sorrow is more strictly a passion than rejoicing.[34]

The primary attribute of the passions qua passion is their aspect of receptivity. Passion in a stricter and more idiosyncratic sense also involves suffering, and so, according to this schema, sorrow is more properly a passion than joy. This specification, however, does not do much work in Aquinas's system. He does affirm that passion in the strictest sense refers to suffering, and occasionally points out that certain passions are more strictly passions because they involve suffering or the experience of something contrary to nature's most basic inclinations,[35] but this is a linguistic clarification, not a philosophical claim. For Aquinas, love, not sorrow or fear, is the most paradigmatic of the passions. Although he says sorrow and fear are more strictly passions than love and joy, he singles out love as the first of the passions and the source of all the rest.[36] Furthermore, in his discussion of love, Aquinas observes: "The term 'passion' denotes the effect produced in a thing when it is acted upon by some agent," without noting that, in its most strict sense, passion requires suffering.[37] This text seems to supply his actual working definition of passion.

Some scholars interpret the passages discussed above as evidence of a negative view of the passions.[38] Nonetheless, a close reading of the texts in their context suggests the opposite interpretation. First, although he accepts the common meaning of the word "passion" established by centuries of pagan and Christian thinkers (which was more a fact of language than a philosophical axiom), Aquinas subtly shifts its connotation in favor of a more positive signification. By laying out the various meanings of

---

34 "Et his tribus modis contingit esse in anima passionem. Nam secundum receptionem tantum dicitur quod sentire et intelligere est quoddam pati. Passio autem cum abjectione non est, nisi secundum transmutationem corporalem; unde passio proprie dicta non potest competere animae nisi per accidens, inquatum scilicet compositum patitur. Sed in hoc est diversitas: nam quando hujusmodi transmutatio fit in deterius magis proprie habet rationem passionis quam quando fit in melius; unde tristitia magis proprie est passio quam laetitia." *ST* I–II 22.1.

35 *ST* I–II 22.1, 35.1, 41.1. Contemporary use of the word "emotion" seems to involve similar negative associations. While the word "emotion" usually has a neutral connotation, in ordinary language use, we say that someone is emotional if overcome with sorrow or fear or anger—all of which imply something negative—but not so much if filled with joy or energy or hope. We say that someone is emotional when joyful to the point of tears, but even here some latent negative association remains, since such joy implies the loss of self-control and even something phenomenologically similar to sorrow.

36 *ST* I–II 25.2–3.

37 "Dicendum quod passio est effectus agentis in patiente." *ST* I–II 26.2.

38 See, for example, Dixon, *From Passions to Emotions*, 41–42.

passion side by side, as he does repeatedly, he stresses the possible positive connotations of passion and minimizes the negative.[39] In the end, he locates passion's defining characteristic in receptivity rather than suffering.

Second, although Aquinas mentions that passion indicates deficiency (*defectus*), in the context of his metaphysics, or indeed any Aristotelian metaphysics, "deficiency" and "imperfection" are technical terms that do not necessarily have negative connotations. For Aquinas, something can be imperfect and deficient with respect to its ultimate *telos*, or compared to God, but nonetheless entirely intact and morally praiseworthy. Furthermore, imperfection and deficiency in the Aristotelian sense creates the space for movement, dynamism, and some of the more outstanding forms of creaturely excellence. The rational creature is the most dramatic instance of this principle. Unless the rational creature is imperfect—that is, not yet brought to the completion of its being—before it begins to make choices, there would be no room for it to shape its own identity. Lastly, according to Aquinas, God is the only being that does not need anything; every other being is deficient and imperfect insofar as it is dependent on God and other beings. The modern proclivity to interpret dependence as inherently negative can obscure the neutrality of "deficiency" and "imperfection" in Aquinas's metaphysics.

Passion as Movement toward a Telos

Unlike many other forms of passion, the passions of the soul involve more than the experience of being acted upon by some agent; they also move their subject toward its *telos*.[40] As movements of an appetitive power, they are passive and active, not just one or the other.[41] For example, the sense appetite has the capacity to be acted upon by the apprehension of something beautiful (the passive dimension of passion), one consequence

[39] *ST* I 79.2, 97.2; ST I–II 22.1, 41.1. Two of the three meanings Aquinas gives for *passio* have positive or neutral connotations. Sweeney seems to interpret Aquinas's use of the word *passio* in the same way. She suggests that in the *Summa* he employs a rhetorical strategy that downplays the negative connotations of *passio* even while acknowledging them. See Sweeney, "Restructuring Desire," 220.

[40] For a discussion of Aquinas's use of the metaphor of physical movement to describe psychological events, see James, *Passion and Action*, 62–63; Gondreau, *Passions of Christ's Soul*, 209–10; Knuuttila, *Emotions*, 249–51; and especially Carlo Leget, "Moral Theology Upside Down: Aquinas' Treatise *de passionibus animae* Considered through the Lens of Its Spatial Metaphors," in *Jaarboek Thomas Instituut 1999* (Utrecht: Thomas Instituut, 2000), 101–26.

[41] "Appetite both moves and is moved" ("appetitus autem movens motum," *ST* I 80.2).

of which is that the subject may come to desire the beautiful (the active dimension of passion). The words "passion" and "movement" refer to the same reality, but each emphasizes different aspects. The former emphasizes being acted upon; the latter emphasizes moving in such a way that the perfection of the subject is advanced or safeguarded.

Aquinas's account of the passions cannot be understood without reference to both their active dimension and their passive dimension, but their active dimension is primary and more central to his account. Although the sense appetite encompasses the capacity to enjoy (or suffer) present sensible objects, it is principally an inclination toward sensible objects, irrespective of whether they are already possessed or not. "Sense appetite," Aquinas writes, "is an inclination responding to sense apprehension (*apprehensionem sensitivam*)."[42] So too are the passions that are its movements. "An act of an appetitive power is a kind of inclination,"[43] and the passions, insofar as they are acts of the sense appetite, are inclinations toward sensible objects. The primary function of the passions is not to allow sensible objects to act upon us, although of course they do that, but to incline us toward the perfection of our nature. Aquinas's view that the passions are *movements*, rather than *qualities*, was a minority position in his lifetime—Albert the Great among others disagreed with it—and remained a minority position after Aquinas's death.[44]

Disagreement among medieval thinkers about whether the passions constitute movements or qualities, or both, derives in large part from study of Aristotle's *Categories*. In his discussion of the category of quality, Aristotle first names the passions as the third genus of quality, but then he goes on to note that there are some sorts of passions that are not qualities.[45] What Aristotle seems to be getting at is the difference between moods that are more or less stable, and thus qualities, and sudden flashes of passion, which are not qualities. The uncertainty of Aristotle's meaning is heightened by an ambiguous remark by Boethius in his commentary on the *Categories*, which leads many to interpret Aristotle as holding that the passions are always qualities.[46] Albert follows this line of interpretation and argues that the passions are not movements, even though John Damascene imprecisely calls them movements, but rather what are left

42 *ST* I 81.2.

43 *ST* I–II 15.1: "actus appetitivae virtutis est quaedam inclinatio."

44 Knuuttila, *Emotions*, 248–55.

45 *Categories* 8, 9a–10a.

46 Knuuttila, *Emotions*, 237.

from movements.[47] Pleasure, for instance, is not itself a movement, but is left from a movement that alters the soul.[48] Despite Albert's position and the dominant interpretative tradition that he represents, Aquinas holds firmly to a sense of passion as movement and makes it one of the cornerstones of his account of the passions. By thus affirming the literal sense of John Damascene's definition of passion as a movement of the sense appetite, Aquinas seems to be closer to Aristotle's original meaning in the *Categories* than Albert. Whereas Albert's view of the passions as qualities implicitly emphasizes their receptivity and how they color our experience of the world, Aquinas also emphasizes the way the passions carry us toward our *telos*. His commitment to an unpopular position suggests that he found the analogy of movement particularly illuminating, and further indicates that seeing the passions as active expressions of the sense appetite's inclinations is more central to his conception of the passions than their passivity.

Aquinas's attribution of appetite to God also indicates that the inclination toward a *telos* is more essential to the sense appetite than its passivity, because, while he affirms that appetite is found in God, he states that passion is not. God is pure act and perfection itself; passion implies potential not yet actualized and the possibility for improvement; therefore passion cannot be found in God.[49] Passion is present only in creaturely forms of appetite. If passion were more essential to the meaning of appetite than the inclination toward a *telos*, it stands to reason that Aquinas would not have attributed appetite to God.

Nonetheless, some passions considered individually have less of the aspect of movement and consist more in the quasi-contemplative experience of some object, whether that object is perfective of nature or repugnant to it. These passions, such as pleasure and sadness, have more the character of passion (in its most generic sense) than movement (in the sense of moving somewhere) because they are dead ends; they follow the fulfillment or failure of the sense appetite to attain a certain *telos*.[50] Yet even these passions are not without an active element. Pleasure inclines

---

[47] See *De fide orthodoxa* 2.22 and *De bono* III 5.1 ad 8.

[48] *De bono* III 5.3 ad 4.

[49] *ST* I 3.1, 4.1–2, 9.1, 25.1. See also *De potentia* 2.1 ad 1. Regarding Aquinas on the absence of passion in God, see Michael Dodds, *The Unchanging God of Love: Thomas Aquinas and Contemporary Theology on Divine Immutability*, 2nd edn (Washington, D.C.: The Catholic University of America Press, 2008).

[50] Note that, according to this interpretation of Aquinas, pleasure and sadness equally represent the most "passive" of the passions. Contrary to his linguistic clarification in *ST*

the subject toward the maintenance of pleasure, and sadness inclines the subject away from the cause of the sadness. They accomplish this by communicating information insofar as pleasure tells the subject that a *telos* has been attained and sadness indicates that it has not. Sadness, or the experience of the frustration of a given desire of the sense appetite, also inclines the human person to pursue those other desires, including desires of the intellectual appetite, that are still open to fulfillment. Hence the educative and self-transcending consequence often noted about suffering: it inclines us to consider other ways in which fulfillment is still possible despite the suffering. So, in Aquinas's account, even the frustration of appetite (or at least some kinds of frustration of appetite) ultimately moves us toward our *telos*. Taking these resting, quasi-contemplative passions into consideration, we might say that for Aquinas, the passions paradoxically drive us toward passion, that is, toward letting the goods we desire act upon us.

The Passions and Human Flourishing

Aquinas emphatically rejects negative evaluations of the passions, as we see when he disagrees with the Stoic understanding of passion, arguing instead that "the passions are not diseases or disturbances of the soul, unless they are without the moderation of reason."[51] The contrast between Aquinas and some earlier understandings of the passions, both pagan and Christian, is dramatic. Aquinas distances himself from the Stoic view of the passions as intrinsically disordered in favor of the more positive Aristotelian view of the passions as good or evil, depending on whether or not they are guided by reason. However, instead of rejecting the Stoic view outright, he prefers to give their view of the passions a charitable interpretation, suggesting that the difference between the Stoic and Aristotelian views of the passions is more verbal than substantial, even with Cicero's description of the passions as "disturbances of the soul" (*perturbationes animi*, in *Tusculan Disputations*, 3.4). Whatever the validity of his interpretation of Stoic doctrine, Aquinas's intellectual charity should not obscure his firm rejection of the view of the passions as intrinsically disordered. Instead of being obstacles to the *telos* of human existence, the passions

I–II 22.1, sadness is not more passive than pleasure, with respect to the way the passions actually function in his account.

51 "Non enim passiones dicuntur morbi vel perturbationes animae, nisi cum carent moderatione rationis." *ST* I–II 24.2.

are indispensable to its attainment.[52] They are psychic motors driving us toward it.[53]

Numerous modern scholars have made similar observations about the centrality of the passions to human flourishing in Aquinas.[54] The tendency toward specific objects is not an extrinsic feature of the sense appetite; the inclination toward its proper objects "belongs to the very essence of a power."[55] The receptivity of passion is an important aspect of Aquinas's account, but it does not exhaust it, and this receptivity also moves us toward sense goods and their enjoyment.

An important qualification is necessary here. Aquinas does not hold that the fundamental orientation of the passions toward human flourishing implies that each and every movement of the sense appetite reliably directs us toward our proper *telos*. The passions require the guidance of reason, especially in our fallen condition. Paradoxically, however, even when the passions prompt us to act in ways that we ultimately judge inappropriate, in their essential structure, the passions still serve the attainment of our *telos*. The passions require the guidance of reason in order to become virtuous, and thus fully conducive to human flourishing, but virtue also requires the passions. Without the passions, we would not respond to sensible objects, and without this first step toward engaging the world, human flourishing would not be possible. As he argues:

> The moral virtues which are concerned with the passions as their proper matter cannot exist without them. The reason for this is that otherwise it would follow that moral virtue would make the sense appetite indifferent to everything. But virtue does not consist in the passions being subject to

---

52 The placement of the *Treatise on the Passions* shortly after questions 1–5 of the *Prima secundae* (in which happiness is laid out as the end of all human action) manifests the centrality of the passions to human flourishing in Aquinas's anthropology. For a discussion of this point, see Loughlin, "Human and Animal Emotion," 60 n29, and Gondreau, *Passions of Christ's Soul*, 108.

53 The phrase "psychic motors" is taken from Conrad Baars, who uses it to describe the emotions in his Thomistic psychology. See Conrad W. Baars, *Feeling and Healing Your Emotions* (Plainsfield, N.J.: Logos International, 1979).

54 See Pinckaers, "Les passions et la morale;" Thomas Ryan, "Positive and Negative Emotions in Aquinas: Retrieving a Distorted Tradition", *Australasian Catholic Record* 78 (2001): 141–52; Paul J. Wadell, *The Primacy of Love: An Introduction to the Ethics of Thomas Aquinas* (Mahwah, NJ: Paulist Press, 1992), esp. 79–105; Simon Harak, *Virtuous Passions: The Formation of Christian Character* (New York: Paulist Press, 1993); Sweeney, "Restructuring Desire," esp. 218–23; and Gondreau, "The Passions and the Moral Life."

55 "pertinet ad ipsam rationem potentiarum." *ST* I–II 51.1.

> reason, apart from their own proper acts, but rather in the passions executing the command of reason through their own proper acts.[56]

In his view, the function of the passions is not to decide upon a course of action, but to respond to stimuli and prompt the human person to act according to the face value of those stimuli. Then the passions defer to the judgment of reason, because only the rational appetite can command human action, and because the sense appetite naturally tends toward conformity with reason.[57] When rational analysis concludes that acting on a certain prompting of the passions is not conducive to the attainment of our final end, the passions have not failed to offer reliable guidance: they have provided precisely the sort of first-order response and motivation that is their sphere of competence. The passions require education and the elevation of grace for optimal functioning, and various things can warp the passions and their responses to stimuli, most obviously sin and the privation of grace and all their attendant consequences. Nonetheless, in their essential structure, the passions make a crucial contribution in guiding us toward flourishing and happiness.[58]

Aquinas's positive evaluation of the passions and their role in human flourishing pervades his analysis of particular passions. He touts the beneficial effects and inherent goodness of pleasure: it perfects actions,[59] and insensitivity to pleasure is a vice.[60] Unlike some early Christian theologians, Aquinas not only affirms that sexual intercourse was possible in the Garden of Eden, he claims that it would have been more pleasurable, since human nature would have been fully intact and the body more

[56] "virtutes morales quae sunt circa passiones sicut circa propriam materiam, sine passionibus esse non possunt. Cuius ratio est, quia secundum hoc, sequeretur quod virtus moralis faceret appetitum sensitivum omnino otiosum. Non autem ad virtutem pertinet quod ea quae sunt subiecta rationi, a propriis actibus vacent, sed quod exequantur imperium rationis, proprios actus agendo." *ST* I–II 59.5.

[57] For more on the relationship between passion and reason, see Lombardo, *The Logic of Desire*, 94–101.

[58] Gondreau elaborates on Aquinas's view of the passions vis-à-vis our *telos* in "The Passions and the Moral Life," 427–28.

[59] "perficit delectatio operationem." *ST* I–II 33.4.

[60] "Natura autem delectationem apposuit operationibus necessariis ad vitam hominis. Et ideo naturalis ordo requirit ut homo intantum huiusmodi delectationibus utatur, quantum necessarium est saluti humanae, vel quantum ad conservationem individui vel quantum ad conservationem speciei. Si quis ergo intantum delectationem refugeret quod praetermitteret ea quae sunt necessaria ad conservationem naturae peccaret, quasi ordini naturali repugnans. Et hoc pertinet ad vitium insensibilitatis." *ST* II–II 142.1.

sensitive.[61] By contrast, his Franciscan contemporaries Alexander of Hales and Bonaventure argued that the pleasure would have been less.[62] Sorrow can be morally good because, in its inmost nature, it is ontologically good, even though it involves the suffering of an evil.[63]

Aquinas's view of passion and *telos* does not derive from philosophical reflection alone. There is a massive theological premise that is never explicitly stated because it is so obvious: the passions carry us toward our *telos* (and therefore happiness) because they were created by a God who is trustworthy. God is the guarantor of desire. In him, there is a metaphysical basis for welcoming and trusting the passions.[64]

Passion, Reason, and Virtue

Aquinas has a very complex, and fundamentally positive, understanding of the relationship between passion, reason, and virtue as essentially aligned and complementary. Despite the possibility of internal conflict, Aquinas trusts the fundamental orientation of the passions, as well as their capacity to be guided by reason.[65] His positive evaluation becomes more striking when we compare him with his contemporaries and realize that he is consciously staking out a position that stands in opposition to theirs. For example, in the view of Bonaventure, his Franciscan colleague at the University of Paris, the passions lack either an instinctual

---

[61] "fuisset enim tanto maior delectatio sensibilis, quanto esset purior natura, et corpus magis sensibile." *ST* I 98.2 ad 3. See also *Commentaria in quatuor libros Sententiarum*, II 20.1.3.

[62] Bonaventure, II *Sentences* 20, 1.3; Alexander of Hales, *Summa theologiae* I.2 496 (pp. 701–03).

[63] *ST* I–II 39.1–3.

[64] Aristotle was able to arrive at some of these conclusions without theological premises because he sees human fulfillment as the proper operation of all the powers of the human person, and consequently the sense appetite is integral to his understanding of moral virtue. In the *De anima* he discusses the sense appetite and the passions, but his account of the passions is not as systematically related to the sense appetite as Aquinas's, and his lengthy discussion of the passions in the *Rhetoric* is more a phenomenological survey than a discussion of how they lead us toward our flourishing. For Aristotle, the passions should be moderated, not squelched, but not necessarily seen as guiding us toward fulfillment either. Aquinas's faith in a benevolent Creator provides him with theological as well as philosophical reasons to think that our passions, in their inner structure, ultimately guide us toward our *telos*, as long as they are properly moderated by reason. He has more trust in the passions and where they are inclined to take us.

[65] For a similar interpretation of Aquinas's understanding of the passions and their role in the moral life, and how this stems from his view that the passions can be guided by reason, see Gondreau, "The Passions and the Moral Life," esp. 431–42.

drive toward conformity with reason or an intrinsic ordering to human flourishing. They can be forced to submit to reason (*obtemperat rationi*) by an exterior imposition, but their independent dynamism is an inherent threat to virtue.[66] Bonaventure views the autonomy of the passions as a hindrance rather than a help to virtue.

For Aquinas, however, the passions are not a threat to human virtue but an essential component of it, and the ideal relationship between the passions and reason is more fluid. Moreover, while the passions sometimes hinder the use of reason, sometimes they sharpen it, too, since "pleasure that follows the act of reason, strengthens the use of reason," and moderate fear concentrates the mind.[67] Virtue consists not in the forced submission of passion to reason, or the evisceration of passion into something manageable, but the rational ordering of the various faculties toward human flourishing.[68] He builds his account of passion and virtue on this simple but controversial outlook.[69]

For Aquinas, virtue does not involve just reason and will, but also the passions as well. This view crystallizes in the claim that the sense appetite can be the subject, that is, the seat or location, of virtue,[70] which he qualifies by observing that virtue is in the passions only insofar as they participate in reason—"virtue cannot be in the irrational part of the soul, except to the extent that it participates in reason"—and that, therefore,

---

[66] Bonaventure, *Commentaria in Quatuor Libros Sententiarum Magistri Petri Lombardi* (Quaracchi, Florence: Collegium S. Bonaventurae, 1882–89), III 33.1.3 ad 1; Marie-Dominique Chenu, "Les passions vertueuses: L'anthropologie de saint Thomas," *Revue philosophique de Louvain* 72 (1974): 13–16; W. D. Hughes, Introduction, notes, and appendices to *Summa theologiae*, vol. 23: *Virtue* (New York: McGraw-Hill Book Co.; London: Eyre and Spottiswoode, 1969), 245–46; Gondreau, *Passions of Christ's Soul*, 276–81.

[67] Aquinas notes the salutary effects of pleasure in *ST* I–II 33.4 ad 1 and of fear in *ST* I–II 44.4. He discusses how the passions can hinder or sharpen reason in various places, including *ST* I–II 10.3, 33.3, 33.4 ad 1, 37.1, 44.2, 44.4, 46.4 ad 3, 48.3, 77.7. For a discussion of Aquinas's understanding of how passion influences reason, see Uffenheimer-Lippens, "Rationalized Passion and Passionate Rationality," 547–57.

[68] Chenu gives a helpful overview of the importance of the passions to Aquinas and his disagreement with Bonaventure, and also of the neglect and disparagement Aquinas's theories received in his lifetime and afterwards. See Chenu, "Body and Body Politic in the Creation Spirituality of Thomas Aquinas," in *Western Spirituality: Historical Roots, Ecumenical Routes*, ed. Matthew Fox (Santa Fe: Bear and Company, 1981), 193–214.

[69] His outlook remains controversial. It is easy to dismiss Bonaventure as behind the times, but the tendency to regard the passions as *intrinsically* troublesome to rational behavior continues to pervade many ethical traditions, religious and non-religious. For a similar assessment see Chenu, "Body and Body Politic."

[70] *ST* I–II 56.4, 56.5 ad 1.

"reason or mind (*ratio sive mens*) is the proper seat of virtue."[71] He classifies different virtues according to the passions they perfect: "temperance is concerned with the concupiscible passions; fortitude, with fear and daring; magnanimity, with hope and despair; meekness with anger."[72] Even though Aquinas is drawing here on Aristotle, his position was controversial in his time: many of his contemporaries, including Hugh of St. Cher, John of La Rochelle, and Bonaventure, disagreed and located virtue only in the reason and the will.[73] Their position follows from their view of passion as fundamentally irrational, just as Aquinas's more optimistic outlook follows from his view of the passions as fundamentally oriented toward reason's guidance. For them, the various moral virtues describe volitional dispositions to right behavior. For Aquinas, the various moral virtues are holistic character traits with passion and reason inclined (and mutually inclining) toward our *telos*, that is, our perfection as human persons created in the image and likeness of God.

Aquinas rejects the idea that virtue eradicates passion.[74] If disordered, the passions of the soul may incline to sin, "but in so far as they are ordered to reason, they pertain to virtue."[75] Passion is not simply tamed by virtue; ordered passion positively assists the execution of virtuous acts, and "helps the execution of reason's command."[76] Contrary to Stoic philosophy even sorrow can be a mark of virtue when moderate and appropriate.[77] The vehement expression of anger can also be virtuous, as in Aristotle's magnanimous man, "who is open about what he loves and hates and in how

[71] *ST* I–II 55.4 ad 3. Aquinas does not specify much more than this about the precise mechanism by which virtue is present in the passions, but it seems he would hold that it is present especially in the memory, the particular reason, and the body (insofar as the passions affect the body's physical constitution).

[72] "fortitudo est circa timores et audacias; temperantia circa concupiscentias; mansuetudo circa iras." *ST* I–II 60.4. Aquinas's analysis of particular virtues in the *Secunda secundae* includes detailed and interesting discussions of how the virtues intersect with the passions, how one virtue generates passions other than the passions immediately proper to itself (if any), and how the lack of a given virtue has negative consequences in the sense appetite.

[73] See Aristotle, *Ethics* III.10, 1117b23; Chenu, "Les passions vertueuses," 16–18; Hughes, Appendices to *Summa*, 245–46; Gondreau, *Passions of Christ's Soul*, 276–81.

[74] *ST* I–II 59.2.

[75] "passiones animae, inquantum sunt praeter ordinem rationis, inclinant ad peccatum, inquantum autem sunt ordinatae a ratione, pertinent ad virtutem." *ST* I–II 24.2 ad 3. See also *ST* I–II 24.3.

[76] "adiuvat ad exequendum imperium rationis." *ST* I–II 59.2 ad 3.

[77] *ST* I–II 59.3.

he speaks and acts."[78] There is also a sense in which virtuous passions impart "affective knowledge" that assists moral decision making, so that the right choice is selected not just by the judgment of reason, but by the instinctual response of passion.[79] In sum, virtue does not eradicate the passions but produces ordered passions, that is, passions actively oriented toward human flourishing.[80]

Consequently, when it is well-ordered, intense passion is a mark of intense virtue. It indicates that the will is powerfully inclined toward the good, and that the sense appetite has been thoroughly suffused with right reason. "The more perfect the virtue," Aquinas writes, "the more it causes passion."[81]

Christology and the Passions

The portrait of Christ in the Gospels is another important source for Aquinas's evaluation of the passions. In his view, Christ assumed ordinary human affectivity for our instruction (among other reasons), to show us what virtuous affectivity looks like, and therefore what it looks like to be truly human. He takes the instructive role of Christ's affectivity seriously, and sometimes mentions it when discussing the passions. For instance, he argues that sorrow must be compatible with virtue, because Christ experienced sorrow in the Garden of Gethsemane.[82] Elsewhere he argues that anger is not always sinful, because Christ was angry.[83] Christ's example is not the only reason that he thinks sorrow and anger are compatible with virtue, but he sets it forth as particularly authoritative, since he is writing for a Christian audience.

The influence is not unidirectional: his evaluation of Christ's passions often refers back to his *Treatise on the Passions*. At one point, for example, he argues that Christ could experience anger, because anger is praise-

78 "quod est manifestus oditor et amator et manifeste dicit et operatur." *ST* I–II 48.3 ad 2. Aristotle, *Ethics* 4.3, 1124b26.

79 Daniel Maguire and Thomas Ryan give a lengthy treatment of "affective knowledge" and its role in Aquinas's moral theory, especially with regard to the virtues of prudence, fortitude, and temperance, and the gifts of the Holy Spirit. See Daniel C. Maguire, "*Ratio Practica* and the Intellectualistic Fallacy," *Journal of Religious Ethics* 10 (1982): 22–39; Ryan, "Revisiting Affective Knowledge."

80 *ST* I–II 59.5 ad 1.

81 "quanto virtus fuerit perfectior, tanto magis passionem causat." *ST* I–II 59.5.

82 *ST* I–II 59.3.

83 *De malo* 12.1 sc 4.

worthy when reasonably ordered.[84] Furthermore, wrestling with Christ's passions and affections seems to have forced Aquinas to clarify his account of human affectivity in certain respects. For Aquinas, Christ is the model and exemplar of human affectivity—yet, in order to understand Christ's emotions, it is necessary to reflect on ordinary human experience, not just sacred scripture. In short, Aquinas's account of ordinary human emotions is in constant dialogue with his theology of Christ's emotions, and each reinforces the other's positive evaluation of affectivity.

Competing Interpretations of Aquinas on the Passions

The evidence examined so far showing that Aquinas has a remarkably positive evaluation of the passions may need further discussion, given the differing interpretation suggested by historians of emotion like Thomas Dixon.[85] It would be beyond the scope of this essay to provide a detailed analysis of how the seemingly negative interpretations of Aquinas might have been arrived at, and how they might be modified in the light of further evidence from Aquinas. It might suffice to note that the passages that can be used to argue that Aquinas's default attitude toward the passions is negative are vastly outnumbered by other passages (some of which have been cited here) in which he clearly argues for a very positive evaluation of the passions, though it is also helpful to consider why it might easy to misread Aquinas, and why there is any controversy in the first place.

The first thing to understand is that Aquinas bends over and backwards to show continuity with the opinions of established intellectual authorities, whether Jewish, Christian, Islamic, or pagan. In the writings of many pagan philosophers and patristic theologians, the word "passion" has negative connotations, even when these philosophers and theologians manifest a generally positive interpretation of what we would call desire and emotion. But in the Middle Ages these authors were considered authorities. Consequently, even when he is subverting their conceptualization of passion toward a more positive interpretation, Aquinas goes out of his way to show continuity with these authors. In order to read Aquinas correctly, then, it is important to be attentive to his subversive project.

84 *ST* III 15.9.

85 See Dixon, *From Passions to Emotions*, 35–61. Aquinas also has a very positive evaluation of the affections, but there is general agreement on this point.

As Bonnie Kent observes, in his attentiveness to innumerable authorities, Aquinas is

> very much like a host laboring to produce congenial, fruitful conversation among guests deeply at odds with each other. Like all good hosts, he conceals how hard he must work to ensure that conflicts are defused and the party goes well. Sometimes Thomas repeats, approvingly, the words of an authority while giving them a meaning rather different from what the author intended.... Sometimes he sounds as if he agrees wholeheartedly when he actually agrees only with significant reservations. And sometimes his reservations become clear only later in the *Summa*, so that his earlier statements appear, retrospectively, in an altogether different light.[86]

Kent's excellent analogy sheds light on why some recent scholars have misread Aquinas as showing negative understanding of passion. Given that in the Middle Ages originality was not prized in the same way as it is today, we can see why Aquinas is trying to present a radical re-conceptualization of passion while still claiming continuity with earlier theologians. Aquinas is original, and he does not shy away from contradicting authorities when he thinks it is necessary, but he does not advertise his originality, either. To have done so would have left his theological positions vulnerable to criticism from his peers, and in any case it would have run counter to his own theological instincts.

The Emotions and Psychological Health

Aquinas does not invoke the concept of psychological health. Moreover, while he acknowledges the reality of mental illness, he mentions it only in passing. However, Aquinas is very concerned with psychological health, because Aquinas is very concerned with virtue. For Aquinas, virtue is nothing other than the proper functioning of the various powers of the human psyche. So when our emotions function as they were designed to function, then they are virtuous and psychologically healthy. Aquinas's understanding of virtue is much richer than ours; it lacks the moralistic overtones that taint our contemporary notions of virtue. *Virtus*, the Latin word for virtue, literally means "excellence." For Aquinas, virtue is not a matter of getting rid of sadness, anger, fear, or other "negative" emotions. It is a matter of the emotions operating according to their own inner structure, of being an excellent—and emotionally "perfected"—human being.

86 Kent, "Habits and Virtues," 116.

It should be emphasized that Aquinas does not only maintain that virtue involves the emotions operating as they should operate. That would be tautological and any moral philosopher would agree. Rather, Aquinas maintains that virtue involves the emotions operating *according to their own inner nature*. For example, when it comes to anger, Aquinas does not say: here are the circumstances when it is appropriate to get angry. Instead, he looks at how anger works and what kinds of things prompt us to get angry, and he concludes that we get angry when we perceive that we have been treated unjustly. Therefore, according to Aquinas, it is virtuous to get angry when in fact we have been treated unjustly, but not when, perhaps due to an inflated sense of self, we perceive injustice when there is no injustice.

Aquinas's correlation of virtue and psychological health makes for an especially interesting treatment of vice. According to Aquinas, "sins are located mainly in affection."[87] Consequently, his treatment of vice is primarily concerned with its psychology. His main interest is not to offer judgments on innumerable moral decisions, but rather to analyze the structure of vice, especially as it relates to affectivity. He prefers to describe vices in terms of affections and affective dispositions, rather than external actions and behavior patterns (although he discusses these as well). For Aquinas, the key criterion for evaluating a character trait is whether it departs from the inner structure of our desires and emotions.

Aquinas also gives a great deal of attention to the psychological implications of vice, such as how specific vices influence specific passions and affections, and how one vice spawns another. For example, he discusses how pride leads to envy, how greediness leads to internal disorder and excessive anxiety about material concerns, and how gluttony and lust cloud one's judgment.[88] In many ways, his descriptions of individual vices read like clinical descriptions of psychological pathologies. This anthropological focus makes his analysis of specific vices particularly engaging. His approach is a refreshing contrast to those ethical systems that focus almost exclusively on the moral value of particular decisions and, in the process, neglect the psychological context and consequences of those decisions.

---

87 "peccata praecipue in affectu consistunt." *ST* II–II 118.6.

88 *ST* II–II 162.8 ad 3; *ST* II–II 118.1 ad 2, 118.7, 118.8 ad 4; *ST* II–II 148.5–6, 153.5.

The Case of Sadness

Finally, for an example of Aquinas's analysis of a specific emotion, it is helpful to consider the case of sadness and its relationship to psychological health. For the purposes of this essay, it suffices to consider three features of his account of sadness, which, in an impressionistic way, capture much about his views on the emotions and psychological health.

First, Aquinas does not simply think that it is acceptable to be sad; he thinks it is *positively good* to be sad in response to some evil. In the *Treatise on the Passions*, he writes:

> If something saddening or painful is present, it is good if someone becomes sad or feels pain because of it. For if someone does not become sad or feel pain in the presence of an evil, either he does not feel it or he does not count it as something repugnant, and, obviously, both possibilities are evils. Consequently, it is good that sadness or pain follows from the presence of an evil.[89]

The reason that it is good to be sad about an evil is not because there is a moral principle that any sentient creature with a body should feel sad in certain circumstances, but because we have a passion of sadness that operates in certain ways, and it is good for the inclinations of our nature to reach their fulfillment. The measure against which the moral quality of a specific instance of sadness is measured is the internal structure of the passion of sadness itself, not some moral code derived from abstract principles that have nothing to do with it. Consequently, contrary to Stoic philosophy, Aquinas affirms that sorrow can be a mark of virtue—and therefore psychological health—when moderate and appropriate.[90] Thus, even though the virtue of fortitude might reduce feelings of sadness and sorrow, fortitude does not consist in eliminating sadness and pain, but simply in preventing them from overwhelming one's mental state and actions.[91]

Second, while Aquinas acknowledges the goodness of being sad in some circumstances, he also promotes happiness. In the *Treatise on the Passions*, Aquinas devotes a whole question to discussing remedies for

[89] "supposito aliquo contristabili vel doloroso, ad bonitatem pertinet quod aliquis de malo praesenti tristetur vel doleat. Quod enim non tristaretur vel non doleret, non posset esse nisi quia vel non sentiret, vel quia non reputaret sibi repugnans, et utrumque istorum est malum manifeste. Et ideo ad bonitatem pertinet ut, supposita praesentia mali, sequatur tristitia vel dolor." *ST* I–II 39.1.

[90] *ST* I–II 59.3.

[91] *ST* I–II 59.3, *ST* II–II 123.8.

sadness.[92] In the middle of a very technical discussion of the metaphysics of emotion, he suddenly starts to offer practical suggestions for what to do when we are feeling sad. For the modern mind, the seeming incongruity is startling. Even if Aquinas's explanation for why these remedies work is far more technical than anything we would find in a typical self-help book, we are not accustomed to philosophers or theologians bouncing between these sorts of topics. In any case, for those who are wondering, Aquinas prescribes a variety of different remedies for sadness. He encourages us to cry, to talk with our friends, to contemplate the truth (because, for Aquinas, the truth is intrinsically consoling), to take a nap and, finally, to take a good soak. Two things are especially striking about his discussion of remedies for sadness. First, in a particularly obvious way, it shows that Aquinas's interest in the passions is not moralistic. Second, insofar as his remedies for sadness are oriented toward the body as well as the mind, it shows that Aquinas's approach to the emotions is essentially holistic: it embraces both body and soul, not one or the other.

Third, Aquinas distinguishes between the *passion* of sadness and the *intellectual affection* of sadness. Among other things, this distinction leads to a very interesting analysis of the vice of *acedia*, one of the seven deadly sins, often misleadingly translated as sloth. His account of acedia is universally acknowledged as a huge innovation in the history of the concept, and, in my opinion, that innovativeness springs to a large extent from his distinction between these two different kinds of sadness.[93]

Acedia is often seen as a kind of laziness, but Aquinas defines *acedia* as a spiritual sadness, or more specifically, feeling sadness about spiritual goods—that is, things that should be inspiring joy rather than sadness—such as God and the idea of actively loving God and neighbor.[94] Rather than examining his account of *acedia* in detail, it suffices to consider one of the remedies he proposes for *acedia*: namely, he suggests that those plagued by *acedia* to spend more time thinking about spiritual goods.[95]

This solution might seem distinctly unhelpful, almost cruel. If someone finds the idea of loving God and neighbor depressing, why would thinking about them alleviate the vice of *acedia*? But Aquinas is not advocating

[92] *ST* I–II 38.

[93] For more on Aquinas's place in the intellectual history of *acedia*, see Siegfried Wenzel, *The Sin of Sloth: Acedia in Medieval Thought and Literature* (Chapel Hill: University of North Carolina Press, 1967), 64.

[94] *ST* II–II 35.1.

[95] *ST* II–II 35.1 ad 4.

that people chain themselves to church pews until, perhaps out of sheer exhaustion, loving God and neighbor starts to look good. For Aquinas, when spiritual goods are considered properly, they are necessarily attractive. Consequently, *acedia* is not only an affective problem; it is also an intellectual problem. Aquinas is proposing that we first focus on sorting out the intellectual problem, and then the affective problem will be much easier to handle. For example, Aquinas opposes *acedia* to the commandment to keep holy the Sabbath, and he suggests that there is a special link between them. The vice of *acedia* disposes us to see this commandment as burdensome and difficult, but for Aquinas, once the matter is understood properly, what it commands us to do should start to look good.

Aquinas affirms the fundamental goodness of emotion even while maintaining that, in a fallen world, human affectivity is prone to distortions. Consequently, for Aquinas, the operation of the emotions according to their inner structure is essential to psychological health.

TEMPTED TO KILL: MIRACULOUS CONSOLATION FOR A MOTHER AFTER THE DEATH OF HER INFANT DAUGHTER[1]

Nicole Archambeau

In the spring and summer of 1363, papal officials met in the city of Apt, roughly 60 kilometers east of Avignon, to hear witnesses testify about the holy life and miracles of Countess Delphine de Puimichel. Not only was she notable for her chaste marriage to Elzear de Sabran, who was a Provençal aristocrat, count of Ariano, and diplomat for the King of Naples, she had also performed numerous miracles while alive. She had become a protector of her people during the crises of the first wave of plague and the Hundred Years War. And, most importantly for this essay, she healed sufferers' sadness and anxiety.

Some of that sadness and anxiety was related to the large-scale crises of war and epidemic that affected almost every community in the later fourteenth century. But not all witnesses spoke about these well-known events. Several witness related personal moments of sorrow when they and their families turned to Delphine for healing.

One of these personal moments emerged in the testimony of Lady Mathildis de Sault. This Provençal noblewoman described her internal struggle after her infant daughter's death. Her reaction took the form of inconsolable sadness that further expressed itself in a temptation to kill the wetnurse—present when her daughter died—with her bare hands.

While Mathildis' testimony, as we will see below, appears tantalizingly clear and straightforward (a normal human reaction to such a tragedy), modern audiences must keep in mind that her testimony reflected both the dynamic tension of a canonization inquest and the ways available for a fourteenth-century noblewoman to experience and express emotion. In order to study the emotional experience of someone like Mathildis, therefore, we must consider the language she used to express herself, the context within which she spoke, and the cultural options that shaped her expression.

[1] I owe sincere thanks to those who read and critiqued this essay in its many stages, including Peregrine Horden, Elena Carrera, Fernando Salmon, and the anonymous reviewers.

As many scholars have pointed out, what we call emotional expression is not innate and unchanging. It is shaped by language, culture, and time period.[2] Arthur Kleinman and Byron Good captured this in the introduction to their cross-cultural study of depression. "Describing how it feels to be grieved or melancholy in another society leads straightway into analysis of different ways of being a person in radically different worlds."[3] Renato Rosaldo also showed this poignantly in his research on the headhunter's rage: what causes distress and how people choose to heal that distress are culture-specific and can change over time.[4]

Understanding the emotional expression of a woman from the fourteenth century requires us to look at the words she used and the context of those words. At the same time, since we are discussing this in English, an awareness the fact that the modern English lexicon of emotion differs significantly from the medieval also aids our ability to understand medieval usage.[5] For example, one key word in this essay that never appeared in witness testimonies was a general term like 'emotion.' While terms like the passions and the accidents of the soul existed, none were as broad as 'emotion,' which came into general use in the eighteenth century.[6]

Emotion is a word that everyone today recognizes, but few can precisely define, because the boundaries between what is and what is not an emotion remain stubbornly unclear.[7] As an umbrella concept, the word encompasses the primary emotions—e.g., anger, joy, fear, and sadness—and also includes more nebulous concepts like worry, doubt, boredom, and unease. On the outside edges of the umbrella crowd a host of words

[2] See Graham Richards, "Emotions into Words—Or Words into Emotions?," in *Representing Emotions: New Connections in the Histories of Art, Music, and Medicine*, ed. Penelope Gouk and Helen Hills (Aldershot: Ashgate, 2005), 49–68. This idea is common in anthropological studies of affect. For an overview, see Niko Besnier, "Language and Affect," *Annual Review of Anthropology*, 19 (1990): 419–51. For a thoughtful consideration of emotion, see John Leavitt, "Meaning and Feeling in the Anthropology of Emotions," *American Ethnologist* 23 (1996): 514–39.

[3] *Culture and Depression: Studies in Anthropology and Cross-Cultural Psychiatry of Affect and Disorder*, ed. Byron Good and Arthur Kleinman (Berkeley: University of California Press, 1985), 3.

[4] See Renato Rosaldo, *Ilongot Headhunting 1883–1974: A Study in Society and History* (Stanford: Standford University Press, 1980).

[5] For a discussion of English emotion terms in relation to Romance languages, see Rosenwein, "Emotion Words," *Le sujet des émotions au Moyen Âge*, ed. Piroska Nagy and Damien Boquet (Paris: Éditions Beauchesne, 2009), 93–106.

[6] See Barbara Rosenwein, *Emotional Communities in the Early Middle Ages* (New York: Cornell University Press, 2006), 53.

[7] For a discussion of the difficulties of identifying emotions, see Rosenwein, "Emotion Words."

that could be emotions or perhaps not. For example, are morally loaded words like loyalty, lust, and greed emotions or are they virtues and vices? The word 'emotion' can stretch to include almost everything that goes on inside our heads. Or the word can contract to just a few core emotions and ignore everything else.[8] The same warning holds true for particular emotion words. This essay especially concerns *tristitia*, what I and many other scholars translate as sadness. But the modern meaning of sadness does not include many of the concepts, particularly the ideas about how sadness might influence the brain, which were common in the fourteenth century.

Historians of emotion in the Middle Ages have developed several methods of working with this slippery concept. On the one hand, Barbara Rosenwein has developed a methodology for studying emotion that includes looking for specific words in written texts that relate to a recognizable emotional state, words like *tristitia* (sadness) or *gaudium* (joy).[9] This approach provides a useful base of language that people did use and builds a lexical context in which those words appeared.[10] Other approaches that emphasize language look at one emotion, like sadness or anger, across a range of surviving sources or focus on philosophical approaches to the passions.[11] Other approaches push past the boundary of

---

[8] For a discussion of different ways of viewing what is and is not an emotion, see Antonio Damasio, *The Feeling of What Happens: Body and Emotion in the Making of Consciousness* (New York: Harcourt Brace and Company, 1999).

[9] Barbara Rosenwein, "Problems and Methods in the History of Emotions," *Passions in Context: Journal of the History and Philosphy of the Emotions* 1 (2010): 1–32. Pedro Gil Sotres, "Modelo teórico y observación clínica: Las pasiones del alma en la psicología médica medieval," in *Comprendre et maîtriser la nature au Moyen Âge: Mélanges d'histoire des sciences offerts à Guy Beaujouan* (Genève: Droz, 1994), 181–204.

[10] For sets of emotion words from ancient and early medieval texts including the texts they came from and an analysis of their use, see Rosenwein, *Emotional Communities*, 32–99.

[11] The bibliography of historical studies of specific emotions is extensive, but for examples of different approaches to specific emotions see, Sigfried Wenzel, *The Sin of Sloth: Acedia in Medieval Thought and Literature* (Chapel Hill: University of North Carolina Press, 1960); Raymund Klibansky, Erwin Panofsky and Fritz Saxl, *Saturn and Melancholy: Studies in the History of Natural Philosophy, Religion, and Art* (New York: Basic Books Inc., 1964); Mary Francis Wack, *Lovesickness in the Middle Ages: The Viaticum and Its Commentaries* (Philadelphia: University of Pennsylvania Press, 1990); and *Anger's Past: The Social Uses of an Emotion in the Middle Ages*, ed. Barbara Rosenwein (Ithaca: Cornell University Press, 1998). For philosophical approaches, see Damien Boquet, *L'ordre de l'affect au Moyen Âge: Autour de l'anthropologie affective d'Aelred de Rievaulx* (Caen: Publications du CRAHM, 2005), Simo Knuuttila, *Emotions in Ancient and Medieval Philosophy* (Oxford: Clarendon Press, 2004) and Na'ama Cohen-Hanegbi, "The Matter of Emotion: Priests and Physicians on the Movement of the Soul," *Poetica* 72 (2009): 21–42.

words and look at events that would have caused emotional reaction and then analyze people's reactions to those events as emotional expression.[12] All of these methods avoid the trap of forcing medieval views into a modern framework, and thereby judging medieval emotional expression by modern criteria.[13]

In studying Mathildis' distress at the death of her infant daughter, I combine multiple approaches. I explore the language Mathildis used in the context of Delphine's inquest, especially how the requirements of a canonization inquest might both limit her expression and free her to speak.[14] I also look at her description of the event—the loss of her child—and her multi-layered reaction. The loss caused her sadness, which led to homicidal temptation and seeking out a saint for consolation. Her reaction allows modern scholars a chance to see some of the ways Mathildis had available in her culture to express her sadness.[15] This does not mean she consciously chose any one way or another to express her sadness, but, like the headhunter in Rosaldo's study, her historical moment offered frameworks for her to experience and express her emotion that might not appear in other cultures at other times. These frameworks help us see Mathildis' sadness and homicidal temptation not simply as general human reactions, but as experiences of the fourteenth century, which included spiritual homicide, madness, and vengeance.

---

[12] For example, see Jeroen Deploige, "Meurtre Politique, Émotions Collectives et Catharsis Littéraire: Guibert de Nogent et Galbert de Bruges Faces aux Révolts Urbaines de Laon (1111–1112) et de Bruges (1127–1128)," *Politques des émotions au Moyen Âge* (Florence: Sismel, 2010), 225–54.

[13] For a clear argument against studying emotion as part of a civilizing process, see Rosenwein, *Emotional Communities*, 5–10.

[14] The most nuanced studies of the impact of the inquest procedure on testimony concern heresy inquests. See for example, John Arnold, *Inquisition and Power: Catharism and the Confessing Subject in Medieval Languedoc* (Philadelphia: University of Pennsylvania Press, 2001).

[15] Others have used miracle collections and inquest testimony for similar purposes. See Sharon Farmer, *Surviving Poverty in Medieval Paris: Gender, Ideology, and the Daily Lives of the Poor* (Ithaca: Cornell University Press, 2002); Didier Lett, *Un Procès de Canonisation au Moyen Âge: Essai d'Histoire Sociale, Nicolas de Tolentino, 1325* (Paris: Presses Universitaires de France, 2008); Gérard Veyssière, *Vivre en Provence au XIVe siècle* (Paris: Éditions l'Harmattan, 1998); Sari Katajala-Peltomaa, *Gender, Miracle, and Daily Life: The Evidence of Fourteenth-Century Canonization Processes* (Turnhout: Brepols, 2009). For other kinds of inquests, see Carol Lansing, *Passion and Order: Restraint of Grief in the Medieval Italian Communes* (Ithaca: Cornell University Press, 2008).

Mathildis as a Witnesses in a Fourteenth-Century Canonization Inquest

Roughly sixty-eight witnesses gathered to testify about the life, living miracles, and posthumous miracles of the holy Countess Delphine de Puimichel. This was not a large number for a fourteenth-century inquest, but by 1363, when the inquest took place, Delphine had only been dead for three years. There had been no time for large numbers of posthumous miracles to occur at her tomb. The witnesses who testified tended to have been part of her communities—the convent and hermitage she lived in, the political sphere in which she moved, and the city of Apt where she spent much of her later years.

Delphine lived seventy-five years, from 1285 to 1360. Her life spanned the papacy's move to Avignon in 1308, the first wave of the Plague in 1348, the near civil war in Provence in 1348–1349, and the mercenary invasions beginning in 1357. During her life, Delphine upheld ideals of poverty and chastity even though she was a wealthy heiress and was married to Elzear de Sabran, an advisor of King Robert I of Naples. She and Elzear shared a chaste marriage from 1300 until Elzear's death in 1321. Highly influenced by Franciscan ideals, Delphine sold her goods after her husband's death and lived a relatively secluded life. She did not take religious vows, but she often lived at a convent in Apt or at a hermitage in nearby Cabrières.[16]

Mathildis de Sault was a typical witness, part of the pious, mostly socially elite group surrounding Delphine. The fact that Delphine successfully navigated two worlds—the secular and religious—made her special. She had been a married woman and a virgin, an heiress and a pauper, a political force called upon to negotiate between warring Provençal lords and a humble penitent. All of these things, including the fact that her

[16] For studies of Countess Delphine and her husband, St. Elzear de Sabran, see Rosalynn Voaden, "A Marriage Made for Heaven: The *Vies Occitanes* of Elzear of Sabran and Delphine of Puimichel," in *Framing the Family: Narrative and Representation in the Medieval and Early Modern Periods*, ed. Rosalynn Voaden and Diane Wolfthal (Tempe: Arizona Center for Medieval and Renaissance Studies, 2005), 101–16; Florian Mazel, *La noblesse et l'Église en Provence, fin X^e-début XIVe siècle: l'example des familles d'Agoult-Simiane, de Baux et de Marseille* (Paris: CTHS, 2002); and Dyan Elliott, *Spiritual Marriage: Sexual Abstinence in Medieval Wedlock* (Princeton: Princeton University Press, 1993). André Vauchez, however, has emphasized her similarity to thirteenth-century mystics. See his "La religion populaire dans la France méridionale au XIVe siècle d'après les procès de canonisation," in *La religion populaire en Languedoc du XIIe siècle à la moitié du XIVe siècle* (Toulouse: Édouard Privat, 1976), 91–107. Finally, several scholars have studied her inquest. See Pierre-André Sigal, "Les temoins et les temoignages au procès de Dauphine de Puimichel (1363)," *Provence Historique* 195–96 (1999): 461–471, and Veyssière, *Vivre en Provence.*

deceased husband was the subject of his own canonization inquest, made her a conduit of God's grace for the people in her community.

Witnesses frequently remarked on Delphine's gift of clear sight: her ability to see into their hearts and know their feelings, sins, and spiritual state.[17] Not only could she see into hearts, but she could also console the men and women who visited her, transforming their sadness and anxiety into joy and reassurance. Inquest organizers fit her ability to console into a broader ability to heal illness while she was alive—a rare saintly trait by the fourteenth century.

Delphine's inquest, though ultimately unsuccessful, produced testimonies from people who had known her in her later years and experienced her sanctity and healing power. These testimonies are important statements about how people understood their physical illness as well as their emotional distress. But by the fourteenth century, canonization inquests were expensive, long-term efforts often engaged in as much for the political glory of a family as the spiritual glory of a holy person.[18] This makes it difficult to know to what extent witnesses' language reflected the inquest organizers' language or expressed their own ideas.

As a witness, Mathildis' statement about her sadness and temptation was shaped by the requirements of the canonization inquest. By the fourteenth century, witness testimony for a canonization reflected two main requirements. On the one hand, a canonization inquest was a highly controlled, carefully constructed moment of memory. Witness testimony was not spontaneous or naive. Inquest organizers controlled who spoke, where they spoke, and what they were allowed to speak about. We have a testimony that tells us what witnesses wanted the papal commissioners to know about themselves and their holy person. The testimonies were cautious statements, solicited long in advance of the inquest, in response to elaborate summaries of the life moments, sanctity, and miracles of Countess Delphine. Through witness testimony therefore, we cannot directly see what people 'really' thought.

On the other hand, while witnesses perhaps consciously shaped their stories to appeal to the papal commissioners, they were still being given

---

[17] For clear sight see, see Donald Weinstein and Rudolph Bell, *Saints and Society: The Two Worlds of Western Christendom, 1000–1700* (Chicago: The University of Chicago Press, 1982), 147–50. For a more general approach, see Michael Goodich, "The Contours of Female Piety in Later Medieval Hagiography," *Church History* 50 (1981): 20–32.

[18] Gabor Klaniczay, *Holy Rulers and Blessed Princesses: Dynastic Cults in Medieval Central Europe* (Cambridge: Cambridge University Press, 2002).

an opportunity to describe important events from their lives. And the papacy considered it very important that they do so. As André Vauchez explains, according to the innovations of Pope Innocent III in the canonization process, "the depositions of sworn witnesses must be recorded accurately and forwarded as they stood," not summarized as had been the standard practice previously.[19] This meant that the papal court wanted proof of local support in the words of local people. To meet this goal, testimony in Delphine's inquest was taken down by two notaries, a papal-appointed notary and a local notary. Most testimonies included a statement indicating that the person spoke in the common or vulgar tongue, including Mathildis'. Although the testimonies were then transcribed into Latin for the papal court, some words that resisted translation into Latin were left in the Occitan that most of the witnesses (as well as the local notary) would have spoken. Many other words, including words like *tristitia* that are so important to this study, were very similar between Latin and Occitan, so the translation would not have had to be overly intrusive.[20]

The physical location and audience of the testimony also likely influenced what witnesses said. Most witnesses, including Mathildis, testified in front of two papal commissioners—the archbishop of Aix and the bishop of Vaison—in the cathedral of Apt. The cathedral was the town's social center, and the church in which the bishop of Apt said mass. It was an important relic site, housing among other holy objects, the veil of Jesus' grandmother. In other words, witnesses spoke to spiritual authorities, in the presence of notaries, in a place that held spiritual importance for them. This was not a place for foolish talk.

Witness testimonies in Delphine's inquest emerged in a methodical manner. After witnesses were sworn in, a series of summaries called *articuli interrogatori*, what I shall refer to as articles, were read to them. These ninety-one carefully crafted articles summarized Delphine's life

---

[19] André, Vauchez, *Sainthood in the Later Middle Ages*, trans. Jean Birrell (Cambridge: Cambridge University Press, 1997), 37–39. He cites the inquest for Gilbert of Sempringham in 1201 in which Innocent III denied the first application for official sainthood on the grounds that the witness testimonies had been synthesized into one brief report rather than taken down individually.

[20] For examples of many emotion words, see Peter Ricketts, "Prayers in Medieval Occitan: Critical Edition, Translation and Notes," *Studies on Ibero-Romance Linguistics Dedicated to Ralph Penny*, ed. Roger Wright and Peter Ricketts (Newark: Juan de la Cuesta, 2005), 127–51. Syntax variations between witnesses also strongly suggest that the testimonies were not overly latinized.

events and miracles. Witnesses could choose to speak about an article or not. Alternatively they could choose to waive their right to hear all of the articles and speak to only one or two, if their experience of Delphine were limited. After each article, the commissioners asked questions, such as "When did you see or hear this?" "Who was present?" "Where did it take place?" and "Were you requested, paid, or instructed to give this testimony?" At times, the commissioners asked more complex questions about the wording of a vow or how the witness knew a miracle had occurred, but in Mathildis' case they asked only these basic questions.

Some witnesses in Delphine's inquest repeated much of the language that appeared in the articles. Others, however, differed significantly from the language of the article, suggesting that their word choice was their own, rather than simply following the inquest organizers' formulation. Mathildis chose to testify only to Article 86, which directly concerned her experience, and waived her opportunity to speak to any other article. The article stated:

> Moreover, that the noble lady Mathildis de Sault had a certain temptation from which she was not able to be free by reason or admonishment at any time. And so when it came to her mind that she ought to go to that lady, the Countess [Delphine], she did so immediately; and while she was in Delphine's presence and she disclosed and explained the thing or cause of such temptation with trust, she was freed thoroughly in Delphine's presence of the said temptation.[21]

The article was very general. It did not mention the cause or nature of Mathildis' temptation, nor did it mention the sadness that she experienced. In this simple version of events, Mathildis described the cause of temptation to Delphine and was freed of it.

---

[21] The Latin text comes from the critical edition of Delphine's inquest by Jacques Cambell, O.F.M. *Enquête pour le Procès de Canonisation de Dauphine de Puimichel Comtesse d'Ariano* (Turin: Bottega d'Erasmo, 1978). Cambell used two main copies of Delphine's inquest, including Bibliotheque Méjanes, ms. 355 in Aix-en-Provence, France and, what was then St. Leonard College Library, ms.1 in Dayton, Ohio. See Cambell, *Enquête,* pp. xx–xxii. My translations maintain the meaning and structure of the testimony without the many repetitions and formalized identifying phrases of the original. Page references in this article will refer to the critical edition. See Article 86: "*Item,* quod nobilis Matheldis de Saltu habuit quandam temptacionem a qua liberari minime poterat inductionibus et monicionibus quibuscumque. Unde cum semel sibi in sua mente venisset ut ad dictam dominam comitissam deberet accedere pro premissis, statim nunc; et dum fuit ad eius presenciam et rem sive causam temptacionis huiusmodi cum confidencia aperuisset et enarrasset, fuit ibidem in eius presencia a dicta temptacione penitus liberata, nec postea ad eandem temptacionem reversa fuit ullo modo." *Enquête,* 90.

As we will see below, there are significant differences between the article and Mathildis' testimony. The differences show that, while she likely chose her words carefully in the setting of the canonization inquest, she did not repeat the article as if it were a prepared statement. Her description of herself as a pious noblewoman who could visit Delphine when she was unable to control her sadness and temptation was her own.[22]

Therefore, although Mathildis spoke in a setting with very real constraints, her testimony can still reveal her perspective, which included the emotions she felt, her struggle to control her sadness and temptation to kill. She experienced a Christian moral framework that rewarded certain kinds of thought and punished others. Her testimony also reveals how she tried to change her internal state by meeting with Delphine, a holy woman who had led an exemplary life of Christian faith. Through Delphine's sanctity, the holy Countess could act for Mathildis as a conduit of God's grace.

Resisting the Temptation to Kill

The noble lady Mathildis de Sault was an unlikely murderer. She came from the Agoult family that ruled the region around Sault and often served as seneschals of Provence.[23] Delphine and her husband had strong ties to the family. For example, when Delphine and Elzear were first married, they lived in Sault with his grandmother Cecilia and his uncle, Raimon IV d'Agoult.[24] After Elzear's death, Delphine continued to interact with the Agoult family on a political and spiritual level. According to her inquest,

---

[22] For the creation of social relationships through witness testimony, see Laura Smoller, "Miracle, Memory, and Meaning in the Canonization of Vincent Ferrer, 1453–1454," *Speculum* 72 (1998): 429–54. For the public presentation of self and others in medieval courts, see Daniel Lord Smail, "Telling Tales in Angevin Courts," *French Historical Studies* 20 (1997): 183–215. For a broader look at written constructions of self in the early modern period, see Natalie Zemon-Davis, *Fiction in the Archives: Pardon Tales and Their Tellers in Sixteenth-Century France* (Stanford: Stanford University Press, 1990).

[23] For the importance of the Agoult family to Provence, see Mazel, *La noblesse et l'Église en Provence*. For their ties to the Angevin kings, see Thierry Pécout, "Les mutations du pouvoir seigneurial en Haute-Provence sous les premiers comtes angevins, vers 1260—début du XIVe siècle," in *La noblesse dans les territoires Angevins à la fin du Moyen Âge*, ed. Noel Coulet and Jean-Michel Matz (Rome: École Française de Rome, 2000), 71–87.

[24] For their early life together see Jacques Cambell, ed., *Vies Occitanes de Saint Auzias et de Sainte Dauphine* (Rome: Bibliotheca Potificii Athenaei Antoniani, 1963) and Voaden, "A Marriage Made for Heaven." Elzear even had his first ecstatic vision of the Holy Spirit in Sault.

she helped negotiate a famous peace in 1349 between the warring lords Hugo X de Baux and Raimon VII Agoult, then the senechal of Provence.[25] Florian Mazel saw Elzear and Delphine as able to limit the violence around them because of their sanctity.[26] The local aristocracy of Provence, especially the Agoult family, deeply respected the couple's sanctity, and saw in Delphine a peace-bringing negotiator like her husband.

A more personal link existed between Mathildis and Delphine, however. Mathildis' relatives, Beatrice and Rostagna, had both been nuns at the Holy Cross convent in Apt where Delphine lived for years at a time. Rostagna had been one of Delphine's closest associates. She had cared for Delphine during bouts of illness and had spoken to many about Delphine's vigils and various forms of penitence.[27]

Mathildis' testimony in Delphine's inquest reads:

> On a certain day, Mathildis rose from her bed to hear mass after giving birth. Her daughter—who was [Mathildis'] first child—was discovered to have died during the night in her wetnurse's bed. From the death of her daughter, the witness speaking felt great sadness and great sorrow, so much so that she was not able to find any consolation, especially because she did not hope to have another child. And from this sadness and sorrow, she had the strong temptation to kill the wetnurse with her own hands. And in this temptation for many days (from the middle of Lent continuously until the day after the feast of Pentecost), if she had been able to grasp the said wetnurse, she would have killed her.
>
> The day following the feast of Pentecost, the witness speaking and her husband went up to the convent of the Holy Cross in the diocese of Apt, where the lady Delphine then was, in order to see the lady Delphine and speak with her. Mathildis hoped to receive consolation from her for the sadness which she had, and that, through the good and holy words and examples of the lady Delphine, the evil temptation which she had might withdraw from her.
>
> While she was in the convent and in the presence of lady Delphine, because of the great sadness that she had, it was as if she could not speak. Nonetheless she placed the cause of her sadness and her sadness before lady Delphine, and she lay her head in the lap of that lady. And then lady Delphine spoke many good, consoling, and devout words to her, saying to her among other words, "Daughter, trust in the Lord, because this sadness and temptation will not remain in you!" Thus, suddenly, when she withdrew

[25] For this event, called by some the War of the Seneschals, see Émile Léonard, "Un Ami de Petrarque, Seneschal de Provence: Giovanni Barrili," *Études Italiennes* 9 (1927): 109–42.

[26] Mazel, *Noblesse et l'Église*, 534.

[27] Cambell, *Enquête*, 244; 252–55. Rostagna did not testify because she died before Delphine.

> from the presence of lady Delphine, she was completely consoled and all the previously mentioned sadness and wicked temptation withdrew from her, so much so that, if she were to see the wetnurse afterwards or at some other time, she would do no harm to her, on the contrary she would be sparing.
>
> Having been asked about the year [this happened], she said that seventeen years had elapsed, as it seemed to her. She did not recall the month or day. Having been asked who was present, she said that lady Raynauda and a certain woman named Raybauda de Menerbes were present when she learned her daughter was dead. And when she was in lady Delphine's presence, lady Rostagna de Sault was present, the sister of the witness speaking.[28]

Mathildis' social status and personal links to Delphine shaped her presentation of her reaction to the death of her daughter. In starting her narrative by recounting how, when she went to mass after giving birth, she found out that her daughter was dead, Mathildis established her own piety and clearly set the events in her testimony in a Christian moral framework. The death of her daughter caused her inconsolable sadness, from which emerged a desire to kill the infant's wetnurse. After suffering for two months, she and her husband went to Apt to visit Delphine.

[28] "... cum quadam die qua ipsa testis loquens surrexerit de puerperio et debebat audire missam, quedam eius filia, que fuit prima proles V septimanarum, fuisset reperta mortua de nocte iuxta nutricem ipsius in lecto et ipsa testis loquens ex morte dicte filie magnam concepisset tristiciam et magnum dolorem, in tantum quod consolacionem aliquam non poterat reperire, presertim cum non speraret aliam prolem habere; et ex tristicia et dolore huiusmodi habuit temptacionem vehementem dictam nutricem interficiendi suis propriis manibus; et in huiusmodi temptacione pluribus diebus, videlicet a media Quadragesima usque in crastinum post festum Penthecostes tunc proxime futurum fuisset et esset sic quod, si potuisset dictam nutricem tenere, ipsam interfecisset. Et die sequenti post dictum festum Penthecostes ipsa testis loquens et vir suus accesserunt ad monasterium Sancte Crucis, Aptensis diocesis, in quo dicta domina Dalphina tunc erat, causa dictam dominam Dalphinam videndi et cum ea loquendi, quia sperabat ab ea consolacionem recipere de tristicia quam habebat et quod per bona et sancta verba et exempla ipsius domine Dalphine dicta mala temptacio quam habebat recederet ab eadem. Que cum fuit in dicto monasterio et in presencia dicte domine Dalphine, pro tristicia magna quam habebat quasi loqui non potuit; nichilominus tamen exposuit causam tristicie sue et tristiciam suam eidem domine Dalphine, et reclinavit caput suum in sinum dicte domine Dalphine. Et tunc dicta domina Dalphina loquuta fuit sibi multa bona verba et consolatoria et devota, dicens sibi inter alia verba, 'Filia, confide in Domino, quia non durabit tibi tristicia et temptacio ista!' Ita quod, statim quod de presencia ipsius domine Dalphine recessit, fuit totaliter consolata et omnis tristicia et mala temptacio predicta recesserunt ab eadem, in tantum quod, si vidisset tunc dictam nutricem vel postea quandocumque, nullum malum fecisset eidem, ymo pepercisset. Interrogata de anno, dixit quod sunt bene XVII anni elapsi, ut sibi videtur; de mensibus et die non recordatur. Interrogata de presentibus, dixit quod fuerunt presentes domina Raynauda et quedam appellata Raybauda de Menerbia, quando fuit reperta dicta filia sua sic mortua; et quando fuit coram dicta domina Dalphina, fuit presens dicta domina Rostagna de Saltu, soror ipsius testis loquentis." Cambell, *Enquête*, 458–59.

Her testimony reveals what she expected of the encounter. She hoped that the holy woman would console her sadness and remove the temptation.

The moment of consolation in Mathildis' testimony is suggestive. Mathildis was one of many witnesses who expressed the belief that Delphine could transform her internal state. Most of the witnesses testified to the wondrous power of Delphine's voice. As they had heard her speak about God and about the importance of leading a holy life, they had felt transformed.[29] But some, like Mathildis, also touched the holy woman. Given that physical touch played an important role in miraculous healing, particularly for a holy person like Delphine, who performed healing miracles while alive, we can see how, when Mathildis laid her head in Delphine's lap, coming into physical contact with Delphine, the transformation of her sadness and temptation took on a new significance as a miraculous cure.

We get a sense of how Mathildis understood her sadness and temptation from the words she remembered Delphine saying. Delphine told her to trust in God, because the sadness and temptation would not remain in her. On the one hand, this might be a generic admonishment. But on the other hand, it suggests that Mathildis did not trust God and she felt that Delphine intuited this. Her sadness and the following temptation to kill made her question even her basic faith. This is not so farfetched when we consider that this pious woman was struggling with a desire to kill another human being with her own hands.

Finally, what happened when Mathildis left Delphine's presence was exactly what she had hoped for. Her sadness was consoled and her temptation to kill was gone. Instead of a desire to kill, Mathildis felt sparing toward the wetnurse, though she did not see the woman again.

Mathildis' experiences expose cultural frameworks of sin, sickness, and crime. Mathildis clearly understood her temptation to kill as sinful. Although the noble lady did not act on her murderous temptation, by desiring to kill she had already sinned in thought.[30] In confessors' manuals, like Raymond of Penaforte's *Summa* for confessors, she had committed a mortal sin called spiritual homicide, which was understood in terms

[29] I deal with this extensively in my present book project, *Body and Soul under Siege: Surviving Plague, War, and Anxiety in Fourteenth-Century Southern France.*

[30] For an awareness of sinning in thought, see Ricketts, "Prayers in Medieval Occitan," 149.

of criminal behavior even though it was not legally a criminal act.[31] While she did not use this learned phrase for her experience, she knew that what she was tempted to do was wrong and even the experience of temptation—the desire to kill—was wrong in a Christian moral framework.

If we consider her suffering from the standpoint of sin, however, two complications emerge in her testimony that would have added to her suffering. The first problem involves her feeling in Delphine's presence as if she could not speak, which happened to several witnesses in Delphine's inquest who experienced extreme emotions. This would have limited their ability to confess their sins and receive absolution.[32] Although Mathildis eventually seems to overcome her inability to speak, as we can infer from the verb *exposuit* in her testimony, her initial feeling that she could not speak could have posed a problem. Perhaps visiting Delphine and being able to speak to her was a prelude to visiting a confessor. The idea of confession is strengthened here by Mathildis laying her head in Delphine's lap. While this may be a comforting gesture, it also evokes the kneeling posture of the penitent before the priest.[33]

Another problem with sin for Mathildis appears in the idea that she was not able to overcome her sinful temptation to kill. One of the core components of a successful confession was the desire not to sin again.[34] This was exactly what Mathildis could not do. Her sinful desire to kill stayed with her until Delphine miraculously consoled her and helped her feel merciful. Only at that point could she experience an effective confession.

31 According to Raymond of Penaforte, "species homicidii sunt plures, nam aliud spirituale, aliud corporale. Spirituale, quo quis spiritualiter et quadam iuris fictione occiditur. Quod fit quinque modis: odiendo, detrahendo, male consulendo, nocendo, victum subtrahendo. Quodlibet istorum est mortale." Raymond of Penaforte, *Summa de Paenitentia*, Volume I, Tome B, ed. Xaverio Ochoa and Aloisio Diez (Rome: Commentarium pro religiosis, 1976), col. 442. For a discussion of spiritual homicide see Judith Shaw, "Corporeal and Spiritual Homicide, the Sin of Wrath, and the Parson's Tale," *Traditio* 38 (1982): 281–300.

32 See for example, the witness Cecilia Baxiana, discussed in Nicole Archambeau, "Healing Options during the Plague: Survivor Stories from a Fourteenth-Century Canonization Inquest," *Bulletin of the History of Medicine* 85 (2011): 531–59, esp. 537–539. This was a well-known difficulty in confession and appeared in preachers' sermons, particularly those given during Lent. See also Sigfried Wenzel, *Latin Sermon Collections from Later Medieval England: Orthodox Preaching in the Age of Wyclif* (Cambridge: Cambridge University Press, 2005), 363.

33 For example, see London, British Library, MS Yates Thompson 31, f. 167v. Matfré Ermangau of Béziers, Breviari d'Amor, 14th century Catalan.

34 See Thomas Tentler, *Sin and Confession on the Eve of the Reformation* (Princeton: Princeton University Press, 1977), 104–22.

But sin was only one cultural avenue open to Mathildis for both understanding and expressing her sadness and temptation to kill. Her extreme reaction to her daughter's sudden death also evokes the pattern of mania brought on by a powerful emotional trigger like grief or fear seen in other miracle stories and in medical texts.[35]

Like other miracle stories in canonization inquests, Mathildis' experience took the form a healing narrative. Although she did not claim that her sadness or temptation to kill was mania, and she did not lose her senses, her experience was strikingly similar to that of sufferers in other canonization inquests who suddenly lost their minds in response to a shock. A representative example from the inquest of Saint Louis of Anjou, which took place in Marseille in 1308, helps locate Mathildis' temptation in the framework of mental illness at the time. In this miraculous healing, a woman named Beatrix, who lived in Nice, lost her senses after her mother became ill on pilgrimage and failed to return with the group she had traveled with. Beatrix became convinced that her mother was not sick, but dead. In response, Beatrix, who had been a wise and humble wife, lost her senses. She became blasphemous, tried to cut people with knives, and her hands had to be restrained with ropes. She suffered until her husband, Leo, convinced her to make a vow to St. Louis.[36]

Mathildis' story has strong parallels to Beatrix's story, including the sudden shock of the death of a loved one and her temptation to kill. Although Mathildis did not lose her senses and did not act on her desire to kill, madness was a cultural framework available to her; it was a familiar part of canonization inquests, and it hovers on the edge of her testimony. It also appears obliquely in the language of the article that summarized her experience, which described her temptation to kill as "a certain temptation from which she was not able to be free by reason or admonishment at any time."[37]

---

[35] See Stanley Jackson, "Unusual Mental States in Medieval Europe. I. Medical Syndromes of Mental Disorder: 400–1100 A.D.," *Journal of the History of Medicine* 28 (1972): 262–97; see esp. pp. 288–89 for a discussion of grief in psychological illness. See a discussion of both medical and theological understandings of this kind of melancholy in Judith Neaman, *Suggestion of the Devil: The Origins of Madness* (New York: Anchor Books, 1975), 17–65. For more examples of legal texts in which people lost their senses after a sudden shock or change in their lives, see Aleksandra Pfau, "Crimes of Passion: Emotion and Madness in French Remission Letters," in *Madness in Medieval Law and Custom*, ed. Wendy J. Turner (Leiden: Brill, 2010), 97–122.

[36] "Processus canonizationis et legendae variae Sancti Ludovici, O.F.M., episcopi Tolosani," *Analecta Franciscana* 7 (1951). For Beatrix's healing miracle, see 218–21.

[37] Cambell, *Enquête*, 90.

Beatrix was not punished for her blasphemy and violence, but was seen instead to be suffering from an illness.[38] It is useful, therefore, to consider medieval medical conceptions of madness and its effects on the body. This will help us approach how Mathildis may have understood her experience as an illness and presented it to the commissioners.

Fourteenth-century medical compendia located mania as an illness of the head. Mania could be triggered by an emotional shock, usually grief or fear, which then caused an imbalance of humors resulting in too much dryness. This caused vapors to rise to the head, impeding a person's imaginative faculty.[39]

People suffering from mania could display diverse behavior, but many scholars agreed they could be "aggressive and so dangerous to themselves and others that they should be tied."[40] Mania was often linked in medical compendia to melancholy and described in similar ways, particularly in terms of how they could become chronic illnesses. If sufferers did not break the cycle of sad or frightening thoughts, the humors could become severely imbalanced causing a continuous buildup of vapors in the brain.

Medical doctors considered sadness one of the accidents of the soul that could influence both the heart and the brain.[41] The accidents of the soul were one of the six non-naturals that were not part of the body, like an organ or blood, but that were necessary for the body to function.[42]

---

[38] For a discussion of miraculous healing of mental illness, see Vauchez, *Sainthood in the Later Middle Ages*, 468–72 and 495.

[39] See Luke Demaitre, *Medieval Medicine: The Art of Healing, from Head to Toe* (New York: ABC-CLIO, 2013), see esp. ch. 4, "Head Problems, from Hair to Epilepsy." See also Jackson, "Unusual Mental States," 275–77.

[40] Demaitre, *Medieval Medicine*, ch. 4. For more on the experience of madness as described in medical texts, see Fernando Salmon, "From Patient to Text? Narratives of Pain and Madness in Medical Scholasticism," in *Between Text and Patient: The Medical Enterprise in Medieval and Early Modern Europe*, ed. Florence Eliza Glaze and Brian Nance (Florence: Sismel/Edizioni del Galluzo, 2011), 373–95.

[41] For an overview of the processes of the brain, see Ruth Harvey, *Inward Wits: Psychological Theory in the Middle Ages and Renaissance* (London: The Warburg Institute, 1975). For a broad study of the illness melancholy, see Klibansky, Panofsky and Saxl, *Saturn and Melancholy*. For a specific explanation of the effects of emotion on the heart and brain, see Nancy Siraisi, *Taddeo Alderotti and His Pupils: Two Generations of Italian Medical Learning* (Princeton: Princeton University Press, 1981), 233. For the function of imagination, see Angus Gowland, "Melancholy, Imagination, and Dreaming in Renaissance Learning," in *Diseases of the Imagination and Imaginary Diseases in the Early Modern Period*, ed. Yasmin Haskell (Turnhout: Brepols, 2011), 53–102.

[42] See Peter Neibyl, "The Non-Naturals," *Bulletin of the History of Medicine* 45 (1971): 468–492 J. L. Rather, "The 'Six Things Non-Natural': A Note on the Origins and Fate of a Doctrine and Phrase," *Clio Medica* 3 (1968): 337–47; Saul Jarcho, "Galen's Six Non-Naturals:

The six included: air and breathing, food and drink, repletion and excretion, motion and rest, sleeping and waking, and the accidents of the soul. The most basic list of accidents of the soul were sadness, fear, anger, and joy, but some lists included others. At the risk of oversimplifying a complex issue, the accidents of the soul involved the most rarified spirits of the body, refined in the heart and moving up to the brain where they could affect behavior and thought.[43]

Medieval medical doctors wrote about using the six non-naturals to promote and maintain health.[44] In order to control the body's internal workings, especially to balance the humors in relationship to the entire body, doctors suggested changes in a person's air, food and drink, exercise, sleep, and emotion-causing experiences.[45] When illness severely disrupted a person's health, doctors then turned to various forms of therapy such as a strict diet, purging, drugs, and surgery.[46] In the case of an illness like mania or melancholy, doctors often tried to manipulate the accidents of the soul via the senses.[47] For example, in the *Lilium Medicinae*, Bernard de Gordon suggested that the sufferer's room ought to be brightly lit and have good smells. The sufferer should also have the company of lovely and happy people and instrumental music.[48]

a bibliographic note and translation," *Bulletin of the History of Medicine* 44 (1970): 372–77; Jerome Bylebyl, "Galen on the Non-Natural Causes of Variation in the Pulse," *Bulletin of the History of Medicine* 45 (1971): 482–85.

[43] Siraisi, *Taddeo Alderotti*, 227–28.

[44] For a discussion of the non-naturals in the regimens of health, see McVaugh, *Medicine Before the Plague*, 144–50. See also Gil Sotres, "The Regimens of Health," in *Western Medical Thought from Antiquity to the Middle Ages*, ed. Mirko Grmek (Cambridge: Harvard University Press, 1998), 313–14. See also Siraisi, *Taddeo Alderotti*, 226–36.

[45] For more information on regimens in Southern France in particular, see Luis Garcia-Ballester, "Changes in the *regimina sanitatis*: The Role of the Jewish Physicians," in *Health, Disease, and Healing in Medieval Culture*, ed. Sheila Campbell, Bert Hall and David Klausner (New York: St. Martin's Press, 1992), 119–31.

[46] For a discussion of these therapies see McVaugh, *Medicine Before the Plague*, 150–65; *Western Medical Thought*, 259–318.

[47] Demaitre, *Medieval Medicine*, ch. 4.

[48] "et ideo domus debet esse clara luminosa sine picturis et debent ibi esse multa odorifera et omnis habitantes cum eo debent esse pulchri aspecta et homines quos timeat et de quibus verecundetur si enorma egerit aut fatua loqueretur. Et ipsi debent multa permittere et in multis iocalia pulcherima presentare. Debent etiam ibi esse instrumenta musicalia. Et breviter omnia que letificant animam. Autem si perveniant ista egritudo ex nimio gaudio et repentino ut quia fuit nunciatum quam ipse indignitate erat maxime sublimatus aut amicus suus tunc bonum est quam de illo eodem tristicia inducatur [...]." Bernard de Gordon, *Lilium Medicinae*, Book 2, fol. 64v, col. 2. Bernard's suggestions are similar to other physicians' remedies; see, for example, Siraisi, *Taddeo Alderotti*, 234.

Although the behavior of mania and melancholy were often regarded as an illness, as we saw in Beatrix's case, and medical doctors had a developed understanding of mania and melancholy, medical treatment for mania was uncommon in the fourteenth century. For example, Michael McVaugh's research into the Crown of Aragon revealed little evidence "to show that people thought of mental disorder as a medical problem—or at least as a problem that physicians could relieve."[49] Stanley Jackson's overview of treatment for mental disorders also argues that people did not turn to doctors to treat mental illness, but instead turned to family and religious figures. Although he does not state why sufferers might have made this choice, he implies that medieval people understood mental illness as a moral phenomenon that could be treated by a religious practitioner better than by medical doctors, even when possession by demonic spirits was not suggested.[50]

It is no surprise, therefore, that Mathildis did not seek out a medical doctor for her mental disturbance—her great sadness her temptation to kill—even though her experience as she presented it to the papal commissioners had strong similarities to medical understandings of mania. Instead she sought a holy woman who was also a friend of the family, well-known for consoling and transforming the internal state the people around her.[51]

A third cultural framework existed within which Mathildis' experience of sadness and temptation to kill can be understood. Because Mathildis' internal feeling took the form of wishing to kill a person who had harmed her family, her experience fit into a framework of vengeance and mercy.[52]

---

[49] For more on doctors' reactions to psychological disorders, see McVaugh, *Medicine Before the Plague*, 230–35, and Siraisi, *Taddeo Alderotti*, 233.

[50] Jackson, "Unusual Mental States," 262–63. This view is substantiated by Professor Heidi Marx-Wolf at the University of Manitoba, who analyzed the treatment of sufferers of mental illness in many canonization inquests in "Insanity and Demon Possession in Medieval Canonization Inquests", unpublished paper, University of California, Santa Barbara, 2003.

[51] For the use and awareness of the non-naturals, especially the accidents of the soul, outside medical texts, see Peregrine Horden, "A Non-natural Environment: Medicine without Doctors and the Medieval European Hospital," in *The Medieval Hospital and Medical Practice*, ed. Barbara Bowers (Aldershot: Ashgate, 2007), 133–45.

[52] Although not stated directly in the testimony, there is the assumption that the wetnurse rolled over onto the child in her sleep. Called 'overlaying,' this problem appeared in legal and penitential literature of the time. However, Barbara Hanawalt, in her study of coroners' inquests in fourteenth and fifteenth-century England, found only one case. See Barbara Hanawalt, *The Ties That Bound: Peasant Families in Medieval England* (Oxford: Oxford University Press, 1989), 178. For a Provençal example of legal complications

By the fourteenth century, these were legal categories in Provence, but they also reflected long-term ways in which aristocratic families pursued justice.

As Daniel Lord Smail points out in his article on late medieval hatred, when one person wronged another in the way the wetnurse wronged Mathildis, an enmity grew between them and could be expressed (at times appropriately) through violent behavior. These wronged persons used emotion words like 'enmity', 'anger', and 'rage' that had legal weight in fourteenth-century courts, though, as Smail emphasizes, this type of violent revenge usually occurred between relative social equals and was similar to a system of aristocratic honor that had existed for much longer than the legal courts.[53]

While Mathildis' experience evoked a cultural script of vengeance, it differed significantly from the legal examples Smail analyzed. Mathildis did not name her emotion as rage, anger, or enmity, which might have put her legally into the position of a wronged person and justified her desire to kill. Also, the wetnurse was not Mathildis' social equal. So killing her would not only have been against Christian ideals, but also outside the bounds of socially acceptable vengeance. It would have made Mathildis a criminal.

By resisting her desire to kill, Mathildis evoked an alternative 'script' of honor—the script of mercy. Mercy played an important role in Mathildis' testimony. When Mathildis' sadness was consoled, the wicked temptation to kill left her and she claimed that she would not have harmed the wetnurse, instead she would have been sparing—she would have shown the woman mercy. Mercy appears to be is unique to Delphine's inquest, though it was a common framework in other kinds of sources, such as sermons.

One brief exemplum from the *Fasciculus Morum*, a fourteenth-century Franciscan preachers' treatise on the seven deadly sins, can help us better

surrounding childbirth, see Monica Green and Daniel Lord Smail, "The trial of Floreta d'Ays (1430): Jews, Christians, and obstetrics in later medieval Marseille," *Journal of Medieval History* 34 (2008): 185–211. For a discussion of homicide between Christians, see p. 193.

53 Daniel Lord Smail, "Hatred as a Social Institution in Late-Medieval Society," *Speculum* 76 (2001): 93–94. For issues of honor and violence in Provence, see Ronald Gosselin, "Les hommes et l'honneur: injures et violence à Manosque," *Vie privé et ordre public à la fin du Moyen Âge: Études sur Manosque, la Provence et la Piémont (1240–1450)*, ed. Michel Hébert (Aix-en-Provence: Université de Provence, 1987), 53–64. For customs regarding vengeance in Apt, see Fernand Sauve, "La vie Apténsienne d'autrefois," *Mercure Apténsien* (Sunday June 30, 1907).

understand the framework of mercy that Mathildis' testimony evokes. This exemplum appeared in a sermon on wrath and encapsulated how mercy worked in social relationships. The anonymous author wrote:

> Notice also the story about the knight who on Good Friday forgave another knight the death of his father, out of love for Him who died on that day for all mankind. When the two knights went together to worship the cross and bring their offerings, the Crucified detached His arms and embraced the one who had acted so mercifully, and he then heard a voice speaking of forgiveness.[54]

This story shows that mercy helped one avoid the dangers of the deadly sin of wrath. The injured party appeared magnanimous and was rewarded by God through a miracle, while the offending party was integrated back into society through forgiveness of his/her crime or sin.[55]

While Mathildis did not use the word wrath, she expressed her response to sadness as a desire to kill the wetnurse—which could appear to be vengeance. Like the knight in the short exemplum, she ultimately forgave the wetnurse. But unlike him, she needed help to transform her sadness and remove the temptation to kill. The miracle in Mathildis' story was the transformation of her internal state.

Conclusion

The historian who wants to understand emotion in the past must understand both the language of emotion people used and the social constructions that gave the language meaning. Mathildis' description of her temptation and Delphine's help placed her experience in the frameworks of sin, sickness, and crime in the fourteenth century. Her temptation to kill was a sin called 'spiritual homicide' by confessors at the time. Her inability to control her own thoughts in response to the sudden shock caused by her infant daughter's death echoed the causes of madness or mania found

---

54 *Fasciculum Morum: A Fourteenth-Century Preacher's Handbook*, ed. and trans. Sigfried Wenzel (University Park: The Pennsylvania State University Press, 1989), 125, his translation. For an example of the impact of sermons on audiences, see Nirit Ben-Aryeh Debby, "The Preacher as Women's Mentor," in *Preacher, Sermon and Audience in the Middle Ages*, ed. Carolyn Muessig (Leiden: Brill, 2002), 229–54.

55 M. T. Clanchy explores this kind of arbitration in his essay, "Law and Love in the Middle Ages," *Disputes and Sentiments: Law and Human Relations in the West*, ed. John Bossy (Cambridge: Cambridge University Press, 1983), 47–67. As he points out, most of these negotiations took place outside official legal court structures and were therefore rarely documented.

in other canonization inquests and described in medical texts from the time and region, like that of Bernard de Gordon. Her inappropriate desire to kill was transformed into the experience of mercifulness, which was more appropriate for a woman of her social class.

Perhaps the most interesting element of Mathildis' testimony was her self-awareness. Her self-awareness of her problem—not just her sorrow at her daughter's death, but her inappropriate desire to kill with her own hands—separated her from many sufferers at the time. While other sufferers mentioned in canonization inquests behaved erratically, Mathildis never lost her senses. She remained aware that her temptation to kill was wrong in her moral framework, and she sought help. This in-depth analysis of one woman's exploration of her sadness and homicidal temptation reveals just how complex the context of emotion can be, but also opens up a path to understanding her within her context rather than judging her from a twenty-first-century perspective.

FEAR, FANTASY AND SLEEP IN MEDIEVAL MEDICINE

William F. MacLehose

Among the many miracles attributed to Thomas Becket and collected soon after the archbishop's violent death in 1170, the story of a wealthy knight named Stephen of Hoyland stands out as a narrative describing the healing of an unusual affliction. Stephen was said to have suffered for thirty years from nightly attacks by a demon, during which assaults he felt himself being crushed or suffocated so ferociously that he imagined he would die.[1] In response to these recurring nocturnal onslaughts, Stephen would call for his servants and beg them to wake him, by raising him to a seated or standing position and even by "violently shak[ing] him by his hair." In requesting this odd remedy, he seems to have believed that, since the attack arose during sleep, the only solution was to awaken him lest he be killed by the demon in his sleep vision.

While suffering from this intolerable *phantasia* for decades, the knight had sought out the advice of physicians and offered them many rewards, but despite their efforts, the attacks persisted. The doctors declared that the condition was *ephialtes*, a Greek term of little significance to the twelfth-century west, and thus requiring the miracle writer's intervention: "It is what we in Latin can interpret as 'that which lies on top of something'" or, glossed in a different manuscript, "what is vulgarly [i.e. commonly] known as the incubus, or 'the crusher' [*oppressor*] in Latin."[2] But the long-suffering Stephen rejects the diagnosis made by the learned physicians: "to those who say it is ephialtes, he constantly asserts that it is a demon." The stalemate between sufferer and medical practitioners simply continues Stephen's torment and the need for his servants' interruption of his sleep.

The remainder of the story relates the inevitable failure of all measures to remove the demon, until he seeks religious intervention. The details of this narrative of healing through the intercession of Thomas Becket follow

---

[1] Miracula S. Thomae, Auctore Benedicto, in James Robertson, *Materials for the History of Thomas Becket* (London: Longman, 1876), 2: 44–45.

[2] "quod nos Latine superincumbentem interpretari possumus." Or "quod vulgus incubonem, Latini oppressorem appellant." Miracula S. Thomae, 44.

well-worn and predetermined patterns established in the genre of miracle tales and are of little concern for the present discussion. The physicians' views are proven to be false and their advice ineffectual, as the demonic force is conquered by the power of the martyred archbishop. Pious prayer does what the medical art could not do: it provides relief to the sufferer by overwhelming the demon's power.

This rich and remarkable narrative introduces the topic under discussion in this essay, the condition known as the incubus, and identifies some of the difficulties medieval doctors faced when dealing with the phenomenon. Although the patient rejects their interpretation, the physicians in the miracle tale have identified Stephen of Hoyland's affliction as an illness with a lengthy and complex past (and future) in medical literature: the incubus. The physicians in the Becket miracle tale call it by its Greek name,[3] but the more common term for the condition is incubus, a name which, as we shall see, brings with it considerable baggage. This study seeks to explore the disease category of the incubus in relation to two topics: the importance of 'emotional' reactions, particularly fear, and the role of the imagination or fantasy in the medical discussion of the condition.

This essay focuses on discussions of the incubus in the medical literature written between the late eleventh and early fourteenth centuries in the Latin west. During this formative period in the history of medieval medicine, as the learned traditions of the ancient and Islamic worlds were rediscovered and explored in Salerno, Paris, Montpellier and elsewhere, the incubus[4] became firmly established as a disease in learned medicine. The incubus is an exceptional category as understood in the medical discourse, in that it straddles the divides between learned and popular, theological and medical, religious and secular.[5] It also provides a

[3] It is highly unusual that physicians in the miracle tale use the Greek term; with rare exception, the medical materials consistently refer to the disease by its Latin name.

[4] Given the lack of definite articles in Latin, it is difficult to know if the term should be translated "the incubus" or just "incubus." This becomes an issue when dealing with the problem of the disease as a personification or as an abstract medical category. For the latter, the use of a definite article would appear awkward in modern English usage, and might distinguish the disease from the demonic figure.

[5] Maaike van der Lugt, "The Incubus in Scholastic Debate: Medicine, Theology and Popular Belief," in *Medicine and Religion in the Middle Ages*, ed. Peter Biller and Joseph Ziegler (Woodbridge: York Medieval Press, 2001), 175–200, provides an excellent study of this particular aspect of the medieval incubus. See also her monograph, *Le ver, le démon et la vierge: Les théories médiévales de la génération extraordinaire* (Paris: Les Belles Lettres, 2004), esp. ch. 4.

very important example of the interplay of the physiological and the mental states, as understood in medieval medicine. Central to this particular interaction of body and mind were the medical understanding of terror and the structure of the mental processes, particularly the fantasy.

* * *

Although the incubus as a premodern demonological category is relatively well known, the historical medical significance of the term remains obscure. The demon known as the incubus is most familiar from folkloric traditions, particularly in early modern witchcraft accusations and in Fuseli's painting of 1781, the Nightmare.[6] The incubus is the nightmare in an entirely literal sense: while the term *incubus* comes from the Latin for "that which lies upon," it has often been connected with our term nightmare, with "maere" referring to a supernatural female creature who sits on a person's chest and crushes him. The modern French *cauchemar* and Spanish *pesadilla* have similar connotations, indicating that which steps or weighs down on something else. Both the Greeks and Romans had their versions of a dangerous spirit creature, *ephialtes* ("that which leaps upon," the term used by the doctors in the Becket miracle) and the *incubo* (later incubus). By the late fifteenth century, if not earlier, the concept became associated with the old hag, and thus became an essential part of western demonology and witchcraft, paired with the succubus. While the demonological aspects of the incubus have been studied, the medical attempts at explaining the incubus in natural terms remain underexplored, and reveal much about medieval notions of medicine, body and emotions.

The medieval world inherited from the classical pagan and Judaeo-Christian traditions the notion of a nocturnal visitation by a spirit. In particular, the twelfth century witnessed a revival of interest in the incubus, as seen in discussions found in theological debates and in courtly literatures of northern Europe.[7] While the Greco-Roman incubo was some sort of supernatural being or lesser god of ambivalent morals, the medieval incubus was a demon with purely evil intentions. What links the two is the association of the incubus, who was generally male, with sleep, dreams

[6] An excellent study of the folklore on the incubus is Owen Davies, "The Nightmare Experience, Sleep Paralysis, and Witchcraft Accusations," *Folklore* 114 (2003): 181–203.

[7] Nicolas Kiessling, *The Incubus in English Literature: Provenance and Progeny* (Pullman, WA: Washington State University Press, 1977), 2, 11–12, 48–50. See also George Kittredge, *Witchcraft in Old and New England* (Cambridge, Mass.: Harvard University Press, 1929), 115–19.

and sexuality. A common element of the myths of the ancient world, tales of the early Christian period, and courtly narratives of the central middle ages lies in the belief that the incubus inhabits the realm of sleep and sexually assaults his female victim. Perhaps the most famous example of this phenomenon from the twelfth century onward can be found in the tales of Merlin's birth. The Arthurian histories and romances often relate the tale that an incubus (sometimes just a devil) either assaulted Merlin's mother or beguiled her in the form of a handsome youth. In Geoffrey of Monmouth's *History of the Kings of England*, a Welsh princess conceives the child Merlin through intercourse with one of those "spirits who live between the moon and the earth, whom we call incubus demons,"[8] sharing the natures of both humans and angels. Similar tales of such marginal, violent and sexualized creatures who sire unusual progeny with women appear often in the literature of the later middle ages.

The courtly romances' association of the incubus's attack with sexual intercourse finds parallels in contemporary scholastic debates over the possibilities of conception from these encounters with an incubus. Van der Lugt has identified very clear associations of theological debates on demonic generation with the tales of Merlin, and agreement by some thinkers that such conception was possible but uncommon, comparable to monstrous births.[9] By the end of fourteenth century, the incubus was firmly established in the spiritual landscape of western Europe, as seen in the Wife of Bath's reference to incubi alongside faeries and elves. For Chaucer's spirited widow, the incubus exhibited impish and destructive traits that interfered with human life.[10] Essential to the central and late medieval understanding of the incubus are aggression, violence and sometimes sexuality, all happening at night in and out of sleep.

---

[8] Geoffrey of Monmouth, *Historia regum Britanniae*, 6.18. See Jeff Rider, "The Fictional Margin: The Merlin of the 'Brut'," *Modern Philology* 87 (1989): 1–12, at 3. Note that William of Auvergne argues that incubi cannot on their own impregnate women, so they must imitate generation, collect seed from a human male and implant it in the woman's womb; he explains Merlin's birth by these means. See Kiessling, *The Incubus*, 25–26 and van der Lugt, "The Incubus," 253–60.

[9] Van der Lugt, *Le ver*, ch. 5, passim, esp 353–7.

[10] Kiessling, *The Incubus*, 43–50, and Dorothy Yamamoto, "Noon Oother Incubus But He: Lines 878–81 in the "Wife of Bath's Tale," *The Chaucer Review* 28 (1994): 275–78.

The Creation of a Disease Category

In comparison with these views of the incubus in the romances and theological discussions, medical understandings of the same term present a very different, even contradictory picture. The medical incubus inhabits a world which is at times explicitly opposed to the demonic incubus, particularly in the medical rejection of any supernatural or sexual aspects to the phenomenon. But the medical incubus is a highly unusual disease, one which raised many questions and objections among physicians. As we shall see, medical experts found it difficult to classify, and argued over its basic taxonomy and etiology, leading to some discussion of whether it should even be a medical issue at all.

How did a supernatural phenomenon of myth and legend become an object of medical interest? If indeed it is true that the supernatural incubus of mythological and folkloric tradition inspired the medical authorities to respond, then what was retained and what disappeared when doctors conceived of the incubus as an illness?

On the most rudimentary level, medical writers who chose to take up the topic felt compelled to argue that it truly was a medical topic, and their defensiveness on this point appears across many centuries of medical writing. The first line of defence lay in the argument that the origins of the phenomenon known as the incubus lay not in the supernatural realm but in the sufferer's body and mind. Such wholesale rejection of a demonological source allowed medical theorists to fill the causal lacuna with an explanation that was both physiological and psychological: a somatic disorder led to the illusion of a creature and the response of fear. A brief definition of the disease in a reference manual notes: "the incubus is a disease in which sleepers seem to be suffocated and crushed by demons,"[11] a description which indicates a direct link with the demonological tradition. But most medical texts approach the subject from an internal, physiological perspective, rather than the patient's point of view identified here. Medical authorities recognized the role of the imagination, which invoked such terrifying creatures, but attributed it, as we shall see, to corporeal and terrestrial causes. The disease that the doctors discussed was one that was inherently associated with fear, confusion, and a loss of control of

[11] Glossarium MSS Alexandrum Iatrosophistam, quoted in Charles Ducange, *Glossarium mediae et infimae latinitatis* (Niort: L. Favre, 1884), at "incubus".

the body. As such, the medical language interacts with and even accepts some of the terminology, but contests many of the interpretations, of the demonological tradition.

The first surviving instance of the incubus in medical literature appears in early imperial Rome, with the *Recipes* of the physician Scribonius Largus, ca. 40 AD. He refers to the *incubo* only in passing, in relation to dangerously deep breathing and choking during sleep.[12] But the incubus only comes into its own as a clearly identifiable disease, with its own etiology, symptoms and cure, in the late antique period. A century and a half after the death of Galen, who does not mention the phenomenon in any of his surviving works, his ideas became increasingly the central authority on things medical, pushing out the many other schools of thought that had proliferated in the Greek and Roman worlds. The late antique authors in the Greek-speaking world sought to systematize medicine, under a Galenic framework, into a coherent whole with claims of universal applicability.[13] Late antique authors composed encyclopedias in which diseases were categorized and analyzed, and it is through these books that the incubus enters the medical canon as a legitimate disease category.

Oribasius of Pergamum, physician to Julian the Apostate in the mid-fourth century, includes a chapter on the disease *ephialtes* in his discussion of diseases of the nerves. From the very first phrase of the entry, Oribasius affirms that this is not a demon but a serious disease, in which the sufferer experiences suffocation and an inability to speak at night.[14] This emphasis on the physiological rather than demonological interpretation of the phenomenon appears in other late antique medical encyclopedias. In his treatise on Acute and Chronic Diseases, written around 400, Caelius Aurelianus also emphatically denies a divine association. Caelius quotes the earlier methodist writer Soranus (2nd century AD) as arguing that "it is not a god, a demigod or a cupid."[15] For Caelius and his source, and for all later medical authorities this phenomenon can be understood in purely natural, physiological ways. The sufferer may feel something rising in his body from his feet toward his head, sense something sitting on his chest and even see "the form or image of a man" or some other fantasy,

[12] *Scribonii Largi Compositiones*, 100, ed. Sergio Sconocchia (Leipzig: Teubner, 1983), 53.

[13] Owsei Temkin, *The Double Face of Janus* (Baltimore: Johns Hopkins University Press, 1977), 167–97.

[14] *Oeuvres d'Oribase*, ed. Charles Daremburg and Ulco Cats Bussemaker (Paris: J.-B. Baillière & fils, 1873), 5: 402–403, and 6 (ed. A. Molinier, 1876): 205–206.

[15] Roscher, *Ephialtes*, 109.

but all of this is explicable as part of a larger disturbance of sleep due mostly to indigestion, drunkenness or some humoral imbalance. The sufferer's inability to speak or move, his mental confusion, and the sensation of being crushed to death are simply consequences of a somatic process.[16] There is no need for any recourse to the supernatural here, in an echo of the Hippocratic critique of epilepsy as a divine disease.[17]

The late antique writers established the basic parameters of the disease, all of which would be inherited by the Arabic and Latin traditions: ephialtes or incubus is a unique disease, and a serious one at that, with no connection to the supernatural; its etiology lay primarily in a disturbance of the digestive process; its basic symptoms included a feeling of suffocation and heaviness, an inability to move and speak, and its occurrence during or around sleep. The Byzantine encyclopedists continued the late antique acknowledgement of the disease as an independent category.[18] The later Latin translations of the encyclopedias faithfully reproduce their sources, but with an increasingly confused terminology.[19] The key terms become *epehaltu, inquibus, incybus, incivo*,[20] which may suggest a decreased familiarity with the Greco-Roman tradition, or at least terminology, of the supernatural creature. If western medical authors wished to distinguish the disease incubus from the creature of the spirit world, it would be logical to use the more foreign ephialtes. Instead, the Latin term, incubus, dominates most of the western literature of the early and later middle ages, potentially reaffirming the associations with a demonological force. Even in the *Passionarius*, an early medieval Latin text overflowing

---

16 Wilhelm Roscher, *Ephialtes: Eine pathologisch-mythologische Abhandlung über die Alpträume und Alpdämonen des klassischen Altertums* (Leipzig: Teubner, 1900), 108. Roscher includes an appendix with editions of the appropriate passages in Caelius Aurelianus and other Late Antique and early medieval sources.

17 See Owsei Temkin, *The Falling Sickness: A History of Epilepsy from the Greeks to the Beginnings of Modern Neurology*, 2nd edition (Baltimore: Johns Hopkins University Press, 1994). For the famous Hippocratic treatise, see Hippocrate, *La maladie sacrée*, ed. Jacques Jouanna (Paris: Les Belles Lettres, 2003), esp preface, liii–lxxiv, and "The Sacred Disease," in *Hippocratic Writings*, ed. G. E. R. Lloyd (Hammondsworth: Penguin, 1978), 237–51. As we shall see, the connection with epilepsy is reinforced by the argument that the incubus is a precursor of apoplexy, epilepsy and mania.

18 See Paul of Aegina (ca. 630), *The Seven Books of Paulus Aegineta*, trans. Francis Adams (London: Sydenham Society, 1844), bk 3, sect. 15, 1: 388.

19 Such confusions in terminology, often complications in transliterating foreign terms or reproducing unfamiliar terms, is common in the early medieval Latin manuscript tradition. See Monica Green, "The Transmission of Ancient Theories of Female Physiology and Disease through the Early Middle Ages," Ph.D. thesis, Princeton University, 1985.

20 *Oeuvres d'Oribase*, 6: 205.

with diseases whose names are transliterated directly from the Greek, the term for this condition is incubus, rather than ephialtes.[21] Similarly, in the Arabic world, although they borrow one term, *ifyaltis*, from the Greek, as might be expected in the translation movements from Greek to Syriac and Arabic, the Islamic medical writers often use a term which seems to be taken from the Latin: *al-kabus* appears in Ibn Sina's *Qanun* and elsewhere.[22] The old name for a malevolent Roman spirit dominated several medieval medical traditions, and ensured that the connections with demonology and with fantasy, imagination and fear would endure.

Medieval Learned Medicine and the Physiology of the Incubus

The core of the remaining discussion here focuses on medical writings produced in western Europe between approximately 1070 and 1310. With the return of major urban centres and long-distance trade in Latin Christendom, the translation movements of southern Italy in the late eleventh century and of Spain, especially Toledo, in the mid-twelfth century introduced the west to the far more expansive and complex medical literature of the Arabic world. The importance of the transmission of Greco-Arabic knowledge to the west is well known.[23] With the rise of universities in the thirteenth century, the new, more theoretical materials played an essential role generally in the organization of medical knowledge, and specifically in the understandings of the brain and its pathologies. While earlier medical authors, especially Galen, certainly expressed interest in the functioning of the brain and pathologies they could connect to it, it is with the Arabic tradition that we find a concerted effort to create a coherent theory of mental order and disorder.[24] Taking up Platonic and Aristotelian programmes, figures such as Ibn Sina sought to map out the

[21] Passionarius Garioponti, *Galeni Pergameni Passionarius, a doctis medicis multum desideratus, egritudines a capite ad pedes vsque complectens* (Lyons: In edibus Antonii Blanchardi, sumptu Bartholomei Trot, 1526), fol. 61vb, ch. 17, De incubo.

[22] Ibn Sina, *al-Qanun fi'l-tibb* (Beirut: Manshurat Muhammad Ali Baydun, Dar al Kutub al-Ilmiya, 1999), 1: 239. Ibn Sina also mentions several other terms (*al-jathum wa al-nidalan;* in Gerard of Cremona's translation, *albodilem* and *alcharon*, fol. 191vb) that have no known connection to the Greek or Roman traditions.

[23] See the voluminous work of Danielle Jacquart, particularly her study, with Françoise Micheau, *La médecine arabe et l'Occident médiéval* (Paris: Maisonneuve et Larose, 1990) and collected essays, *La science médicale occidentale entre deux renaissances (XIIe s.–XVe s.)* (Aldershot: Variorum, 1997).

[24] See Stanley Jackson, "Galen—On mental disorders," *Journal of the History of the Behavioral Sciences* 5 (1969): 365–84.

connections between body and soul, corpus and anima. The tendency of Ibn Sina and other Arabic authors to focus on the soul and the moral as well as the natural philosophical works of Aristotle ensured that diseases of the brain, the seat of the soul,[25] would be among the topics of greatest concern for western medical writers as the influence of Islamic thought triumphed in Salerno, Toledo, Paris, Bologna and Montpellier. With the interest in mental processes came a parallel concern over the emotions, known to the medieval learned world as the accidents of the soul.[26]

The most extensive discussions of the incubus occur in materials from the second half of the thirteenth and early fourteenth centuries, when the influence of Aristotle, via Ibn Sina (Avicenna) and other Arabic natural philosophers and physicians, was being felt most strongly. Following the pattern of the late antique and Islamic worlds, medical authors usually associated with the universities composed new, often massive compendia surveying the art of medicine or more specific treatises on diseases.[27] In the process, western medicine elaborated upon earlier understandings of the condition and more closely scrutinized the mental and emotional states that it inspired. Much of what follows will focus on the works of four medical writers connected to universities: Gilbertus Anglicus, active on the continent around 1250;[28] William of Saliceto, associated with Bologna and Piacenza, active in the 1270s;[29] Arnald of Villanova, associated with Montpellier, active around 1300, died 1311;[30] and Arnald's contemporary,

[25] *Avicenna Latinus: Liber de anima seu Sextus de naturalibus*, ed. S. Van Riet (Louvain/ Leiden: E. Peeters and E.J. Brill, 1968–1972), 2 vols.

[26] The history of this aspect of medieval medicine is still being written. See Jole Agrimi and Chiara Crisciani, "Medicina del corpo e medicina dell'anima: note sul sapere del medico fino all'inizio del sec. XIII," *Episteme* 10 (1976): 5–102 and Mark Jordan, "The Construction of a Philosophical Medicine: Exegesis and Argument in Salernitan Teaching on the Soul," *Osiris* 2nd series, v. 6: *Renaissance Medical Learning: Evolution of a Tradition* (1990): 42–61, and Gerald Grudzen, *Medical Theory about the Body and the Soul in the Middle Ages: the First Western Medical Curriculum at Monte Cassino* (Lewiston, NY: Edwin Mellen Press, 2007).

[27] Aleksandre Birkenmajer, "Le role joué par les médecins et les naturalistes dans la réception d'Aristote au XIIe et XIIIe siècles," in *Studia Copernicana I: Etudes d'histoire des sciences et de la philosophie du moyen âge* (Warsaw: Zaklad Narodowy im. Ossolinskich, 1970), 73–88.

[28] Gilbertus Anglicus, *Compendium medicine Gilberti anglici tam morborum vniuersalium quam particularium nondum medicis sed et cyrurgicis vtilissimum* (Lyons: J. Saccon for V. de Portonariis, 1510).

[29] William of Saliceto, *Liber Magistri Gulielmi Placentini de Saleceto in scientia medicinali & specialiter perfectus incipit: qui summa conseruationis & curationis apellatur* (Piacenza: J.P. de Ferratis, 1476).

[30] Arnald of Villanova. *Arnaldi Villanovani philosophi et medici summi Opera omnia* (Basel: ex officina Pernea per Conradum Vvaldkirch, 1585).

Bernard de Gordon, also part of the medical faculty at Montpellier, died toward the end of the 1310s.[31]

In what ways did western medical writers alter or extend the discussion of the incubus in the thirteenth and early fourteenth centuries? With the literary evidence pointing toward a renewed awareness of the demonological tradition by the twelfth century, medical literature continued to argue forcefully against the supernatural explanation of the affliction, as we shall see. With a rich arsenal of late antique and Arabic materials at their disposal, thirteenth-century physicians were more successful at replacing the demonological hermeneutic with a physiological one, gathering together a variety of causes that were entirely natural, that is, devoid of spiritual implications.

Medical authors rejected a monocausal explanation, whether naturalistic or otherworldly, by stressing a multiplicity of causes, even when such a variety of etiologies might create confusion and conflict. Physicians vigorously disagreed with one another over not just the causes but also the essential taxonomic category into which the incubus fit. While the demonological tradition could appear unified in an explanation based in the shadowy realm of fiendish influence, medical experts in the second half of the thirteenth century were torn: was the incubus an "animal" or a "spiritual" illness? The meanings of these two terms reflect the growing technical vocabulary of scholastic natural philosophy in this period: "animal" here refers to a disease of the soul (*anima*) or brain, while "spiritual" refers to an illness centring on problems related to the lungs and respiration (*spiritus*). Most medical writers followed the tradition established in the late antique and Arabic materials, particularly Avicenna, by choosing the head and brain as the primary organ with which the disease should be associated.

To categorize the incubus as a disease of the lungs makes some sense when one considers the heavy emphasis on breathing—or more accurately the inability to breathe—as perhaps the primary indicator of the disease. Following Avicenna, William of Saliceto identifies an alternative name for the incubus, "the strangler" (*strangulator*), and views the constriction of the breath as central to the ailment.[32] Yet despite such common observations, only one author places the incubus in the category of

[31] Bernard de Gordon. *Practica Gordinij dicta Lilium medicine* (Venice: J. & G. Gregoriis, 1496).

[32] William of Saliceto, *Summa*, ch. 16, fol. 19va.

respiratory diseases. In the later twelfth century, Roger of Salerno, or of Parma, composed an influential treatise on surgery organized, like many manuals of more general medicine, according to the site of diseases, from the head to the feet.[33] He discusses the incubus in the section on diseases of the heart, lungs and stomach, identifying the condition as "another disease of breathing."[34] It is not clear why Roger breaks with the tradition of the incubus as a disease of the brain, but the early date of the text, before the clear impact of the Toledan translations was felt in medical circles, suggests that the taxonomy was not fully established in some medical circles. William of Saliceto refers to some who believe the incubus to be connected to the heart or lungs rather than the brain, and provides a counterargument to this claim.[35]

Although the consensus was generally that the incubus was a disease that affected the brain most of all, medical authors took a multifaceted approach to its etiology and progress. The disease was thought to attack many parts of the body, including the stomach, heart, lungs, brain, vocal cords and nerves throughout the body. But its origins, like those of many other diseases in the medieval medical canon, were perceived to be multiple, mostly based in the bodily processes of digestion. Sometimes the cause lay in excess consumption: too much food or drink could wreak havoc on the stomach and lead to the incubus. At other times the source was too little food, with fasting in particular identified as a cause of the incubus, especially for those with overly hot stomachs.[36]

Gilbertus Anglicus identifies a chain reaction of physiological processes that explains the course of the disease and its symptoms. When the stomach is overly full of food and drink, the diaphragm presses against the lungs, which then press against the heart. Or air (*ventus*) that ordinarily leaves the lungs and brain via the nose and mouth cannot do so, and presses on the heart, "whence out of sympathy (*ex compassione*) the whole body appears to be pressed."[37] The emphasis on the heart relates to both the Aristotelian heart-centred system and the Platonic-Galenic tradition

33 On the uncertainties over Roger's life, see Mario Tabanelli, *La chirurgia italiana nell'alto medioevo* (Florence: L.S. Olschki, 1965), 1: 5–15.

34 *Cyrurgia Guidonis de Cauliaco. Et Cyrurgia Bruni, Theodorici Rogerij Rolandi Bertapalie Lanfranci* (Venice: Bonetus Locatellus for Octavianus Scotus, 1498), fol. 214vb, ch. 26 De incubo.

35 *Liber Magistri Gulielmi Placentini de saleceto… summa conseruationis*, ch. 16, fol. 19vb.

36 Arnald, *De parte operativa*, col. 290.

37 Gilbertus Anglicus, *Compendium*, fol. 113vb.

of a tripartite view of bodily functions: the brain controls the senses, the heart controls movement, and the liver controls digestion. Pressure on the heart, accordingly, could cause the cessation of all movement, as is the case with the incubus.

Whether due to surfeit or want, indigestion was often identified as the most common cause of the incubus. Central to this argument is the medieval medical consensus that one of the basic functions of sleep is the proper and complete digestion of food. While to the modern world, the repose of the body and a general lack of exertion during sleep acts as a replenishment of the body's energy, the medieval medical view saw this refilling of the body's strength as a result of the internal digestive activity during sleep. The period of slumber was considered a very productive and essential phase, as the food consumed during waking hours travelled through multiple stages of concoction, a heating or cooking of the nourishment as it descends through the digestive organs. The least useful foods went through only the first concoction and left the body as excrement, while the later concoctions rarified and purified the nourishment, ending with the third concoction, which produced blood in its purest form.[38] In a healthy individual who has eaten the food most appropriate to his or her constitution, this process should succeed in producing a balanced, healthy body. Many factors, including the quantity and quality of the food consumed, can alter this system and lead to disorder, imbalance and disease. Digestion and proper sleep were thus intimately connected, and any disturbance to one could symbiotically affect the other. Thus raw foods could create a "fatty smokiness" or a "non-poisonous vapour," which would rise within the body and block the heart or brain, thus inducing an attack of the incubus.[39]

The multiplicity of causes that is so typical of scholastic medicine allows for a complex classification of types of the condition, with their consequent individualized prognoses and cures. Various authors divide the etiologies into internal and external categories, so that factors such as the temperature of the sleeping chamber or the position of the sleeper can have as much of an impact as an excess of wine or a general imbalance of the humours. Avicenna notes that the incubus can arise from a pathological vapour made of sanguine, phlegmatic, or melancholic matter,

---

[38] See John Wilkins, introduction, *Galen, On the Property of Foodstuffs* (Cambridge: Cambridge University Press, 2002), 13–18.

[39] Arnald, *De parte operativa*, col. 290; Gilbertus Anglicus, *Compendium*, fol. 113va.

leaving only yellow bile out of the list of possibilities. The *Passionarius* is even less precise by attributing the night-time ailment to a "bad humour" (*cacochimia, id est malo humore*).[40] An overabundance of phlegm appears often, and connects the incubus with epilepsy, which was understood from the Hippocratic corpus onward to be a phlegmatic disease.[41] The sufferer's sleeping position could also induce the incubus, particularly the often-mentioned dangers of the supine position, as noted from Avicenna onward in the medical literature and even in twelfth-century glosses on Macrobius.[42]

From the late antique period, medical authorities drew a parallel between the incubus and a number of other diseases of the brain, but most importantly the falling sickness, epilepsy.[43] While Caelius Aurelianus associated it only with epilepsy, Oribasius began a long-standing tradition that saw the incubus as a condition that could lead to more serious diseases such as apoplexy, epilepsy and mania. We encounter this same equation in Avicenna and Bernard de Gordon, who adds abscesses, paralysis, spasms and even sudden death to the list of prognostic possibilities.[44] What most connects Oribasius' triad and the incubus is the categorization of all as illnesses of the brain. More specifically, they all deal with a lack of control of one's body and/or mind, due mostly to an inability of the nerves to function properly.

Medical authorities saw many connections between epilepsy and the incubus, and used them to reinforce their opposition to a supernatural interpretation of either condition. Both diseases had been associated for centuries with the divine or demonic, a tradition against which medical experts could argue and thus display their knowledge of the inner workings of the human body. The frequency with which medical writers

40 Avicenna, *Liber canonis*, fol. 192ra; *Passionarius*, ch. 17, fol. 61vb, also quoted (as Papias) in Vincent of Beauvais, *Speculum majus* (Douai: Beller, 1624), *Speculum doctrinale*, bk 15, ch. 58, col. 1318C.

41 Hippocrate, *La maladie sacrée*, ed. Jouanna, ch. 3: 11; *Hippocratic Writings*, trans. Lloyd, 241.

42 Avicenna, *Liber canonis*, 1.3.2.9, fol. 61vb. For the natural philosophical discussion of the incubus and dreams, see Thomas Ricklin, *Der Traum der Philosophie im 12. Jahrhundert: Traumtheorien zwischen Constantinus Africanus & Aristoteles* (Leiden, Boston, Cologne: Brill, 1998), 456–57, and Stephen F. Kruger, *Dreaming in the Middle Ages* (Cambridge and New York: Cambridge University Press, 1992), 70–75.

43 Temkin, *Falling Sickness*, esp. 108. See also William G. Lennox, "Bernard of Gordon on Epilepsy," *Annals of Medical History* 3 (1941): 372–383.

44 *Oeuvres d'Oribase*, 5: 402 and 3: 205; Avicenna, *Liber canonis* (Hildesheim: Georg Olms, 1963, facsimile of Venice 1507 edition), 3.1.5.5, fol. 192ra; Bernard de Gordon, *Lilium*, part 2, ch. 25, fol. 74va.

lambasted the supernatural view of these diseases (and to a lesser extent mania) demonstrates their commitment to a vision of medicine and natural philosophy as systems of thought that could explain God's plan in naturalistic terms.[45]

But medical authorities disagreed on the connection between epilepsy and the incubus. Gilbertus Anglicus argues that the incubus is a disease "in a certain way contrary to epilepsy." He notes that the disease *epialtes* or the incubus involves a diminution of movement but not of the senses: instead of epileptic convulsions, a type of paralysis ensues.[46] Others made it clear that the parallels were strong, since, according to William of Saliceto, "it arises out of every cause or matter from which epilepsy arises." He goes on to observe that the incubus is nothing other than a minor or imperfect epilepsy.[47] Contemporary with William's surgical treatise, the translation of Rhazes's *al-Hawi*, known to the west as *Continens*, claims that the incubus is the beginning of epilepsy, a gateway to the more severe and better-established condition, and warns the reader not to neglect the disease for this reason.[48] By connecting the incubus with a well-known condition with a long medical pedigree going back to the Hippocratic corpus, the Arabic and Latin writers underscored the appropriateness of this condition to the field of learned medicine and physiological pathology.

The most revealing connection between epilepsy and the incubus comes in the writings of al-Majusi, known to the west as Haly Abbas. His *Complete Book of Medicine* (*Kitab kamil al-sina'ah al-tibbiyah*) was translated as the *Pantegni* by Constantinus Africanus in the late eleventh century and translated for a second time by Stephen of Antioch in the twelfth century. In both translation, the symptoms appear as a variant of epilepsy, added at the end of a chapter on apoplexy and the falling sickness. Haly Abbas does not fully differentiate the disease—in Constantinus' translation, it is not even named—, but simply connects it with the sensation of constriction felt by epileptics.[49] Similarly, Rhazes's *Continens* intersperses

[45] This was not necessarily incompatible with the miraculous or divine intervention; physicians sought to identify patterns which could define the normative and the pathological, which could be distinguished from the miraculous.

[46] Gilbertus Anglicus, *Compendium*, fol. 113va.

[47] William of Saliceto, *Summa*, fol. 19va.

[48] Rhazes, *Continens*, bk 1, ch. 6, fol. 13rb ("incubus est principium epilepsie"), 13vb.

[49] Constantinus's translation: *Omnia opera Ysaac in hoc volumine contenta . . . Pantechni decem libri theorices . . .* (Lyons: Jean de La Place for Barthélémy Trot, 1515), bk 9, ch. 6, fol. 42rb. Stephen of Antioch's translation: *Haly filius abbas, Liber totius medicine necessaria continens quem sapientissimus Haly filius abbas discipulus abimeher moysi filii seiar edidit:*

references to the incubus within the lengthy discussion of epilepsy, blurring the distinction between the two. Paul of Aegina had, in the early seventh century, made a claim that the characteristics of the epileptic during the day are the same as those of the incubus sufferer at night.[50] Whether they were synonymous or they coexisted on a continuum of related conditions, the incubus and epilepsy were paired together within late antique and medieval medical literature.

This discussion has, up to this point, concentrated on the somatic symptoms of the incubus, rather than the cognitive consequences of the condition. The immediate causes of the condition, like those of epilepsy, are based in the torso—stomach, lungs, and heart—and in the economy of liquids and vapours that permeate the body in medieval medicine. But while the etiology may be located below the head, it is the impact of this condition on mental and sensory functionings that fascinated medical authorities. While some provided only a cursory understanding of the brain's function,[51] other medical authorities used this disease as an opportunity to discuss the impact of the body on the mental processes. Sleep and its pathology provided a very potent combination through which medical authors could explore and try to explain the irrational and the fantastic.

The Demon in the Mind

All medieval medical discussions of the incubus acknowledged the patient's belief that the condition was an attack by some sort of creature, as described so vividly in the miracle of Stephen of Hoyland. The very fact that they placed the incubus among diseases of the brain indicates that medical theorists viewed the patient's belief in a nocturnal attack to be a consequence of a pathology affecting the mental process. To understand the logic of the physicians' interpretation, it is necessary to understand the medieval theories of the brain's structure and processes. Indeed,

---

regique inscripsit unde et regalis dispositionis nomen assumpsit (Lyons: J. Myt, 1523), bk 9, ch. 6, fol. 104ra.

50 Rhazes, *Continens*, 12vb–13vb; *The Seven Books of Paulus Aegineta*, bk 3, section 17; 1: 388.

51 For parallel discussions in the Regimen of health literature, see the commentary by Pedro Gil-Sotres in *Regimen sanitatis ad regem Aragonum. Arnaldi de Villanova opera medica omnia*, X.1, ed. Luis García-Ballester and Michael McVaugh (Barcelona: Seminarium Historiae Scientiae Barcinonense, 1996), 736–40.

the medical sources argue their case from a theoretical understanding of the geography of the brain that had come into prominence in the twelfth century.

According to the dominant theory of the twelfth and thirteenth centuries, the brain is divided into three compartments (*cellulae, ventriculi*), each of which contains and commands one or two faculties or functional properties. The first compartment contains the "common sense" and the "imagination" or "fantasy." The former gathers together the information that comes in from each of the five external senses, which are then interpreted by the imagination, which as its etymology suggests is able to synthesize and retain images as well as sensations entering into the common sense. Slightly less crucial for our discussion, the second compartment contains the ability to think rationally (*cogitatio*) and to act instinctively (*estimatio*), while the third or posterior compartment houses the memory, more enduring than the imagination's ability to recollect images and sensations.[52] This quick overview of the mental landscape developed out of a fusion of very divergent systems advocated in the ancient and Arabic worlds. Aristotle had argued for the common sense and imagination without specifying where these mental processes took place.[53] The notion of the three chambers seems to appear first in Latin literature with bishop Alfanus' mid-eleventh-century translation of Nemesius' *On the Nature of Man*, and received further validation a generation later in Constantinus' *Pantegni* and *Ysagoge*, both translated from Arabic writers, al-Majusi (Haly Abbas) and Hunain ibn Ishaq (Johannitius).[54] Despite the many variations, the model for human perception is relatively consistent: information from the external world is brought by the senses to the common sense, which synthesizes it, and then to the imagination, which stores and further interprets it, with the assistance of the rational faculty in the middle ventricle and the long-term memory in the posterior ventricle.

---

[52] See Simon Kemp and Garth J. O. Fletcher, "The Medieval Theory of the Inner Senses," *The American Journal of Psychology* 106 (1993): 559–76; Simon Kemp, *Cognitive Psychology in the Middle Ages* (Westport, CT and London: Greenwood, 1996), 51–57; and E. Ruth Harvey, *The Inward Wits: Psychological Theory in the Middle Ages and the Renaissance* (London: Warburg Institute, 1975), esp. 43–45.

[53] Murray Wright Bundy, *The Theory of Imagination in Classical and Mediaeval Thought* (Urbana: University of Illinois Press, 1927, rprt. Norwood Editions, 1978), esp. 189–93, Michael Wedin, *Mind and Imagination in Aristotle* (New Haven: Yale University Press, 1988) and Pavel Gregoric, *Aristotle on the Common Sense* (Oxford: Oxford University Press, 2005).

[54] Ynez Viole O'Neill, "William of Conches' Description of the Brain," *Clio medica* 3 (1968): 203–23.

While the healthy, sane adult's brain should function in this way during the waking state, the same was not at all true of the sleeper, whose perception was impaired. The medical understanding of the mental world of the sleeper derives from a fusion of Aristotelian views of cognition with the just-mentioned theories outlining the physiological geography of the brain.[55] During sleep, the senses and the rational faculty are inactive because the passageways by which they would normally function have been clogged by a smokiness that rises from the liver and heart as a consequence of the digestion or concoction of food. The inactivity of the common sense and temporary lack of the capacity to reason were considered nonpathological and normative during sleep, although the latter could lead to difficulties, particularly of a moral nature.[56]

For medieval physicians and natural philosophers, the danger of the sleeping state lay in the ability of the imagination to continue to function, producing images and attempting to interpret phenomena without the use of reason. In terms of the incubus, there was the added complication that the senses were not entirely cut off. In the natural philosophical tradition stemming from Macrobius' *Commentary on the Dream of Scipio*, the incubus is simply a phantasma or apparition which enters the individual's mind in the confusing period between sleeping and waking.[57] Gilbertus argues that the incubus is "a diminution of movement but not of the senses in sleep," thus identifying both the paralysis and intense sensations of the condition as pathological deviations from the normal state of the sleeper, during which the senses should be inoperative.[58] Accordingly, the physiological chain reaction of pressure on the internal organs and the nerves' responses to that pressure seem to have allowed the imagination to interpret the sensations improperly, as an attack by some external entity.[59]

---

[55] Aristotle, *On Sleep*, 453b12–458a32, and the analysis by H. Wijsenbeek-Wijler, *Aristotle's Concept of Soul, Sleep and Dreams* (Amsterdam: Adolf M. Hakkert, 1978).

[56] Concerns over nocturnal emissions and sexual dreams demonstrated the moral dangers made possible by the sleeping state. I pursue this issue in another part of an ongoing study of sleep and irrationality.

[57] Macrobius, *Commentarii in Somnium Scipionis*, ed. James Willis (Leipzig: Teubner, 1963), 1.3.7: 10 and *Commentary on the Dream of Scipio by Macrobius*, trans. William Harris Stahl (New York: Columbia University Press, 1952 and 1990), 89. See Alison M. Peden, "Macrobius and Mediaeval Dream Literature," *Medium Aevum* 54 (1985): 59–73, esp. 64–65 on William of Conches' use of Macrobius and physiological theory.

[58] Gilbertus Anglicus, *Compendium*, fol. 113va.

[59] O'Neill, "William of Conches," 212–14, and Bundy, *Theory of Imagination*, 189–93. For an example of a slightly different theory, see Ronald H. Nash, *The Light of the Mind: St. Augustine's Theory of Knowledge* (Lexington, University of Kentucky Press, 1969).

What was the apparition that sufferers imagined in their sleep, and what caused it to appear? Seeking to explain the folkloric in somatic and naturalistic terms, Gilbertus Anglicus mentions a fatty smoke or windiness (*fumositas* or *ventositas*) that rises to the fantasy, i.e. the mental functions associated with the anterior ventricle of the brain, which produces apparitions. Bernard de Gordon similarly refers to a "corrupt vapour" that obstructs and weighs down on the brain and heart, creating the pathological condition that affects the imagination.[60] But it is Bernard's contemporary Arnald of Villanova who provides the most extensive analysis of the physio-psychology of the incubus. In the midst of an attack of the incubus, the sufferers seek to explain their predicament:

> They know that they cannot speak nor freely make a sound, they attempt to remove the perceived impediment, for they strive to rise up, call out and speak, and because they cannot, they exert themselves but find themselves constrained. They perceive the cause of the impediment [...]. With their spirits bound in a light sleep [and] because their imagination and estimative faculty have not yet been bound by that sleep, since it is light and has just begun, they observe in a shape preserved in the repository of the imagination [*in thesauro imaginativo*] the shape of that thing which most closely signifies the cause of the impediment. Thus, since the chest and throat are prevented from expanding, they see through their imagination the shape of someone lying upon and strangling them.[61]

The passage is obscure and presents many problems, but the larger point is clear: those who experience the incubus find themselves in a helpless state and so search for an explanation, which the imagination readily supplies. Arnald clearly identifies the movement from physical sensation to mental process, with the crucial active role given to the imagination. By referring to this part of the brain as a storehouse or treasure trove of images or forms, Arnald suggests that the imagination has multiple options from which to choose, and from those it selects the image or shape (*forma*) that seems most apposite to the bodily sensations experienced by the sufferer.

It is thus not surprising that those who experience the incubus do not always see a demon, at least in the descriptions given by medical authors. Instead, the sources describe a wide variety of attackers imagined by the

[60] Gilbertus Anglicus, *Compendium*, fol. 113vb; Bernard de Gordon, *Lilium*, fol. 74va.

[61] Arnald of Villanova, *De parte operativa*, col. 290. The estimative faculty is usually associated with an innate or instinctual ability to interpret a situation, as when a sheep instinctively fears a wolf. See Kemp, *Cognitive Psychology*, 56–58.

patients: they can be men in Haly Abbas and the *Passionarius*, demons or beasts in Gilbertus Anglicus, even old women in Bernard de Gordon.[62] But perhaps the medical discourse includes these alternative interpretations in order to undermine the validity of any such perceptions by the sufferers, and further underscores the critique of the disease's origins in an external attack by describing the perceived invader as a *phantasma* or *phantasia*, an apparition, a mere product of fantasy and the imagination. Sometimes the medical sources depict the patient's perspective as particularly vague: something or someone is aggravating, or weighing down on, the body. Here the supernatural is not necessarily the only option for the sufferer to accept: the patient may perceive the culprit to be human, perhaps an enemy or some unknown but not demonic assailant. Gilbertus Anglicus emphasizes the variety of interpretations: a smokiness obstructs the brain and "rises to the fantasy and gives birth to images of various bodies,"[63] which lead to very different responses by individual patients, some of whom may seem to be suffocated and unable to speak while others freely tell tales and dispute with the images they see. Linking all of these possible interpretations is the central argument that, for the medical world, the patient's imagination is functioning wrongly because the sufferer is asleep and suffering from physiological pathologies.

The patient's (mis)interpretation lies at the heart of the medical dilemma over the incubus: a false belief by the sufferer and others derives from a false understanding by the temporarily nonrational brain, specifically by the imagination as it seeks to explain the physiological and nervous actions and reactions of the patient's body. The sensation that the pressure was moving rapidly from the lower extremities up the torso reinforced the imagination's interpretation that an assault from without was underway.[64] We encounter a complex interplay of the "real" and the "imagined": the constriction is identified by physicians as valid and concrete, while the idea that it is an external weight or a violent touch moves beyond the realm of the real into overly-imaginative interpretation. This is further complicated by the sufferer's reactions to the imagined attack: fear, sweat and paleness, discussed in the final section below, all of which are recognized as "real" phenomena, despite their origins as a response to a false vision. The folkloric incubus blurs the line between physiology

[62] Haly Abbas, *Liber totius medicine*, fol. 103va; *Passionarius*, fol. 61b; Gilbertus Anglicus, *Compendium*, fol. 113vb; Bernard de Gordon, *Lilium*, fol. 74rb;

[63] Gilbertus Anglicus, *Compendium*, fol. 113vb.

[64] Bernard de Gordon, *Lilium*, fol. 74va, et al.

and fantasy (in both the medieval and modern senses of that word), thus allowing the opportunity for medical authors to assert their truth claims: they can discern the difference between somatic reality and false apparition, and can consequently help to heal the sufferer through proper identification of the condition.

Of all the aspects of the folkloric incubus, the characteristic that is most consipcuous by its absence in this literature is the sexual component of the demonological tradition. From the Greco-Roman world onward, there were often indications that the incubus' attack involved both violence and sexuality. The stories of intercourse and even insemination found most prominently in the Merlin tales of the twelfth century and later, are generally absent from the medical narratives. But this is not entirely the case. The early nosological descriptions of the incubus refer explicitly to sex and violence.[65] While the violence and speed of the onslaught remain as characteristics of the disease and the phantasm it causes, the sexual component seems to have disappeared from the medical literature of the early and central middle ages, with one exception. In al-Majusi's tenth-century medical encyclopedia *Complete Book of Medicine*, the patient tries but fails to cry out because he imagines a man is sexually assaulting him. In the second, twelfth-century Latin translation of this text, by Stephen of Antioch, the section on epilepsy and the incubus concludes with the following words: "it sometimes happens that he sees a violent man having intercourse with him."[66] This brief statement remains unexamined within the text and seemingly ignored by medical writers of the next few centuries. It remains a mystery why this aspect of the incubus tradition was almost always excluded from the medical discourse, when it was present in contemporary literary and theological accounts of the demonic incubus.[67]

There remains the unanswerable question of why physicians would choose to use the word *incubus*, a term not of their own making, especially one that holds within it an interpretation rejected by medical theory. Both Bernard de Gordon and Arnald of Villanova recognized the dangers inherent in the term incubus due to its broader cultural connotations. Arnald acknowledged that the term was a partial misnomer: "The disease incubus

[65] Caelius Aurelianus, in Roscher, *Ephialtes*, 109: "... et se videre credant irruentem sibi et usum tuprissimae libidinis persuadentem ..." It is not clear if Caelius is, at this moment, quoting from the lost text of Soranus (2nd century AD).

[66] Ali ibn al-ʿAbbas [Al-Majusi], *Kamil al-Sina'ah al-tibbiyah* (Cairo: Bulaq, 1877), 1: 332; *Haly filius abbas, Liber totius medicine*, ch. 6, fol. 103va. The gender of the attacker and attacked, both male, is made explicit in both the Arabic and Latin.

[67] Kiessling, *The Incubus*, ch. 4; van der Lugt, *Le ver*, 273–91.

in Latin and ephialtes in Greek is so called from an *accidens*, since the patient believes that something crushing has lain down or cast itself over him while he is sleeping."[68] The term *accidens* here follows the Aristotelian meaning, of something which is not intrinsic to or causative of the condition but merely a consequence or secondary characteristic of it. For Arnald, there is no reason to define this disease by the sensation of being crushed or suffocated, let alone (he implies) by some external, supernatural creature seeking to strangle the afflicted person. The former is simply one of several possible outcomes or sensory reactions to the disease, and the latter Arnald simply ignores or refers to as imaginary forms.

Bernard makes an even more explicit reference to the incubus as a disease encumbered by a variety of interpretations, learned and popular. In contrast to Arnald, Bernard begins the disease's entry in the *Lilium medicinae* by stating that it is the name of a demon and is a "phantasm in sleep that presses and weighs down on the body and disturbs motion and speech."[69] As van der Lugt has noted, Bernard then distinguishes opposing views of the condition based on three groups: theologians, popular understandings, and doctors. The theologians seem to be focused on the incubus as something that suffocates sucklings (*pueris lactantibus*), in a phrasing that seems to suggest a naturalistic rather than demonological understanding of the condition. In contrast, the second interpretation is clearly supernatural: "the common people (*vulgares*) say that it is some little old woman (*aliqua vetula*) stomping and pressing on bodies."[70] Before turning to what he identifies as the more correct view of the doctors, Bernard rejects the vulgar interpretation in its entirety. Yet Bernard's report of the popular belief is striking for its novelty: the demon—mentioned only a few lines earlier by Bernard in his description of the patient's point of view—has been gendered female and turned into an elderly but seemingly fully human aggressor. The passage contains a report that may reflect the early stages of the transformation of the figure of the "old hag" into a problematized, even demonized character, a pattern which becomes more pronounced in later witchcraft accusations.[71]

The incubus thus stands in a unique position as a personified or demonized condition. Because the incubus demon was well known in the central middle ages and because sufferers often imagined such a creature,

68 Arnald, *De parte operativa*, cols. 289–90.
69 Bernard, *Lilium*, bk 2, ch. 24, fol. 74rb.
70 Bernard, *Lilium*, bk 2, ch. 24, fol. 74va. See van der Lugt, "Incubus," 176.
71 See Kiessling, *The Incubus*, ch. 4: esp. 28.

it is worth noting that the medical terminology describing the condition seems at times to attribute an ontological reality to the disease that parallels the demon's supposed reality. The disease, like the demon, "rushes on," "overcomes" or "quickly attacks" the patient, further reinforcing the patient's experience but with a medical interpretation.[72] The terminology is relatively rare in medical nosology, and may reflect an acknowledgement of the demonological tradition or of the sufferer's experience. But it also has implications for the ontological status of the disease called the incubus: like the demonic incubus, it acts through a sudden ambush-like assault, although its origins lie within, rather than without, the body.

Whatever its physiological origins in the lower parts of the body, the incubus brought medical attention to the cognitive and sensory processes inside the brain, and problematized the role of the imagination. What should simply assist, structure and retain the brain's understanding of external sensations, has become a source of further pathology acting in response to the internal constrictions of the heart, lungs, vocal cords and motor abilities. Instead of receiving and interpreting outside stimuli—the sensations gathered by the common sense—, the imagination reverses the process and interprets processes inside the body as if they were caused by an outside source. Medical theorists, particularly by the late thirteenth century, when interest in psychological issues was becoming more prominent,[73] began to elaborate upon the processes involved in the fantasy and imagination and recognized the pathological potential in mental processes during sleep.[74] In this instance, the imagination compounds the pre-existing imbalances in the body with an interpretive framework of aggressive assault which leads to further complications to the body and to the accidents of the soul.

---

[72] Arnald, *De parte operativa*, col. 290; Gilbertus, *Compendium*, fol. 113vb.

[73] See esp. Luis García-Ballester, "Arnau de Vilanova (c. 1240–1311) y la reforma de los estudios médicos en Montpellier (1309): El Hipócrates latino y la introducción del Nuevo Galeno," *Dynamis* 2 (1982): 97–158, and, with some reductions and alterations, idem, "The New Galenism: A Challenge to Latin Galenism in Thirteenth-Century Montpellier," in *Text and Tradition: Studies in Ancient Medicine and its Transmission*, ed. Klaus-Dietrich Fischer, Diethard Nickel and Paul Potter (Leiden: Brill, 1998), 55–83. The sleepwalker had been discussed in the Salernitan materials of the years around 1200 (Prose Salernitan Questions, Urso of Salerno's Aphorisms) and exhibited similar problems, which again were taken up with greator rigour by Bernard de Gordon around 1300.

[74] Kruger, *Dreaming*, 116–22, discusses the writings of natural philosophers such as Albertus Magnus in relation to this issue. In my current study of sleep pathologies, I analyze this material in relation to the nosological sections of medical texts of the twelfth and thirteenth centuries.

The Incubus and the Accidents of the Soul

One of the more exceptional aspects of the medical incubus is the recognition of emotive responses, and particularly terror, as a constituent part and signifier of the disease. The role of fear, and references to other accidents of the soul, further illustrates the connections between body and mind that are so prominent with this disease. More so than diseases of other parts of the body, diseases of the brain were assumed to be more prone to influence, and be influenced by, the accidents of the soul, especially anger, joy and sadness, but to a lesser extent fear.[75] It is relatively uncommon in medical literature for a patient's emotional reaction to a disease to be noted, but here the accidents of the soul play an important part in the understanding and progress of the condition.

When the patient perceives that the weight on his body is aggression by a demon or human, he reacts with a number of further physiological and emotional responses. Bernard de Gordon notes that the patient takes up the idea that he is being attacked by a demon, and tries to beg for assistance from the creature. The temporary muteness brought on by the disease, or in the patient's mind brought on by being suffocated, prevents him from making any more than a lowing sound like a cow, further increasing the feeling of incapacity and powerlessness. Bernard notes that the sufferer is then "thoroughly terrified on account of the increased heaviness of the burden."[76] Although Bernard reiterates the humoral and internal origins of the weight on and in the body, he makes it clear that the affective response is a consequence of the weight, and of the patient's understanding of its cause.

The *Passionarius* identifies the psychological and physiological reactions to the incubus: "they see or are terrified by [*paveant*] a variety of different dreams, that is a phantasy."[77] The text later notes that sufferers can be both terrified (*pavidi*) and pale in the face (*pallido vultu*) as a response to the perceived assault. Two centuries later, Gilbertus Anglicus seems to paraphrase this passage from the *Passionarius*, and simplifies it

[75] See Simo Knuuttila, "Medieval Theories of the Passions of the Soul," in *Emotions and Choice from Boethius to Descartes*, ed. Henrik Lagerlund and Mikko Yrjönsuuri (Dordrecht: Kluwer Academic Publishers, 2002), and Barbara Rosenwein, ed., *Anger's Past: The Social Uses of an Emotion in the Middle Ages* (Ithaca: Cornell University Press, 1998).

[76] Bernard de Gordon, *Lilium*, fol. 74va; Arnald, *De parte operativa*, col. 290.

[77] *Passionarius*, fol. 61vb. The printed edition has "sonorum," sounds, while Wellcome MS 133, twelfth century, has "sompnorum;" which seems to blur sleeping (somnus) with dreaming (somnium).

into a pithy and alliterative phrase: *pavor et palor*, terror and paleness, are among the consequences of the incubus. The term *pavor* can mean not just terror but its physical manifestations, i.e. trembling or dread. Similarly the light hue of the face indicated by the term *pallor* often refers to a somatic response to fear.[78] In these two words we find a clear medical awareness of the association of bodily sensation and the accidents of the soul.

The connections between the somatic, the mental, and the emotional were never fully elaborated in the medical literature of the medieval period, but were discussed indirectly, as is the case here, if at all. Medieval theories of the accidents of the soul consist of a synoptic fusion of Platonic and Aristotelian thought, transmitted through the Islamic natural philosophers, particularly Avicenna and Averroes.[79] The medical tradition in the twelfth- and early-thirteenth-century west at first followed the description of the motions or movements of the soul found in Haly Abbas's *Pantegni*: six accidents of the soul were identified, both arising from and consequently affecting the physiology of the body. Joy, sadness, fear, anger, anxiety and shame were all associated with the vital spirit, which either moved outward from the heart to the extremities or, in the case of fear, centripetally from the extremities to the heart.[80] The heart-centred model received greater complexity in Avicenna's influential treatment of the subject in his *De anima*.[81] With Avicenna's views on psychology, which gain prominence only in the thirteenth century in the west, we find a closer connection between the accidents of the soul and the brain, cognition and perception.

The accidents of the soul appear in a variety of contexts within medical writings, particularly in discussions of the six non-naturals.[82] In this context, the accidents of the soul take on an active role as one of the

78 *Thesaurus lingae latinae*, at *paleo* and *paveo*.

79 Domenico de Maio, *La malattia mentale nel medioevo islamico* (Milan: Edizioni del Corriere medico, 1993); Ján Bakoš, ed. and trans., *Psychologie d'Ibn Sina (Avicenne) d'après son oeuvre as-Sifa* (Prague: Editions de l'Académie tschécoslovaque des sciences, 1956). Very little of Galen's psychological thought was known directly in the medieval west; see *Galen on the Passions and Errors of the Soul*, trans. Paul W. Harkins and Walther Riese (Columbus: Ohio State University, 1963).

80 *Omnia opera Ysaac*, bk 4, ch. 8–9.

81 *Avicenna Latinus: Liber de anima*, bk 5, ch. 8, 176–77.

82 Luis García-Ballester, "On the Origins of the Six Non-natural Things in Galen," in García-Ballester, *Galen and Galenism: Theory and Medical Practice from Antiquity to the Eruopean Renaissance* (Aldershot: Ashgate Variorum, 2002), IV.

six non-intrinsic categories—alongside environment, food, sleep, exercise and evacuations—that can affect the health of each individual. Discussions of the impact of the non-naturals appear consistently and prominently in the literature on regimens of health from the thirteenth century onward.[83] Fear in particular appears in relation to a number of medical conditions, but most commonly, like the other accidents of the soul, it is connected to the various diseases of the brain, such as melancholia, mania and epilepsy, adding to the associations between the last two diseases and the incubus. It is also associated with sleep, fevers, and children. In the pediatric literature, children's slumber is often interrupted by fears and anxieties, for which various ointments are recommended.[84] For adults, fear can lead to ephemeral fevers,[85] as can lack of sleep, too much work, and other accidents of the soul, particularly joy, anger, and anxiety. However, the medical description of the incubus reverses this notion of terror as an agent causing disease, and has given to fear a dual role, first as a reaction to a medical condition—more correctly, a reaction to a cognitive reaction to a somatic condition—and then as causative of paleness, sweating and other somatic signs.

Awareness of the impact of the accidents of the soul also surfaces in the discussions of treatment and cure. Attention to the affective state of the patient can be found in two areas here, as with other diseases of the brain: the reduction of hazardous affections, and the use of positive affections to reduce physical or mental pathologies. Among the pharmacological cures for the incubus—most of which seek to treat the indigestion or humoral imbalance that led to the constriction—, there appear medicines that could comfort or strengthen [*confortant*] the brain and the heart, the

83 See the extensive study of regimen literature in *Regimen sanitatis ad regem Aragonum. Arnaldi de Villanova opera medica omnia* X.1, ed. Luis García-Ballester and Michael McVaugh (Barcelona: Seminarium Historiae Scientiae Barcinonense, 1996), 803–27, at 823–4; Pedro Gil-Sotres, "Modelo teórico y observación clínica: Las pasiones del alma en la psicología médica medieval," in *Comprendre et maîtriser la nature au moyen âge: Mélanges d'histoire des sciences offerts à Guy Beaujouan* (Geneva: Droz and Paris: Champion, 1996), 181–204, at 199–200; and idem, "The Regimens of Health," in *Western Medical Thought from Antiquity to the Middle Ages*, ed. M. D. Grmek and M. Fantini (Cambridge, MA and London: Harvard University Press, 1998), 291–318, at 313–14.

84 *De cura puerorum*; Samuel S. Kottek, " 'Mater Puerorum': A Medieval Naming for an Engimatic Children's Disease," *European Journal of Pediatrics* 137 (1981): 75–79.

85 Roscher, *Ephialtes*, 121; Serapion, *Practica Jo. Serapionis dicta breuiarum* (Venice: Bernardinus de Vercellensis for R. Toresanus de Asula, 1503), tract. 6, ch. 7: De febre effimera facta ex festinatione anime, fol. 50vb.

two areas singled out as centres of the emotions, as well as, respectively, the senses and movement.[86]

One of the most striking passages concerning treatment of the incubus invokes the connection between the affective and the physical. Bernard de Gordon provides information on the usual combination of treatments, including massage, ointments, and purgatives, but begins it with a highly unusual comment: "First, he who is used to occurrences [of this disease] should have a beloved friend who, upon hearing him calling out and almost lamenting, should wake him" and then provide the various medical treatments.[87] This insistence that a familiar and close friend should take the role of caregiver is rare in the medical literature, which, with the exception of wetnurses, usually avoids any precision in identifying who would care for the sick. It is not at all unusual to assume that many curative procedures were performed by laypeople, but it is unusual to find the individual identified in such a manner. The affective bond between the sufferer and his caregiver, as specified here, perhaps reflects the psychological nature of this disease of the brain and provides reassurance and calm to the distressed sufferer. Here Bernard combines relief of body and accidents of soul: the beloved friend wakes and calms the sufferer, both physiologically and affectively. Some of the actions performed by the beloved friend parallel Stephen of Hoyland's temporary solution to his nightly visitor: both most importantly involve waking the sufferer and doing so with some force (*multum fortiter*). While such parallels exist, the general thrust of Bernard's therapeutics is twofold: to reduce the causes, whether they be indigestion or other imbalances in the body, and to calm the patient's mind.

Diseases of the brain and the nerves often received treatment that involved the manipulation of the accidents of soul. The melancholic and the maniac were seen to be particularly prone to the influence of the accidents of the soul in both positive and negative ways. As with the incubus sufferer, the melancholic's affective extremes could be allayed and balance could be restored to the physiological and mental processes. For the patient who endures the incubus, as with others suffering from diseases of the brain, we find statements like Gilbertus Anglicus's: "they should strive to rejoice and be wary of anger and worry." Bernard de Gordon presents

[86] The history of the term "conforto" is not entirely clear, specifically when its meaning broadened from its etymological origins in strengthening to a meaning closer to its modern cognate, comfort.

[87] Bernard de Gordon, *Lilium*, fol. 74va.

a variation on this theme, emphasizing the health-bringing potential in certain affective states: "he should live in joy and happiness and avoid all sadness."[88] We find parallels in the treatment of melancholy, with the suggestions that music, light, conversations with friends, and other social interactions would help to revive the patient's spirits.[89] Emotional and mental states come into focus as areas of medical interest and relevance: plans to alter the accidents of the soul sit comfortably next to plans to restore the patient's physiological balance.

Conclusions

Among the many issues that arose out of their discussions of the incubus, medical writers of the thirteenth and early fourteenth centuries chose to emphasize concerns over the imagination, the accidents of the soul, bodily sensations, and the close connections between them. The physiology and psychology of the incubus were separated and the former was given priority in terms of initial causality but not necessarily in terms of importance. Medical authors of the thirteenth and early fourteenth centuries incorporated the cognitive processes in their discussion as a means of differentiating the medical incubus from its demonological namesake. They thereby established the relevance of the condition to the field of medicine and affirmed their abilities as healers and interpreters of psychic and somatic disturbances. The disease category called the incubus raised large questions concerning the processes of the imagination and sensation, the nature of sleep and non-rational cognition, and even the epistemology of learned medicine, as theorists sought to distinguish between the real and the imagined.[90]

It is perhaps best not to view this as a conflict between a demonological or spiritual interpretation and a medical or naturalistic hermeneutic. Instead, we find a fundamental difference in viewing cause and effect: the move from an external assault to somatic reactions stands in contrast to the medical move from an internal pathology toward the imagination and

88 Gilbertus Anglicus, *Compendium*, fol. 114ra; Bernard de Gordon, *Lilium*, fol. 74ra.

89 See, inter alia, Bernard de Gordon, *Lilium*, part 2, ch. 19: De mania et melancolia, fol. 68rb–70va.

90 In fact, Aldobrandino of Siena, writing for the French nobility in the mid-thirteenth century, refers to this condition as "fantosme, que li phisitien apelent incubus, c'est à dire en françois apesart." See *Le Régime du corps de maître Aldebrandin de Sienne, texte français du XIIIe siècle*, ed. Louis Landouzy and Roger Pepin (Paris: Honoré Champion, 1911), 22.

subsequent reactions of both nerves and passions. In both models, fear acts as a consequence and sign of disorder and disruption of the norm. While no one but the patient could see the apparition, any onlooker could witness the sufferer's fear and its physical manifestations. Recognizing the importance of fear in the disease, medical authorities identified it as further evidence that the non-rational state of the sleeper and the excessive power of the imagination during sleep caused the patient to misinterpret the disease itself. For medieval medical writers, the relation between physiology, fantasy and fear explains the disease, the individual patient's emotional and physical reactions to it, and the wider cultural acceptance of the fiction of a demonological attack.

Expanding upon late antique and Arabic precedents, western writers of the central middle ages sought to explain the "supernatural" through bodily processes. Much remains unanswered or underexplored in the medical materials: there is no thorough treatment of the brain's processes and their relations to the functions of the rest of the body. However, in expounding upon the disease category of the incubus, medical authors of the thirteenth and early fourteenth centuries explored various borderlands: between the popular and the learned, between somatic reality and fantastic images, and between the body and the accidents of the soul.

ANGER AND THE MIND-BODY CONNECTION IN MEDIEVAL AND EARLY MODERN MEDICINE

Elena Carrera

A recent trend within intellectual history has focused on emotions as categories of study and shown that they have been variously understood since Antiquity as having an anomalous ontological status in being located in the body, while affecting and being affected by thought.[1] In some of the most influential studies on the emotions in post-Cartesian thought, Robert Solomon, Jon Elster and Thomas Dixon have shown the prevalence of the Platonic separation of mind and body, rationality and irrationality. Dixon has enriched and successfully challenged the simplified accounts provided by Solomon and Elster, demonstrating that, in the influential theological traditions developed by Augustine, Aquinas, and a number of eighteenth- and nineteenth-century English-speaking psychological writers, the passions, affections and sentiments were not always presented as irrational. However, the writers Dixon has discussed tend to emphasize the separation between mind and body, and thus (with the exception of Charles Bell (d. 1842)) see the passions, affections and sentiments as either mental or bodily states.[2]

In this essay, I seek to contribute to the current understanding of the historical categories related to the modern term 'emotions' ('passions,' 'accidents of the soul,' 'affections of the mind,' 'perturbations') by focusing

[1] Robert C. Solomon, *The Passions* (Garden City, NY: Anchor Press/Doubleday, 1976); Susan James, *Passion and action: Emotions in Seventeenth-Century Philosophy* (Oxford: Oxford University Press, 1999); Jon Elster, *Alchemies of the Mind: Rationality and the Emotions* (Cambridge: Cambridge University Press, 1998), Richard Sorabji, *Emotion and Peace of Mind: From Stoic Agitation to Christian Temptation* (Oxford: OUP, 2000); Martha Nussbaum, *Upheavals of Thought: The intelligence of Emotions* (Cambridge: Cambridge University Press, 2001); Thomas Dixon, *From Passions to Emotions: the Creation of a Secular Psychological Category* (Cambridge: Cambridge University Press, 2003); Simo Knuuttila, *Emotions in Ancient and Medieval Philosophy* (Oxford: OUP, 2004); David Konstan, *The Emotions of the Ancient Greeks: Studies in Aristotle and Classical Literature* (Toronto: University of Toronto Press, 2006).

[2] "'Emotion': The History of a Keyword in Crisis," *Emotion Review* 4:4 (2012): 338–44. I thank my colleague Thomas Dixon for letting me read a copy of this article in advance of its publication. I would also like to thank Vivian Nutton for his very helpful comments on an earlier draft of this essay, and to Colin Jones for his encouraging feedback on the final draft.

on the period 1250–1700, not covered in Solomon's, Elster's and Dixon's account, and using entirely different sources: medical texts. My sources emphasize the mind-body connection to such an extent that, even when they refer to anger, joy, fear or sadness as being caused by evaluative perceptions, they present these as physiologically-based processes, manifesting as movements and alterations of the spirits in the brain. As I will show, they tend to draw on an Aristotelian understanding of the passions which is at odds with Solomon's portrayal of a historical binary opposition between emotion and rationality.

In what can be seen as one of the most influential recent attempts to do away with the Cartesian separation between rationality and emotion, and between the mind and the body, Antonio Damasio evokes folk-wisdom ideas (which we might have heard from "our grandmothers"), such as that "grief, obsessive worry, excessive anger, and so forth would damage hearts, give ulcers, destroy complexions, and make one more prone to infections," arguing that, rather than rejecting them as "folksy," it is worth considering and investigating in scientific ways the "basis for such human wisdom."[3] In focusing on the non-Cartesian scientific explanations of the harmful and beneficial effects of anger on health which prevailed in medieval and early modern medicine, I seek to respond to Damasio's suggestion that we need to understand the circumstances and the extent to which psychological disturbances can cause diseases in the body. I hope that my discussion of medieval and early modern medical sources will help to counteract the limited knowledge shown in modern debates on emotions of how similar categories were explained in pre-modern science.

I will show the pervasive influence prior to 1700 of the Aristotelian definition of the passions as movements of the embodied soul causing alterations in the body in response to a perceived good or evil.[4] Such understanding of the passions as cognitive-physiological events, located in the mind and the body simultaneously, is found not only in the seminal writings of Thomas Aquinas (discussed in Lombardo's essay in this

[3] *Descartes' Error* (London: Vintage, 2006 [1994]), 256.

[4] I use the term 'embodied' to convey the Aristotelian view that the soul does nothing without the body. In *De anima* (1.1, 403a16–18), Aristotle emphasizes the importance of the material state of the body by noting, for instance, that we are more prone to experience passions at the faintest stimulation, if our "body is already in a state of tension resembling its condition when we are angry." See *The complete Works of Aristotle*, ed. Jonathan Barnes, 2 vols (Princeton: Princeton University Press, 1984), I, p. 643. David Konstan aptly translates Aristotle's definition of the passions in *De anima* (1.1.403a25) as "reasonings set in matter." Konstan, *The Emotions of the Ancient Greeks*, 44.

volume), but also in the texts of a variety of influential medical authors I examine in this essay. Among them, Arnald of Villanova (d. 1311) played a significant role in the development of medical theory in the Latin West as a prominent figure in the medical school of Montpellier in the 1290s, as a translator of Avicenna's *De viribus cordis* and as an author of medical works which were widely disseminated in manuscript form, and had numerous editions in Latin from the late fifteenth to the late sixteenth century. Bernardino Montaña de Montserrate (d. 1558), court physician and surgeon to Emperor Charles V and a professor of anatomy at the University of Valladolid, was the author of the first anatomy treatise written in Spanish. The French royal surgeon Ambroise Paré (d. 1590) wrote on a range of topics, including surgery, the plague and monsters; his medical works had a wide circulation (in Latin, French, English and Italian) well into the eighteenth century. The physician Nicolas de la Framboisière (d. 1640), who taught at the University of Reims, wrote a number of popularizing medical works which were available both in French and English in the late seventeenth century.[5]

I compare these authors' definitions of the passions, accidents of the soul and affections of the mind, and also look specifically at their descriptions of anger and its effects on health, in conjunction with the medical advice on the need to regulate or stimulate anger found in the *Consilia* of Taddeo Alderotti (d. 1296, a Florentine who taught at the University of Bologna in the late thirteenth century) and in the very popular regimens of health and plague tracts circulating in Latin, English, Spanish, French, German, Catalan and Portuguese between 1250 and 1700. I examine, for instance, the regimen written by Maino de Maineri (Magninus Mediolanensis, d. 1368), who was regent master of the University of Paris and later became court physician to the Visconti rulers of Milan.[6] I also look at some of the earliest regimens published in the vernacular, such as the *Regime tres utile* attributed to Villanova (1491), Bartholomäus Scherrenmüller's *Gesundheitsregimen* (1493, a translation of William of Saliceto's regimen)

[5] Laurence Brockliss notes that La Framboisière departed from the practices of his medical colleagues in publishing in the vernacular for those who had no access to university medical training. See Laurence Brockliss and Colin Jones, *The Medical World of Early Modern France* (Oxford: Oxford University Press, 1997), 99.

[6] Though far less known than Villanova, Maineri has been identified as one of the court physicians of the Scottish King Robert I (d. 1329), and his work has been seen as an example of the transmission of medical knowledge in medieval Europe. See Caroline Proctor, "Physician to The Bruce: Maino De Maineri in Scotland," *The Scottish Historical Review* 86:1 (2007): 16–26.

and Thomas Elyot's *Castel of Helth* (1539), as well as the less-known regimens written in Latin, such as that of the German Jacob Joseph Joepser (d. 1695), which combined Hippocratic-Galenic ideas with the more recent theories of chemical medicine.

In the period covered in this essay, 1250–1700, Aristotelo-Galenism was the medical approach predominantly taught at universities, despite serious challenges to Galen's anatomical model (such as the publication of Andreas Vesalius's anatomical treatise in 1543 and of William Harvey's demonstration of the circulation of blood in 1628).[7] The majority of the medical authors I discuss in the essay wrote within a Galenic framework, though they belonged to a wide diversity of historical and geographical contexts, in which understandings of health and disease emerging from multiple learned perspectives (including alchemy, moral philosophy, astrology and, from the sixteenth century onwards, chemical medicine) co-existed with a variety of empirical, spiritual, magical and folk healing practices. The only non-Galenist I consider is Thomas Willis (d. 1671), who taught natural philosophy at Oxford, worked as a physician both in Oxford and London, and became well-known for his significant contributions to the anatomical understanding of the brain. I include Willis to illustrate the argument that there was no discontinuity between Aristotelo-Galenism and the 'new philosophy,' since he drew on the new mechanical philosophy's explanations of the world as composed of particles in motion, but also used old categories of pathological conditions in his medical practice.[8]

My selection of medical texts is intended to show the widespread influence and endurance of two particular aspects of pre-modern medicine: the Galenic notion of 'spirit' as a subtle material substance, and the Hippocratic-Galenic theory of the six non-naturals (i.e., non-organic causes of health and disease). Thus, rather than looking at the diverse sociocultural contexts in which the texts were written, I focus on significant

[7] Vesalius sought to correct Galen's anatomical errors, while still endorsing Galenic physiology. Harvey maintained an Aristotelian view of the soul as responsible for the functioning of the body. Mary Lindemann sums up their impact as opening "few cracks in the Galenic system." See *Medicine and Society in Early Modern Europe*, 2nd edn (Cambridge: Cambridge University Press, 2010), 99.

[8] Like Galenists, Willis explained empirical findings as signs of things happening inside the body, and speculated about the effects of remedies on the inner workings of body, which were not accessible through the senses. On Willis's integration of new ideas and old categories and narratives, see Andrew Wear, *Knowledge and Practice in English Medicine, 1550–1680* (Cambridge: Cambridge University Press, 2000), 434–73.

continuities and changes in their discussions of spirit and of the impact of anger on health.

At a time when Damasio has urged neuroscientists to find ways of explaining why strong emotions may cause physical diseases only in some circumstances, it seems particularly relevant to consider how medieval and early modern medical authors saw each person's physiological disposition or temperament as a unique, though fluctuating, mixture of primary qualities (hot, cold, wet and dry).[9] I will show how, in seeing temperaments as changeable physiological dispositions (rather than as a set of fixed innate 'personality' traits), medieval and early modern authors were able to conceptualize how each of the passions—e.g., hot and dry anger, warm and moist joy, and cold and dry fear and sadness—could have a different impact on each individual, either bringing an unbalanced temperament further out of balance—causing disease—or, more surprisingly, as I will also show, restoring balance and health.

In discussing anger and other passions as recurrent themes in regimens of health, I aim to shed some light on how the Hippocratic-Galenic interpretations (enduring cultural constructs) might have informed the ways in which the passions were understood by medieval and early modern people, who would have also drawn on other relevant interpretations (based, for instance, on their spiritual or social function).[10] As Strier has suggested, when early modern people got angry, they might not have thought about the impact of anger on their liver, but would have focused rather on what made them angry and on what they were going to do about it.[11] Since the medical sources do not provide direct evidence of the causes of anger, its experience, social dimension or expression, I leave aside any consideration of its social meanings, or the culture-specific values and assessments through which its expression might have been interpreted. Such endeavour was the focus of the seminal studies on medieval anger

---

[9] The doctrine that everything in the physical world is a mixture of the four primary qualities, dating back to Empedocles (d. 435 BCE), was adopted both by Aristotle and by Galen, and was still widely accepted in the seventeenth century.

[10] For a recent study on eighteenth-century uses of Galenic theories of the passions and temperaments co-existing with Lutheran interpretations, see Allan Sortkaer, "The Little Girl who Could not Stop Crying: The Use of Emotions as Signifiers of True Conversion in Eighteenth-Century Greenland," in *A History of Emotions*, ed. Liliequist, 167–79.

[11] Richard Strier and Carla Mazzio, "Two Responses to 'Shakespeare and Embodiment: An E-Conversation'," *Literature Compass* 3:1 (2005): 15–31. For a discussion of changes of emphasis in early modern representations of anger as a painful bodily experience oriented towards a goal, see Kristine Steenbergh, "Green Wounds: Pain, Anger and Revenge in Early Modern Culture," in *The Sense of Suffering*, ed. van Dijkhuizen and Enenkel, 165–87.

edited by Barbara Rosenwein, and of Gwynne Kennedy's monograph on the representation of anger in Early Modern England.[12]

In dealing with the relatively little known medieval and early modern views on the effects of anger on bodily and mental health which circulated in Latin and vernacular languages, I intend to bridge some of the gaps in the existing scholarship by crossing boundaries between disciplines such as history of medicine, medieval studies, cultural history and Renaissance studies. The few pages which have been hereto published on medieval views on health and emotions (other than lovesickness) have focused primarily on Islamic authors writing prior to 1200, though they include Pedro Gil Sotres's study of emotions in Arnald of Villanova and Maino de Maineri, and a brief reference by Jürg A. Bosshard to Henri de Mondeville's views on joy.[13]

---

[12] Rosenwein, ed., *Anger's Past: The Social Uses of an Emotion in the Middle Ages* (Ithaca: Cornell University Press, 1998); Kennedy, *Just anger: Representing Women's Anger in Early Modern England* (Carbondale, IL: Southern Illinois University Press, 2000). See also Linda Pollock's study on the significance of anger in letters exchanged between elite men and women in early modern England, "Anger and the Negotiation of Relationships in Early Modern England," *The Historical Journal* 47 (2004): 567–90.

[13] J. C. Bürgel, "Psychosomatic Methods of Cures in the Islamic Middle Ages," *Humaniora Islamica* 1 (1973): 157–72; W. Dols, "Galen and Islamic Psychiatry," *Le opere psicologiche di Galeno: atti del terzo colloquio galenico internazionale, Pavia, 10–12 settembre*, ed. Paola Manuli e Mario Vegetti (Napoli: Bibliopolis, 1988), 243–80; Peter E. Pormann and Emilie Savage-Smith, *Medieval Islamic Medicine* (Edinburgh: Edinburgh University Press, 2007), 48–49; Peter E. Pormann, "Melancholy in the medieval world: the Christian, Jewish, and Muslim traditions," in Rufus of Efesus, *Melancholy*, ed. Peter Pormann (Tübingen: Mohr Siebeck, 2000), 179–96; Bosshard, *Psychosomatik in der Chirurgie des Mittelalters, besonders bei Henri de Mondeville* (Zurich: Juris-Verlag, 1963); J. A. Paniagua, "La psicoterapia en las obras médicas de Arnau de Vilanova," *Archivo Iberoamericano de la medicina* 15 (1963): 3–15; Michael R. McVaugh, *Medicine before the Plague: Practitioners and their Patients in the Crown of Aragon, 1285–1345* (Cambridge: Cambridge University Press, 1993), 146–47; Pedro Gil Sotres, "La higiene de las emociones," in *Regimen sanitatis ad regem Aragonum. Arnaldi de Villanova opera medica omnia*, X.1, ed. Luis García-Ballester and Michael McVaugh (Barcelona: Fundació Noguera-Universitat de Barcelona, 1996), 803–27; rewritten as "Modelo teórico y observación clínica: Las pasiones del alma en la psicología médica medieval," in *Comprendre et maîtriser la nature au moyen âge: Mélanges d'histoire des sciences offerts à Guy Beaujouan* (Geneva Paris: Droz/Champion, 1996), 181–204; summarized in Gil Sotres, "The Regimens of Health," in *Western Medical Thought from Antiquity to the Middle Ages*, ed. Mirko D. Grmek (Cambridge, MA: Harvard University Press, 1998), 291–318, at 313–14; Joseph Ziegler, *Medicine and Religion c. 1300: The Case of Arnau de* Vilanvoa (Oxford: Clarendon Press, 1998), 153–57; Naama Cohen, "The Emotional Body of Women: Medical Practice between the Thirteenth and the Fifteentth Century," in *Le sujet des emotions au Moyen Âge*, ed. Piroska Nagy and Damien Boquet (Paris: Beauchesne, 2008), 465–82.

Even fewer pages have been dedicated to the study of emotions and health in the sixteenth and seventeenth centuries.[14] The existing studies on the cultural representation of emotion in Renaissance Europe have tended to explain the impact of temperament on people's tendencies to display anger, sadness, fear or joy, drawing on well-known non-medical writings on the passions such as that of Thomas Wright (d. 1620) and Edward Reynolds (d. 1676), and on the influential treatises on melancholy of Timothy Bright (d. 1615), André du Laurens (d. 1609) and Robert Burton.[15] Nancy Siraisi's claim that "complexion theory usefully accounted for psychological and social as well as physiological characteristics or stereotypes" has been drawn upon to justify modern scholarly views on the prevalence of physiological materialism in medieval and early modern medical thought and in cultural forms such as drama.[16] For instance, in her recent analysis of characterization and interaction in Shakespeare's plays in terms of "psychophysiology" (or psychological materialism) and "humoral inevitability," Gail Kern Paster has argued that behaviours in Shakepeare's age were understood as partly expressing the four humours.[17] In next few pages, I seek to challenge the existing scholarly emphasis on

---

[14] See, for instance, L. J. Rather's brief accounts of the views of Wright, Harvey and Descartes in "Old and New Views of the Emotions and Bodily Changes: Wright and Harvey versus Descartes, James and Cannon," *Clio Medica* 1 (1965): 1–25. See David Gentilcore's suggestive analysis of fear in early modern Italy, "The Fear of Disease and the Disease of Fear," in *Fear in Early Modern Society*, ed. William G. Naphy and Penny Roberts (Manchester: Manchester University Press, 1997), 184–208. See also Ulinka Rublack's study of predominantly German-speaking cultural milieus between 1580–1660 in the light of a wide range of prevailing natural-philosophical, religious and medical ideas, including those of the alchemist Leonhard Thurneisser, "Erzählungen vom Geblüt und Herzen. Zur einer historischen Anthopologie des frühneuzeitlichen Körpers," *Historische Anthropologie* 9 (2001): 214–32; translated as "Fluxes: the Early Modern Body and the Emotions," trans. Pamela Selwyn, *History Workshop Journal* 53 (2002): 1–15, and "Flujos. El cuerpo humano y las emociones en la Edad Moderna," in *Accidentes del alma. Las emociones en la Edad Moderna*, ed. María Tausiet and James S. Amelang (Madrid: Abada Editores, 2009), 99–122.

[15] Among the seminal studies which showed how knowledge of humoral theory could inform literary analysis, see Lawrence Babb, *The Elizabethan Malady: a Study of Melancholia in English Literature from 1580 to 1642* (East Lansing: Michigan State College Press, 1951); Otis H. Green, "El ingenioso hidalgo," *Hispanic Review* 25 (1957): 175–93; Teresa Scott Soufas, *Melancholy and the Secular Mind in Spanish Golden Age Literature* (Columbia/London: University of Missouri Press, 1990).

[16] Siraisi, *Medieval and Early Renaissance Medicine: An Introduction to Knowledge and Practice* (Chicago: University of Chicago Press, 1990), 103.

[17] Paster, *Humoring the Body: Emotions and the Shakespearean Stage* (Chicago and London: University of Chicago Press, 2004), 12–13, 60. See also the suggestive, wide-ranging collection of essays: *Reading the Early Modern Passions: Essays in the Cultural History of Emotion*, ed. Gail Kern Paster, Katherine Rowe and Mary Floyd-Wilson (Philadelphia: University of Pennsylvania Press, 2004).

humoral determinism by re-considering some of the available visual and textual evidence. I also provide an overview of medieval and Renaissance medical notions of spirit, before examining medical explanations of the accidents of the soul (or affections of the mind) as movements of spirit within the body. I then focus on medical accounts on anger, its physiological basis and its impact on health.

Representations of Anger: Beyond Humoral Types

Much of the existing scholarship on emotions in pre-modern culture has drawn on the notion that humoral theory underpinned classifications of psychological types, relating them to specific emotions. This strand of research has perhaps been aided by the power of well-publicized images of the four temperaments, such as the woodcuts included in the 1603 edition and later editions in Italian, French and English of Cesare Ripa's *Iconologia* (originally published without imagery in 1593) and the similar illustrations included in Henry Peacham's *Minerva Britanna* (1612). The representations of the choleric and sanguine temperaments in Peacham's emblem book are closely related to those in the *Iconologia*, though Ripa's text only mentions the choleric type's intrepid/proud look and his readiness to fight ("sguardo fiero [...] prontezza di voler combattere," Figure 1), while Peacham's is more explicit in associating choler with a young man's readiness to fight and with anger: "with Sword a late, unsheathed in his Ire" (see Figure 2).[18] The fact that both Ripa's and Peacham's emblem of the choleric type depict a naked young man who is not carrying his shield can be interpreted as symbolizing the impulsiveness associated with the abundance of bodily heat, which was thought to reach its peak in young males and to decrease as they became older. Some modern scholars, however, seem to understand temperamental types, in anachronistic terms, as enduring 'personalities.' For instance, suggesting that "the choleric temperament is a permanent personality trait," Dirk Geeraerts has interpreted the "impulsiveness of the hot-tempered nature" of the choleric depicted in Ripa's emblem as the "negative side of his personality."[19] His claim that

[18] See Cesare Ripa, *Iconologia, o vero descrittione d'imagini delle virtù, vitij, affetti, passioni humane* (Padua: Pietro Paolo Tozzi, 1611), 84; Henry Peacham, *Minerva Britanna* (London: Walter Dight, 1612), 128.

[19] Dirk Geeraerts, *Words and Other Wonders: Papers on Lexical and Semantic Topics* (Berlin/Boston: De Gruyter Mouton, 2006), 235–36.

"anger is caused by choler" is indicative of the prevalence among modern scholars of the view that early moderns used humoral theory as unidirectional causal explanations.[20]

Likewise, Peacham's emblem representing choler has been reproduced in a number of recent works which explain the emotions in early modern

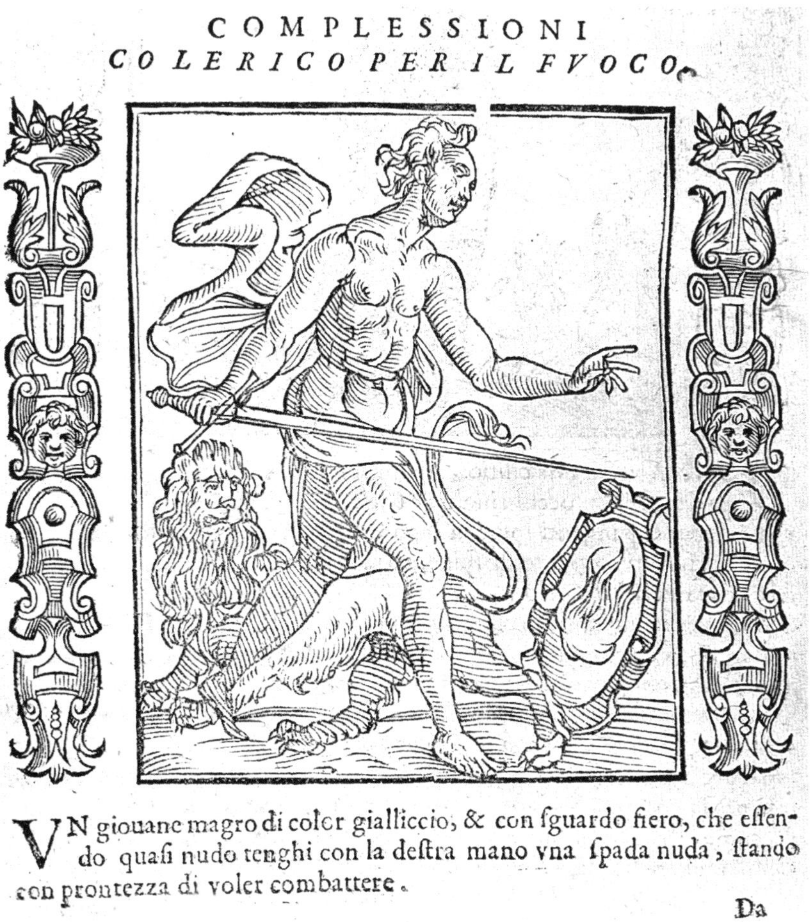

COMPLESSIONI

COLERICO PER IL FVOCO.

VN giouane magro di color gialliccio, & con ſguardo fiero, che eſſendo quaſi nudo tenghi con la deſtra mano vna ſpada nuda, ſtando con prontezza di voler combattere.

Da

Fig. 1. Cesare Ripa, "Complesioni. Colerico per il fuoco." From *Iconologia* (Padua, 1610), 128. Courtesy: Wellcome Library, London.

20 *Words and Other Wonders*, 236.

Cholera. 128

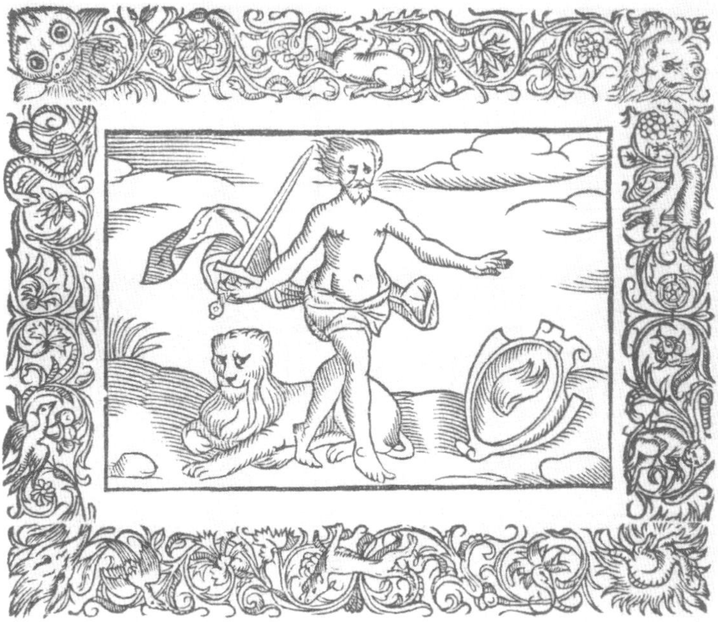

NEXT *Choller* ſtandes, reſembling moſt the fire,
Of ſwarthie yeallow, and a meager face;
With Sword a late, vnſheathed in his Ire:
Neere whome, there lies, within a little ſpace,
A ſterne ei'de Lion, and by him a ſheild,
Charg'd with a flame, vpon a crimſon feild.

We paint him young, to ſhew that paſſions raigne,
The moſt in-heedles, and vnſtaied youth:
That Lion ſhowes, he ſeldome can refraine,
From cruell deede, devoide of gentle ruth:
Or hath perhaps, this beaſt to him aſſign'd,
As bearing moſt, the braue and bounteous mind.

T 2. *Phlegma*

Fig. 2. Henry Peacham, "Cholera." From *Minerva Britanna* (London, 1612), 128. Courtesy: Senate House Library.

English culture in humoral terms.[21] For instance, Paster draws on this emblem to note that for early modern people the "warrior's choler gave him impulsiveness and the capacity for rage."[22] She goes on to quote the explanation of the physiology of the passions provided by Thomas Wright:

> First, then, to our imagination commeth, by sense or memorie, some object to be knowne [...] when we imagine any thing, presently the purer spirits, flocke from the brayne, by certaine secret channels to the heart, where they pitch at the dore, signifying what an obiect was presented, conuenient or disconuenient for it. The heart immediately bendeth, either to prosecute or to eschew it, and the better to effect that affection, draweth other humours to helpe him, so in pleasure concurre great store of pure spirits; in pain and sadness, much melancholy blood; in ire, blood and choller.[23]

Paster quotes this passage twice in *Humoring the Body*. The first time she uses it to illustrate the idea that the pre-modern passions were thought to alter and be altered by the body. The second time she goes on to argue that this description of the relation between perceived sense objects and the passions would have also applied to animals (even though this was not made explicit by Wright).[24] Drawing on Charles Taylor's conflation of early modern psychology and physiology, she argues that "the humours and the emotion that they sustain and move the body to express in action can be lexically distinguished but not functionally separated."[25] She goes from suggesting that the passions are "like liquid states and forces of the natural world" to making the stronger (and somewhat distorting) claim that "the passions actually were liquid forces of nature, because, in this

---

21 As an exception, see Steenbergh's non-humoral interpretation of this emblem as suggesting that, given its association with courage, anger might be "of use to the aristocratic male." Steenbergh, "Green Wounds," 183.

22 *Humoring the Body*, 13.

23 *The Passions of the Minde in Generall*, a facsimile of the 1604 edition, ed. Thomas Sloan (Urbana: University of Illinois Press, 1971), 45.

24 See Paster, *Humoring the Body*, 14, 151–52. Part of the chapter on melancholy cats, in which she discusses how Shakespeare's 'psychological materialism' applied to non-human animals also appears in *Reading the Early Modern Passions*, ed. Paster, Rowe and Floyd-Wilson, 113–29.

25 *Humoring the Body*, 14. Paster cites Taylor's example of how early modern melancholy was thought to reside in black bile, rather than simply be caused by it. See Taylor, *Sources of the Self: The Making of the Modern Identity* (Cambridge: Cambridge University Press, 1989), 188–89. Nonetheless, Taylor's brief account of the inseparability of the 'mental' and the 'physical' in humoral theory does not mention the Galenic emphasis on causal explanations: for instance, while the overabundance of black bile was explained by Galenists as the effect of non-natural causes such as excessive thinking or worrying, it was also thought to cause alterations in the brain spirit, affecting cognitive functions such as the imagination.

cosmology, the stuff of the outside world and the stuff of the body were composed of the same elemental materials."[26] In seeking to illustrate what she calls 'psychophysiology,' she appears to reduce the passions to their physiological manifestations, thereby understating the two-way causal connections early moderns established between the passions and the embodied cognitions to which they related. Even though she notes that the body's humours would predispose the individual to certain kinds of evaluations and responses, she does not dwell on the cognitive aspects of the passions, but only mentions that they were thought to cause subtle changes in the "color and flow of the animal spirits."[27] She makes passing references to the medical view that the onset of passion would "alter a subject's cognitive powers," and that these relied on the "clear flowing of the animal spirits from the cavities of the brain out to the body's organs."[28] While her materialist account focuses on the humours, it is also worth considering, as I do below, medical ideas on how the passions were evoked through perception, imagination and memory, and how these cognitive powers were thought to affect and be affected by the body's physiological state.

Cultural historians working on the English context have sometimes drawn on catchy phrases such as Wright's "passions ingender humours, and humours breed passions" in trying to reconstruct the Renaissance humoral understanding of the interaction between mind and body.[29] Yet, in so doing, they have tended to overlook the crucial role which medieval and early modern Galenic physicians attributed to the spirits within that interaction. For instance, Stephen Pender uses limited pre-1700 textual evidence, primarily from Wright, Elyot, and Reynolds's *Treatise on the Passions* (1640) to support his view that in the seventeenth-century "new physiology" there is a new emphasis on how, "with the assistance of the imagination, the will controls not only passions but spirits."[30]

---

[26] *Humoring the Body*, 4.

[27] *Humoring the Body*, 64. Her interpretation of the early modern notion of spirit draws on a wide range of sources, which include the plays of Shakespeare, the treatise on the passions of the English Jesuit Thomas Wright and the natural philosophical works of Francis Bacon, and seems to be influenced by the 'retrospective' approach taken in John Sutton, *Philosophy and Memory Traces: Descartes to Connectionism* (Cambridge: Cambridge University Press, 1998).

[28] *Humoring the Body*, 64.

[29] *Passions of the Minde*, 64.

[30] See '"Subverting Disease: Anger, Passions, and the Non-Naturals," *Rhetoric of Bodily Disease and Health in Medieval and Early Modern England*, ed. Jennifer C. Vaught (Burlington, VT: Ashgate, 2010), 193–218, at 214.

This emphasis, however, was not new. The idea that spirit and the passions could be moved through persuasion and through the wilful use of images had been discussed in medical texts throughout the late middle ages and the Renaissance. Wright also drew on widely available Hippocratic-Galenic ideas to stress the ways in which certain representations in the imagination would move the passions and the spirits:

> for the imagination herein (though erroneously, conceiuing things better then indeede and really they are) causeth a vehement passion of Hope, wherewith followeth an extraordinary pleasure in the things: which two Passions awake, or rowze vp the purer spirits, and vnite them together, qualifying and refining them in the best manner; which thus combined, do most effectually co-operate with nature, and strengthen her in the performance of any corporall action or vitall operation.[31]

The role played by the imagination in transforming the quality of the body's spirits and its consequent impact on the workings of the body is not sufficiently acknowledged in Paster's account of the early modern passions as liquid forces.

Furthermore, even though Paster does refer to the early modern idea that the passions altered the body, she does not consider medical views on their long-term impact in causing bodily disease or improving health. Instead, she suggests that the humours were to the body what the passions were to the soul: "just as an imbalance of humours causes bodily disease, so an excess of passions causes disease—distemper—in the soul."[32] This claim is a rewording of a passage in which Wright refers to Cicero's discussion of Stoic views of the passions in *Tusculan Disputations*.[33] However, Wright also referred to other prevailing perspectives, which stressed the effect of intense experiences of the passions on the body:

> if the passion of pleasure be too vehement, questionless it causeth great infirmitie: for the heart being continually inuironed with great abundance of spirit, becomes too hot and inflamed, and consequently engendreth much cholericke and burned blood.[34]

Wright's views on how intense passions could cause bodily diseases were in line with the advice provided in popular regimens of health available in Shakespeare's London, like Elyot's *Castel of Helth* and William Bullein's

31 *The Passions of the Minde*, 66.
32 *Humoring the Body*, 14–17.
33 *The Passions of the Minde*, 17.
34 *The Passions of the Minde*, 60.

Bulwarke of Defence, which I discuss below. Such views have, nonetheless, been overlooked by modern literary scholars and cultural historians who have explained the early modern passions as expressions of the four humours and temperaments, seeing anger predominantly as a sign of being choleric, and joy as a character trait of the sanguine temperament.

In medieval and early modern medicine, anger was not always seen as a sign of choleric temperament or overabundant choleric humour, but was also viewed as a cause of significant temperamental and bodily changes. In turn, temperamental differences were not simply thought to 'cause' different passions (as Geeraerts suggests when he claims that "anger is caused by choler"), but were also associated with distinct ways of experiencing each passion. Thus, rather than focusing on establishing direct correspondences between the passions and the humours, we can look more closely at how the medical texts accounted for the effect of physiological disposition in creating different types of joy, sadness, fear and anger. For instance, the medieval medical text most influential in the Renaissance, the *Canon of Medicine* of Avicenna (d. 1037), explained that physiological disposition would affect the ability to imagine revenge, thus making a difference on whether anger subsided soon or turned into rancor.[35] Seeing temperament as underpinning observable qualitative differences in the ways each of the passions were experienced, Benedictus Reguardatus de Nursia (d. 1469) distinguished between sudden and slow joy.[36] The seventeenth-century Reims professor La Framboisière linked the excess of choleric humour to "swiftness to anger" and to proneness to wrath and revenge, as well as to cheerfulness.[37] Among non-medical Renaissance authors, Wright noted that the phlegmatic could be recognized as being "not so soon angrie, nor yet soon pleased," the sanguine would be expected to be "soone angrie, soone friended," the melancholic would need longer to recover from an episode of anger, "hardly offended, and afterward with extreame difficulty

---

[35] See Avicenna (Abū ʿAlī al-Ḥusayn ibn ʿAbd Allāh ibn Sīnā), *The Canon of Medicine* (*al-Qānūn fī'l-ṭibb*), adapted by Laleh Bakhtiar from translations of Volume I by O. Cameron Gruner and Mazar H. Shah; correlated with the Arabic by Jay R. Crook with notes by O. Cameron Gruner (Chicago, Ill.: Great Books of the Islamic World, 1999), Part 1, Lecture 7, pp. 146–52.

[36] Benedictus de Nursia, *Pulcherrimum & utilissimum opus ad sanitatis conseruationem* (Bologna: Dominici de Lapis, 1477), ch. 96 [p. 246]. The popularity of this work in the late fifteenth century can be judged by its frequent re-editions (e.g., 1475, 1477, 1490, 1493 and 1505).

[37] Nicolas Abraham, sieur de La Framboisière, *An Easy Method to Know the Causes and Signs of the Humour most Ruleth in the Body and to Avoid thereby Things Hurtful* (London: 1640), 4.

reconcile," and the choleric would not simply be quick to anger, but also experience a great desire for revenge: "at every trifle they are inflamed, and, till their hearts be consumed (almost) with choler, they never cease, except they be revenged."[38] In stressing that "the same passion affecteth diuers persons in diuers manners," Wright went beyond simple categories such as anger or joy to suggest that there are different types of anger and joy, and diverse ways of experiencing them.[39]

Nonetheless, we should not lose sight of the fact that the medieval and early modern medical emphasis on different types of anger and their longer-term effects on the body co-existed with other approaches to anger, which emphasized its more generic or generalizable features. Among the best-known early modern attempts to capture visually the relationship between anger and the body's physiology, we find the very popular drawings of the royal painter and director of the Académie Royale Charles Le Brun (d. 1690) which illustrated his 1668 lecture on the passions and were frequently reprinted in various versions throughout the eighteenth century (see Figure 3).[40] In seeking to teach other artists how to portray the passions, he focused on the facial expressions of the most dramatic forms of anger. He explained that anger was a violent passion which would cause considerable commotion of the blood and spirits, making the eyes red and inflamed, the pupils dilated, the eyebrows drawn together in a frown, the forehead deeply furrowed, the nostrils open and enlarged, the lips turned out and pressed against one another (with the lower lip raised over the upper lip and the corners of the mouth slightly open), also

---

38 *Passions of the Minde*, 37.

39 *Passions of the Minde*, 34. Floyd-Wilson cites this passage in passing, but moves on to some of the claims made by Wright in his preface to support her argument that modern perceptions of "how easily one is stirred or calmed" were inextricably linked to ethnic distinctions; see "English Mettle." Fay Bound Alberti refers to the seventeenth-century humoral view that a high level of yellow bile would make people subject to anger, and notes in passing that "then as now, different types of persons experienced greater or lesser degrees of emotion." See "Emotions in the Early Modern Medical Tradition," in *Medicine, Emotion and Disease, 1700–1950*, ed. Fay Bound Alberti (Basingstoke: Palgrave Macmillan, 2006), 1–21, at 7.

40 *Méthode pour apprendre à dessiner les passions proposée dans une conférence sur l'expression générale et particulière. Enrichie de figures gravées par B. Picard* (Amsterdam and Paris, 1698). My references are to *Conférence de Monsieur Le Brun, premier peintre du Roy de France, Chancelier & Directeur de l'Académie de Peinture & Sculpture, sur l'expression générale et particulière des passions. Enrichie de figures grravées par B. Picart*, 2nd edn (Amsterdam: Bernard Picart, 1713). For a modern translation of the text, see Jennifer Montagu, *The Expression of the Passions: The Origin and Influence of Charles Le Brun's "Conference sur l'expression generale et particuliere"* (New Haven: Yale University Press, 1994), 125–40. On the numerous editions of this lecture with its drawings, see pp. 175–87.

making the teeth grind, the hair stand on end, and the veins in the neck and temples swell (see Figures 3 and 4).[41] Le Brun's famous depictions of extremely angry faces, devoid of context, contrast with the rather neutral facial expressions of the choleric figures in Ripa's and Peacham's books of emblems, which emphasized stereotypical bodily gestures and externalized attributes (such as heat, represented by the flame, and courage, represented by the lion). Nonetheless, like the emblems, Le Brun's drawings sought to establish a universally valid paradigm for teaching purposes.

Le Brun's 1668 lecture on the expression of the passions ended with the announcement that his next lecture would be on physiognomy, and on the different effects produced by the passions on the various types of

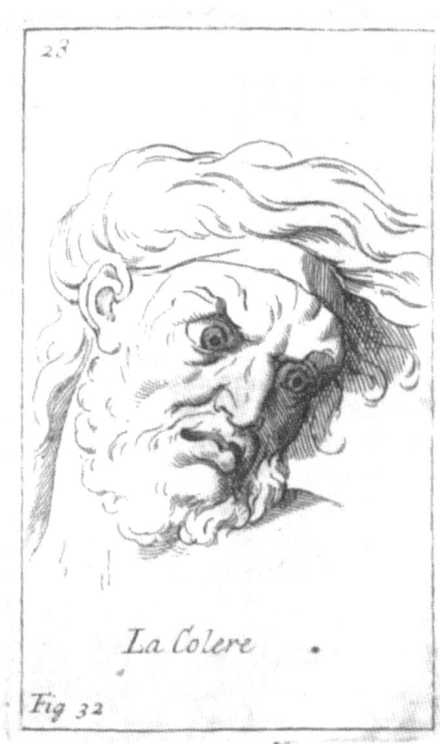

Fig. 3. "La colère." From *Conference de Monsieur Le Brun* (London, 1701). Courtesy: Senate House Library.

[41] Le Brun, *Conférence*, 41–42.

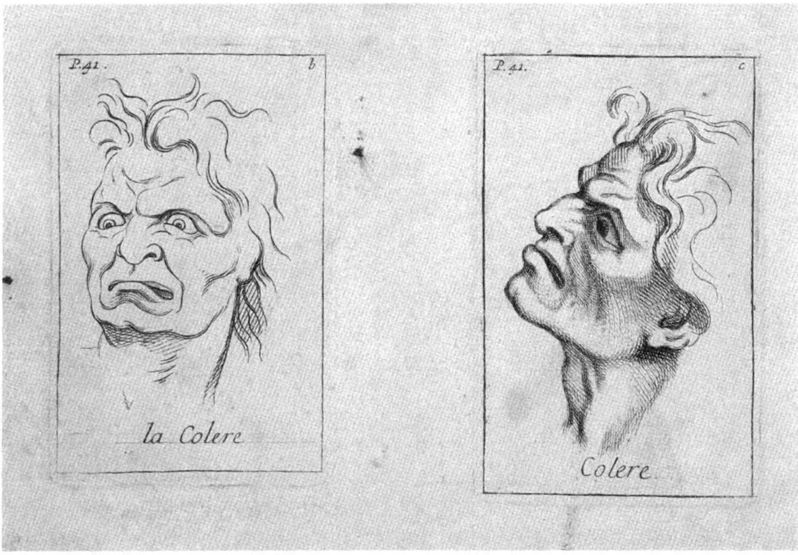

Fig. 4. "La colère" and "colère." A frontal outline and a profile of faces expressing anger. Etching by B. Picart, 1713, after C. Le Brun. Courtesy: Welcome Library.

people subject to them.[42] As a fellow member of the Académie Royale argued, it "is not possible to prescribe precisely all the signs of the different passions, given the diversity of forms and temperaments."[43] In another lecture at the Académie, the sculptor Michel Anguier (d. 1686) suggested that the most significant difference was that choleric types would have a red face when angry because their blood was easily agitated, while the anger of melancholic types would typically be characterized by a gaunt and disfigured face and owl-like eyes.[44] The representations of anger put forward by Le Brun and his fellow members of the Académie show the

[42] "Phisionomie, des effets différents qui causent les Passions selon la diversité des sujets qui la [= les] reçoivent." *Conférence*, 54.

[43] "L'on remarqua pour la fin, qu'il n'est pas possible, de prescrire précisement toutes les marques des différentes passions, à cause de la forme, & du temperament: qu'un visage plein ne forme pas les mêmes plis que celui qu sera maigre, & deseiché [...]. Le bilieaux a les mouvements tout autres que le flegmatique & le sanguin." Henri Testelin, "Sur l'expression générale et particulière," in *Sentiments des plus habiles peintres sur la pratique de la peinture et sculpture* (Paris, 1696), 19–25 (24). See Montagu, *The Expression*, 163–70, at 168–69. For the attribution of the views in this passage to the sculptor Michel Anguier, see Julia Dabbs, "Characterising the Passions: Michel Anguier's Challenge to Le Brun's Theory of Expression," *Journal of the Warburg and Courtauld Institutes* 65 (2002): 273–96.

[44] See Anguier, "Sur l'expression de la colère," cited in Dabbs, "Characterising the Passions," 279.

kind of tensions we still find today between seeing 'anger' as a universal category referring to a type of experience which can be recognized across different geographical, cultural and historical contexts, or focusing instead on specific types of anger. While modern social constructionists have emphasized the importance of paying attention to the specific social contexts in which emotions manifest, theorists like Le Brun and Anguier had the markedly different aim of teaching ways of representing the passions which would be universally valid, or at least generally understood. Yet, in their interpretations of how anger manifests, they were constrained by the cultural paradigms prevailing in their context: Galenic notions of the temperaments and the newer theories of the passions proposed by Descartes.

Even though Le Brun showed awareness of Descartes' classification of the passions and of his notion of the pineal gland, he provided a non-Cartesian account of the passions as movements of the soul manifesting in the body: "the soul receives the impressions of the passions in the brain, and feels its effects in the heart" through the spirits which fill the brain's cavities and are carried by the nerves.[45] This explanation drew on traditional notions of the role of spirit as the material instrument of the soul, to which we now turn.

Mind, Body and Spirit

Medieval and Renaissance Galenism adopted Galen's terminological distinction between 'spirit' (*pneuma*) and 'natural heat' as referring to the two main functions of the same rarefied vaporous substance circulating throughout the body, conveying instructions (spirit) and supplying warmth to the bodily organs and limbs (natural heat).[46] The spirits were

---

45 "par les esprits qui sont contenus par les cavités du cerveau, & le cerveau ne reçoit les esprits que du sang, qui passe continuellement par le coeur, [...]. Le cerveau ainsi rempli renvoie de ces esprits aux autres parties par les nerfs qui sont comme autant de petis filets ou tuiaux qui portent ces esprits dans le muscles [...] l'Ame reçoit les impressions des passions dans le cerveau, & qu'elle en ressent les effects au coeur." *Conférence*, 5–8. Christopher Allen examines the Cartesian and non-Cartesian elements of Le Brun's view of the passions in relation to Aquinas's scholastic definitions in "Painting the Passions: The *Passions de l'Âme* as a Basis for Pictorial Expression." *The Soft Underbelly of Reason: The Passions in the Seventeenth-Century* (London: Routledge, 1998), 79–111, at 96. However, he seeks to explain Brun's reference to 'soul' without taking into account the Galeno-Aristotelian medical ideas on which Le Brun draws.

46 On the medical notion of spirit, or *pneuma*, see Gérard Verbeke, *L'evolution de la doctrine du pneuma du stoicism à S Augustin* (Paris: de Brower, 1945); Owsei Temkin,

seen as material parts of the human body, alongside the humours and the solid parts. The subtle materiality attributed to the spirits meant that they could be considered as a potential locus for sudden, short-term diseases like ephemeral fever, as Bernard de Gordon had noted in the *Lilium medicine* (written 1303–05), drawing on Avicenna and Arabized versions of Galen.[47]

Avicenna had referred to spirit (or breath) as a "luminous substance," a "ray of light" emerging from a mixture of the four primary qualities (hot, cold, wet and dry), and approaching the substance of celestial beings.[48] Writing in the early fourteenth-century, Henri de Mondeville explained that spirit was produced from part of the blood being warmed up, rarefied, digested and purified by the strength of the heart. Like Avicenna, he described spirit as "lighter, more subtle, purer and brighter than all bodily things composed from the four elements," and consequently "closer to the nature of supercelestial things."[49]

Galenic authors often distinguished three types of spirit, depending on their function: natural heat associated with the soul's functions of nourishment and growth, vital spirit associated with movement, and animal spirit used in cognitive function. They thought of vital spirit as circulating throughout the body through the arterial blood, and of "animal spirit" (distilled from it in the brain) as being propelled through the nerves, acting as a transmitting agent between the brain and the rest of the body. The subtle, almost celestial, nature of spirit enabled it to provide "a friendly and suitable link between soul and body," acting as the direct instrument of the soul, bearing its powers (*virtutum*).[50] Spirit had the function of

"On Galen's Pneumatology," *Gesnerus* 8 (1951): 180–89; Rudolf E. Siegel, *Galen on Psychology, Psychopathology and Function and Diseases of the Nervous* System (Basel: S. Karger, 1973), 72–91; Ruth Harvey, *The Inward Wits: Psychological Theory in the Middle Ages and the Renaissance* (London: Warburg Institute, 1975), 5–7.

47 As de Gordon explains, hectic fever originates in the organs and other solid parts, putrid fever originates in the humours, and ephemeral fever in the spirits. We find the same idea in Avicenna's *Canon*, though Gordon claims to have taken it from Galen's book on fevers. See *Practica seu Lilium medicine* (Naples: F. del Tuppo for B. Geraldinus, 1480), book 1, ch. 2. I will cite from the modern critical edition of the Spanish translation published in 1495: Bernardo de Gordonio, *Lilio de medicina*, ed. Brian Dutton and María Nieves Sánchez. 2 vols (Madrid: Arco/Libros, 1993), I, 65.

48 Avicenna, *Canon*, Part I, Lecture 7, "The Breath," 146.

49 *Chirurgie*, 61, 35. See also Marie-Christine Pouchelle, *The Body and Surgery in the Middle Ages*, trans. Rosemary Morris (Oxford: Polity Press, 1990), 116–17.

50 Henri de Mondeville, *Chirurgie*, 35. Seeing the soul in Aristotelian terms as the efficient principle of all activity, Benedictus de Nursia also referred to the spirits of the heart

maintaining the body alive as "the seate and caryer of heate," while acting as the main instrument of the soul in all its operations.[51]

In the seventeenth century, the physiological notions of spirit evolved, beyond Galenism, into more mechanistic models such as the influential one proposed by Descartes, and eclectic models such as Pierre Gassendi's or Thomas Willis's. Like Gassendi, Willis distinguished between an immortal "Rational Soul, Superior and Immaterial," and a corporeal sensitive soul, which depended completely on the body and would be born and would die with it. He propounded that the two souls communicated with each other through the movements of spirit in the nerves. Within the corporeal soul he distinguished between a vital part, which he described as a fire, "either a Flame or a Breath" in the blood (enkindled by sulphur and nitrous particles), and a sensitive part consisting of a heap of lucid or ethereal animal spirits diffused through the brain and the nerves.[52] This conception was indebted to Gassendi's re-elaboration of the Aristotelian faculty psychology distinction between the rational, sensitive and vegetative powers of the soul (with the vegetative function now being ascribed to the mechanical actions of the body).

For Willis, there was only one type of spirit, circulating throughout the body through the nerves (which he still conceived of as hollow), not in the blood. In contrast with the Galenic theory that the animal spirits were distilled at the back of the brain (from the vital spirits), and filled the brain's ventricles and the nerves, Willis provided a more accurate account of the anatomy of the brain. Explaining that they were distilled directly from the blood in the richly vascular cerebral and cerebellar cortex ("the Cortical or Barky substances of the Brain and Cerebel") and carried in the white

(*cordiales spiritus*) and natural heat as the instruments of the soul in its operations. See *Pulcherrimum*, ch. 96 [p. 242].

51 Levinus Lemnius, *The Touchstone of Complexions*, trans. Thomas Newton (London: Thomas Marsh, 1576), 8.

52 I cite from the translation of *De anima brutorum* (1672), *The Soul of Brutes*, Preface, 1–7, in *Dr Willis's Practice of Physick: Being the Whole Works of that and Famous Physician*, trans. Samuel Pordage (London: Printed for T. Dring, C. Harper, and J. Leighm, 1684). For other seventeenth-century notions of physiological spirits, see Roger French, *William Harvey's Natural Philosophy* (Cambridge: Cambridge University Press, 1994), 220–26; John Henry, "A Cambridge Platonist Materialism: Henry More and the Concept of Soul," *Journal of the Warburg and Courtauld Institutes* 49 (1986): 172–95; "Occult Qualities and the Experimental Philosophy: Active Principles in Pre-Newtonian Matter Theory," *History of Science* 24 (1986): 335–81; "Medicine and Pneumatology: Henry More, Richard Baxter, and Francis Glisson's *Treatise on the Energetic Nature of Substance*," *Medical History* 31 (1987): 15–40. See also Simon Schaffer, "Godly Men and Mechanical Philosophers: Souls and Spirits in Restoration Natural Philosophy," *Science in Context* 1 (1987): 55–85.

matter, the brain stem and the nerves, he described animal spirits as a lucid, fiery substance, which, like air or wind, could be altered by becoming disordered in its movement.[53] Thus Willis would explain the most significant changes in the mind-body connection in cognitive function and in the experience of passions in terms of the order or disorder of spirit. We see here a clear change of emphasis, away from the earlier qualitative model of spirit, to a model in which movement (orderly or disorderly) was the main variable.[54] In the long run, this new emphasis on type of movement would gradually lead to changes in the understanding of temperament (seen less and less in terms of 'temperature', or proportion of moisture and warmth) and of the impact of diet and other lifestyle factors on cognitive-affective operations.

However, in the Galenic paradigm prevailing in university medical teaching and in popularizing regimens of health prior to 1700, the functions of the soul and body were still thought to be dependent on the temperature (or temperament) of spirit being moderately warm and moderately moist (i.e., not too thick or wet and not excessively thin or dry). The temperature, degree of brightness and density of spirit were all seen to be crucial factors of good cognitive function, influencing and being influenced by the intensity of the passions.[55] The bodily alterations caused by an inadequate lifestyle (e.g., insufficient or improper diet, or lack of exercise) were believed to have a similar impact on spirit to that of fear, sadness, worrying or anger: making it too scarce, too cold and dark or too hot and dazzling. This explains why fear, sadness, anger and joy had come to be conceptualized as "accidents" of the embodied soul (i.e., movements of spirit) affecting both the body and the mind. It is to such accidents that we now turn.

---

53 *Cerebri anatome* (1664). See the translation *Anatomy of the Brain*, 73–79, 103–104, in *Dr Willis's Practice of Physick*.

54 Despite the widespread influence of quantitative models among natural philosophers, medical practice largely maintained its use of qualitative categories still in the eighteenth century. On the English context, see Andrew Wear, "Medical Practice in Late Seventeenth and Early Eighteenth Century England: Continuity and Union," in *The Medical Revolution of the Seventeenth Century*, ed. Roger K. French and Andrew Wear (Cambridge University Press, 1989), 294–320.

55 As Bernard de Gordon had pointed out, spirit needed to be abundant, warm and luminous for the good working of memory, imagination and thinking. See *Lilium*, ch. 19, on melancholia; *Lilio*, I, 503.

The Accidentia Animae

Anger, fear, sadness and joy were frequently discussed by medieval Muslim and Jewish Galenic authors (such as Joannitius, Isaac Israeli, Haly Abbas and Avicenna) under a category usually translated into medieval Latin as *accidentia animae*.[56] In medieval and early modern medical texts the "accidents of the soul" or "affections of the mind" were normally considered the sixth of the non-natural factors of health and disease, alongside the other five: air, food and drink, movement and rest, sleep and wakefulness, and repletion (or retention) and depletion (or evacuation, including bloodletting and sexual activity).[57] Seen as variable exchanges between the body and the environment, the six non-naturals were differentiated from the natural (organic or material) causes of health: the elements (air, water, earth and fire), the qualities (moist, hot, dry and cold), the humours (blood, yellow bile, black bile and phlegm), the solid parts of the body, the spirits (natural, vital and animal or psychic) and the operations (like appetite, digestion, retention, expulsion or desire).[58] They were also distinguished from the things contrary to nature, known as "contranaturals" (disease and its causes and consequences).[59]

---

56 The phrase *accidentia animae* was used in the most influential medical texts available in Latin from the mid-twelfth century, such as Constantinus's translations of the *Isagoge* and the *Pantegni*, and in the Toledan Latin translations (supervised by Gerard of Cremona) of Avicenna's *Canon*. For a brief discussion of the medieval medical use of the alternative term 'passion,' see Gil Sotres, "La higiene de las emociones," 803–805.

57 This list has been dated back to two Latin manuscript copies from the twelfth and the thirteenth centuries of Joannitius's *Isagoge ad Techne Galieni*: "non naturalia sunt VI: aer, exercitium, optium, cibus et potus, sommus et vigilia, repletio et inanitio, accidentia anime." See G. Maurach, "Johannicius, *Isagoge ad Techne Galieni*," *Sudhoffs Archiv für Geschichte der Medizin* 62 (1978): 148–74. Without using the label 'non-natural,' Galen had referred to similar factors, including mental activity as the sixth, in *In Hippocratis Epidemiarum* VI.5, 483. The *Ars medica* lists as "necessary factors" air, movement and rest, sleep and wakefulness, intake (*quae assumuntur*), evacuation and retention, and affections of the mind (*ex animi affectibus; ek ton psychikon pathon*); *Ars medica*, ch. 23 (Kühn 1: 367). Singer renders rather literally the broader meaning of *ek ton psychikon pathon* and of *accidentia animae* as "what happens to the soul." Galen, *The Art of Medicine*, in *Selected Works*, ed. P. N. Singer, 345–96. By contrast, Culpeper's translation as "affections of the mind" establishes a useful link between Galen's notion of *psyche* in this context and the modern concept of 'mind,' which includes emotional states. See Galen, *Art of Physick*, trans. Nicholas Culpeper (London: Peter Cole, 1652).

58 Among the natural or organic causes of health and disease, the most frequently discussed were the solid parts, the spirits, the humours and the elements; see, for instance, Ambrogio Oderico [da Genova (d. 1505)], *De regenda sanitate consilium*, Italian translation, ed. Fortunato Cirenei (Genova, 1961), 21–22.

59 On the non-naturals see L. J. Rather, "The 'Six Things Non-Natural:' A Note on the Origins and Fate of a Doctrine and a Phrase," *Clio Medica* 3 (1968), 337–47; Saul Jarcho,

The accidents of the soul were believed to have a rather complex impact on health. They were thought to produce alterations in the quality and availability of spirit, thus affecting the degree of nourishment available to the solid parts of the body, but also affecting cognitive function, which, in turn, could also have a deleterious effect on well-being. This can be seen, for instance, in Arnold von Bamberg's suggestion in his early-fourteenth-century *Regimen sanitatis* that the "accidents of the soul" need to be regulated because they might confuse the intellect, which would have a considerable impact on the body because it would disrupt the routines through which people looked after themselves, such as the amount of food and drink they took, whether they exerted themselves or rested excessively, their ability to sleep, and their bodily functions related to evacuation. Von Bamberg also stressed that if people paid insufficient attention to accidents of the soul as part of a healthy lifestyle (preventive care), they would have to resort to curative medical methods (therapeutic care).[60]

Seeing how the accidents of the soul were conceptualized as part of an interlinked set of exchanges between the body and the environment makes it clear that in this context the term 'soul' did not refer to Platonic or theological notions of the soul as an immaterial immortal entity. It referred rather to the states of the embodied soul, which were thought to manifest through the movements of the spirits between the brain, the heart and the outer surface of the body. As the seat of perception, imagination, reason and memory, the brain was seen to have a crucial role in the explanations of the accidents of the soul provided by Avicenna and later authors like Arnald of Villanova. Nonetheless, earlier texts like the *Pantegni* and the *Isagoge* made no reference to the brain and simply

"Galen's Six Non-Naturals: A Bibliographic Note and Translation," *Bulletin of the History of Medicine*, 44:4 (1970), 372–77; Jerome Bylebyl, "Galen on 'the Non-Natural Causes' of Variation in the Pulse," *Bulletin of the History of Medicine* 45:5 (1971): 482–85; Luis García-Ballester, "On the Origin of the 'Six Non-Natural Things' in Galen," in Jutta Kollesch and Kiethard Nickel, *Galen und das hellenische Erbe* (Stuttgart: Franz Steiner, 1993), 105–115; repr. in *Galen and Galenism*, IV.

60 "Et quia inter sex res non naturales circa quarum commensurationem et ordinationem debitam versatur regimen sanitatis accidentia animae turbant ut in pluribus aliqualiter intellectum quo turbato cuiuslibet regiminis executio pariter conturbatur et cum hoc etiam corpus non modicum alterant, cui alterato non iam debetur regimen sanativum sed potius curativum, ideo ut videtur in dicto regimine merito est ab ipsis incipendum." See Arnold von Bamberg, *Regimen sanitatis*, fol. 183r. Günter Kallinich und Karin Figala, "Das 'Regimen sanitatis' des Arnold von Bamberg," *Sudhoffs Archiv: Zeitscrift für Wissenschaftsgeschichte* 56:1 (1972), 44–60.

described the accidents of the soul as movements of natural heat or spirit towards or away from the heart.

The text which offered the most succinct and most frequently cited medieval explanation of the accidents of the soul was the *Pantegni*, one of the medical texts most widely disseminated in the late middle ages and the sixteenth century.[61] Its account focused on the direction of their movement of natural heat: fear and sadness moving it inwards, anger and joy moving it outwards, and anxiety and shame as moving it in both directions. In one paragraph, it captured very effectively Galen's descriptions of the movements of *pneuma* in *On the Causes of Symptoms*, his explanation in the *Commentary on Epidemics* that certain types of excessive mental activity (like anger, fear of death, worry, grief and shame) can cause illness, and his scattered references to joy as being potentially harmful if in excess.[62] The *Pantegni*'s succinct six-partite classification provided a common framework for the medieval and early modern medical discussions of their impact on health.

Equally influential, though less often cited in relation to the *accidentia animae*, was the *Isagoge* (*ad Tegni Galeni*), one of the six medical texts contained in the *Articella*, the collection of authoritative treatises used in medical training in European universities from the mid-thirteenth to the late sixteenth century. Emphasizing differences in speed, the *Isagoge* suggested that anger is sudden, and delight and joy are gentle and slow, though both move natural heat outwards and upwards to the surface of the skin. By contrast, the sudden movement of terror and fear and the

61 *Pantegni*, in Isaac Israeli, *Opera omnia* (Lyons: Jean de La Place for Barthlémy Trot, 1515), Theorica, Bk 5, ch. 109, 25v. Though attributed to Israeli, the *Pantegni* was Constantinus Africanus's translation of the theoretical and most of the practical parts of the medical encyclopaedia of *'Alī ibn 'Abbās al-Maǧūsī*, known in the West as Haly Abbas. On the wide dissemination of this text in the Renaissance, see "A catalogue of Renaissance editions and manuscripts of the *Pantegni*," in *Constantine the African and 'Alī ibn 'Abbās al-Maǧūsī: The Pantegni and Related Texts*, ed. Charles Burnett and Danielle Jacquart (Leiden: Brill, 1994), 316–51.

62 Like García-Ballester, I draw on the German translation of the *Commentary on Epidemics*, rendering "Geistestätigkeit" as "mental activity," though, departing from his distinction between "fear" and "anxiety," I would render both "Furcht vor dem Tode" and "Angst vor dem Tode" as fear of death; see *In Hippocratis Epidemiarum*, VI.1–8, ed. Ernst Wenkebach and Franz Pfaff (Berlin: Academiae Litterarum, 1956), VI.5, 484–86. On the impact of the *Commentary on Epidemics* through medieval Arabic medical writers, see Peter E. Pormann, "Case Notes and Clinicians: Galen's Commentary on the Hippocratic Epidemics in the Arabic Tradition," *Arabic Sciences and Philosophy* 18 (2008): 247–84. The potentially harmful effects of joy were discussed by Galen in *De symptomatum causis*, 2.5 (Kühn 7: 192–93) and *De methodo medendi*, 12.5 (Kühn 10: 841).

gradual movement of distress (*angustia*) are inward movements of natural heat, and sadness (*tristitia*) involves movements in both directions.[63] Nonetheless, the *Isagoge*'s understanding of sadness as a bi-directional movement was not recognized in the most standard medieval and early modern medical accounts, which tended to describe it as an inward movement or contraction.

Drawing on the basic "accidents" listed by the *Pantegni*, though distinguishing, like the *Isagoge*, between different speeds, Avicenna referred to the sudden and forcible outward movement of anger, the gradual outward movement of delight and joy, the sudden inward movement or contraction of acute fear and terror, the gradual inward movement or contraction of sorrow or gloom, and the more complex bi-directional movements. These would typically occur when fear and dread were mixed with anxiety about the future, when anger and gloom were experienced simultaneously, or when shame was produced by a first confinement of spirit in the interior part, followed by a return of the power of reason (*ratio*), which would allow the contracted spirit to expand, bringing heat to the surface, thereby making the skin red.[64]

Avicenna's reference to the role of reason (*ratio*) in reversing the initially inward movement of shame shows how in Galenic medicine reason and passion were not always separable processes. His account appears to have drawn on Galen's description of shame (in *On the Causes of Symptoms* 2.5) as producing an initial sudden inward movement of *pneuma* similar to that of fear, followed by an outward movement caused by reason.[65] The *Pantegni* had made no reference to reason when describing shame as an initial inward movement of fear and an ensuing outward

63 The *Isagoge* was the introduction to Galen's Art written in the ninth century by the Nestorian Christian Hunayn ibn Ishāq, known in the West as Joannitius. I cite from *Liber Hysagoge Joannici*, in *Articella* (Venice: Joannes & Gregorius de Gregoriis, 1502), section 30. Cholmeley translates *angustia* figuratively as "poverty." See "Isagoge," trans. H. P. Cholmeley, in *A Source Book in Medieval Science*, ed. Edward Grant (Cambridge, MA: Harvard University Press, 1974), 705–15. However, in the context of the *accidentia animae* (which Cholmeley translates as "affections of the mind"), it seems more appropriate to translate *angustia* as "distress," "anxiety" or "anguish."

64 See Avicenna, *Canon medicinae*, Bk 1, fen. 2, ch. 14, "Anime accidentia."

65 "ratione vero patibilem animi excitante atque impellente, quae terretur et verecundatur, et redit et foras movetur simillimo motus modo, quo ex frigida lavatione caloris fit revocatio." *De symptomatum causis*, 2.5 (Kühn 7: 192–93). See Johnston's translation: "when reason has stirred up and excited the affective part of the soul, which is what is being afraid and ashamed, it [the *pneuma*] returns and moves towards the outside, predominantly by the same kind of movement in which a recall of heat would occur after bathing in cold water." *On the Causes of Symptoms*, 2.5, p. 259.

movement in preparation for defence, which reddens the skin.[66] By contrast, the explanation provided in Maino de Mainieri's regimen of how reason produces the redness associated with shame, derived perhaps from Avicenna (rather than from the *Pantegni* or from Galen), offers further evidence of the physiological alterations commonly associated with mental processes in medieval medicine.[67]

One of the most comprehensive medieval discussions of the relationship between mind and body in the *accidentia animae* is provided by Arnald of Villanova, who explained them as evaluative perceptions of an object, action or situation as beneficial or harmful, producing physical alterations in the heart and in other parts of the body through their movements and changes in the quantity and qualities of the spirits.[68] As he put it, the accidents of the soul originate in the "inner cognitive reason" (*ratio interior cognitiva*), when its evaluating power (*vis estimativa*) judges an object or action as beneficial or harmful. Once a quick judgment or assessment is made, the accident of the soul produces a number of alterations in the body, starting with the heart area. All accidents of the soul have an extrinsic cause—i.e., the external object perceived by the outer senses or by the imagination—and two types of intrinsic causes: "efficient" and "dispositional." The efficient cause is the cognitive process of knowing or imagining an object or situation as good or bad, even if it is not good or bad in itself. The dispositional cause relates to the physiological alterations in the solid parts of the body (i.e., organs and limbs), the spirits, and the blood (understood as a mixture of humours).[69]

In Villanova's and later Galenic writings, the spirits were attributed a crucial role in states such as worrying, fearing and being angry, sad or happy, as well as in the mental operations associated with them: perceiving, imagining,

---

[66] "Verecundia est cum calor naturalis interiora intret et exterior in vno momento visitet. Calor enim naturalis ad interiora sicut et in timore refugit in verecundia et post memorialiter recurrit ad exteriora ut defendat certis not sibi certa, unde sit cutis rubeat in verecundia." *Pantegni*, 25v.

[67] "& similiter in verecundia spiritus primo movetur ad intra et deinde redit ratio & consilium & dilatat illud quod est constrictum et egreditur exterius et rubificat calorem," Maineri, *Regimen sanitatis* (Paris: Anthonium Bonnemere, 1524), fol. 80r. The earliest extant edition is from 1482.

[68] Villanova, *Speculum medicine*, in *Hec sunt Opera Arnaldi de Villanoua* (Lyons, 1509), fols. 1r–36r, ch. 80, 23v–25v. Villanova used the phrase *accidentia anime* in his medical works, though he also justified the popular use of the phrases "passions of the heart" and "passions of the mind." *Speculum medicine*, 23v. For a brief examination of Villanova's views on the *accidentia anime* in the context of early fourteenth-century preventive medicine, see McVaugh, *Medicine before the Plague*, 146–47.

[69] *Speculum medicine*, 23v.

remembering and thinking. Such mental operations were thought to be performed by the wits or internal senses—imagination, practical reasoning (vis *cogitativa*, in humans) or assessment (*vis estimativa*, in animals and humans) and memory—which, according to the Galenic model developed by Avicenna and widely accepted in medieval and Renaissance faculty psychology, were housed in the brain and its spirit (see Figures 5 and 6). As we can see, for instance, from the fifteenth-century German

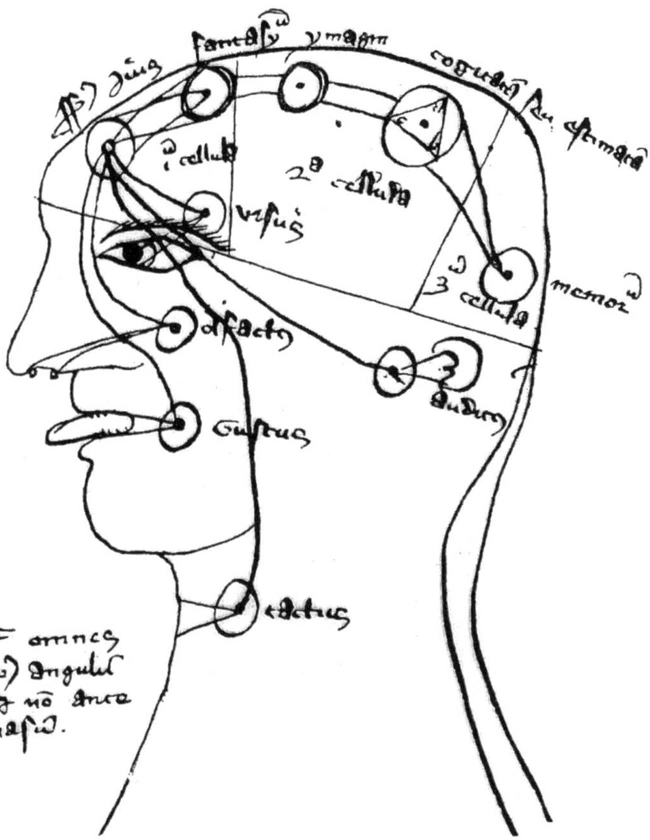

Fig. 5. Drawing of head showing the location of the inner senses in the brain (*sensus communis, fantasia, ymaginativa, cogitativa seu estimativa* and *memoria*). From a manuscript dated 1347 illustrating Avicenna's *De generatione embryonis*. From W. Sudhoff, "Die Lehre von den Hirnventrikeln in textlicher und graphischer Tradition des Altertums und Mittelalters," *Archiv für Geschichte der Medizin* 7 (1913): 149–205. Courtesy: Wellcome Library, London.

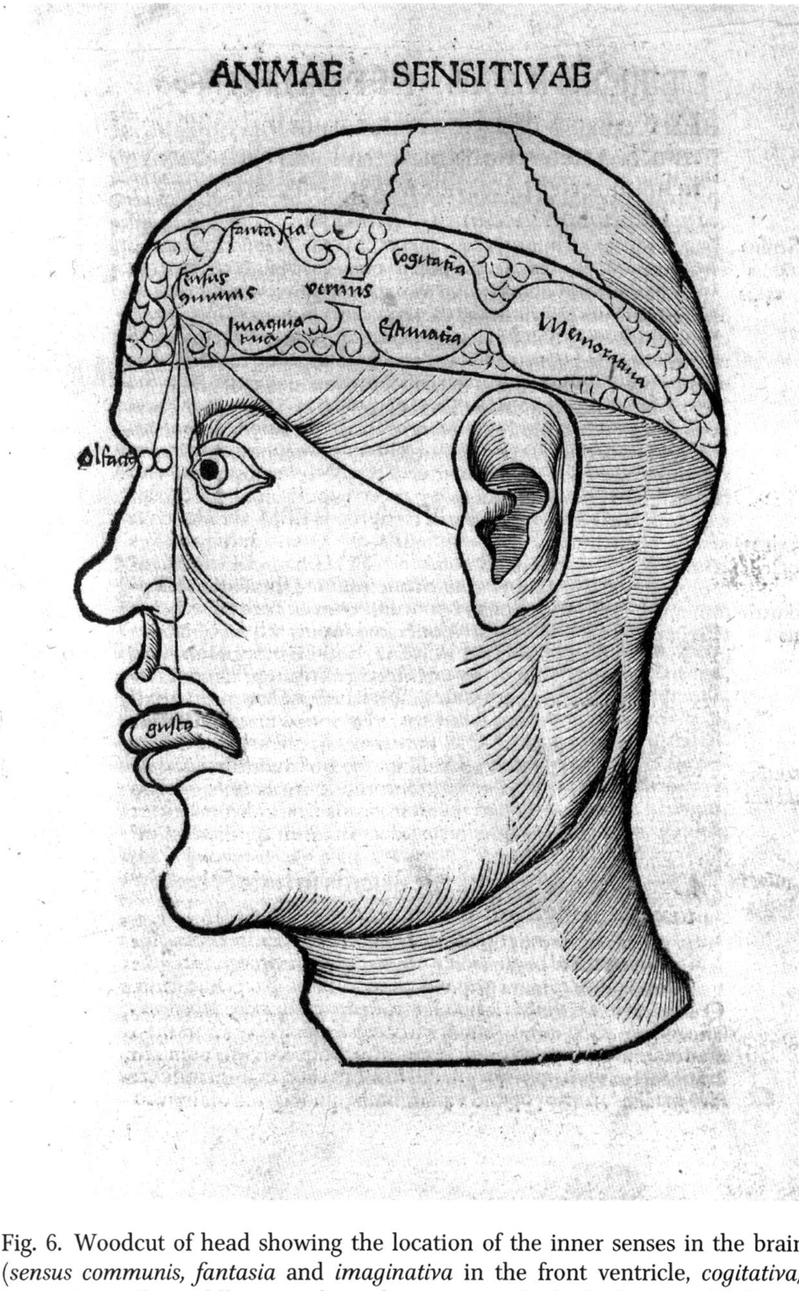

Fig. 6. Woodcut of head showing the location of the inner senses in the brain (*sensus communis, fantasia* and *imaginativa* in the front ventricle, *cogitativa/ estimativa* in the middle ventricle, and *memorativa* in the back ventricle). From: Gregor Reisch, *Margarita philosophica* (Freiburg, 1503). Courtesy: Wellcome Library, London.

translation of *accidentia animae* as "tzufallen dez synnes und dez mutes," the internal senses were considered to be the cognitive functions particularly involved in the accidents of the soul.[70]

Like Villanova, the sixteenth-century Spanish royal physician Bernardino Montaña de Montserrate also stressed the involvement in the accidents of the soul of cognitive operations which were thought to have a physiological impact not only on the spirits of the brain but also on the vital spirits moving in and out of the heart. Defining the accidents of the soul in Aristotelian terms as arising from the knowledge of a present or expected harm or benefit, he explained that they were called "accidents of the soul" because they depended on the soul's knowledge (*conocimiento*), and were also known as "passions of the heart" because they were marked movements of the spirits away from or towards the heart.[71]

Montaña seems to have followed closely Villanova's definition of the accidents of the soul and his justification of the popular use of the phrases "passions of the heart" and "passions of the mind."[72] However, he was closer than Villanova to the emphasis placed by Aristotle (*De anima* 1.1, 403a16–18) on the role of physiological pre-disposition in influencing the degree of stimulation people require in order to experience passions. He thus argued that individual differences in physiological disposition explain why some people are saddened (or experience anger, fear and despair) at the slightest occasion, while others are easily pleased and only saddened by very significant events.[73] His definition of anger was also closer to Aristotle than Villanova's in that it referred to an initial inward movement of sadness followed by the outward manifestation of the pleasure produced by the thought of revenge.[74] However, he did not specify how the soul might arrive at the knowledge of objects as harmful or beneficial.

A more detailed Aristotelian account of the processes of apprehension and evaluation associated with the "Perturbations, or Passions of the

---

70 *Regel der Gesundheit*, edited by Peter Strauss in his PhD Thesis, *Arnald von Villanova deutsch unter besonderer Berücksichtigung der "Regel der Gesundheit"* (Heidelberg: Institut für Geschichte der Medizin, 1963), 86.

71 Bernardino Montaña de Montserrate, *Libro de la anathomia del hombre* (Valladolid: Sebastian Martinez, 1551), 104r.

72 Villanova, *Speculum medicine*, 23v.

73 *Anathomia del hombre*, 106r.

74 "la yra, en la qual al principio la tristeza mueue los espiritus al coraçon y despues el plazer de la esperança de vengarse los torna a boluer a los miembros." *Anathomia del hombre*, 104v.

mind" is provided in the English translation of Paré's manual for surgeons published in 1634:

> For it is first necessary, before wee be moved by any Passions, that the senses in their proper seates, in which they are seldome deceived, apprehend the objects, and strait as messengers carrie them to the common sense, which sends their conceived formes to all the faculties. And then, that each facultie, as a Iudge may a fresh examine the whole matter, how it is, and conceive in the presented objects some shew of good, or ill, to bee desired, or shunned. For what man that was well in his wits, did ever fall into a laughter, unlesse he formerly knew, or saw somewhat said or done, which might yeeld occasion of laughter?[75]

Drawing on the kind of explanations which had prevailed in medieval and Renaissance faculty psychology, this passage reinforces the role attributed to the internal senses in judging the practical value of sense images—i.e., as to be desired or avoided. It also agrees with the causative role given to practical evaluations in Villanova's and Montaña's definitions of the passions.

As Villanova and Montaña had done before him, Paré drew on Avicenna's account of the accidents of the soul, in which Aristotle's model of sense-perception was merged with Galen's attribution of the functions of perception and judgement to the brain's *pneuma*, and with Galen's descriptions of the movements of *pneuma* in and out of the heart. He urged surgeons to try to understand the effects of the passions of the mind, suggesting that they did not always cause diseases, and that they could even have a positive impact on the mind and body: in stirring up the spirits, some passions could make the bodily heat and the blood flow better, thus refreshing and quickening all the faculties. He noted, for instance, that joy, hope and love could move heat and the spirits "sometimes gently, sometimes violently diffused over all the body, for the enjoying of the present, or hoped for good."[76]

Nicolas de La Framboisière also relied on medieval and Renaissance Galenic views on the passions as factors of health and disease, referring to them in his regimen of health, *Le Gouvernement* (1608), as agitations arising from judgments or evaluations of present or future good or evil, which

[75] *An Introduction or Compendious Way to Chyrurgerie*, 39; in *The Workes of that Famous Chirurgion Ambrose Parey*, trans. Thomas Johnson (London: Thomas Cotes and R. Young, 1634); hereafter, *Chyrurgerie*. This passage is not in the French version, *Introduction a la Chirugie*, in *Les œuvres de M. Ambroise Paré* (Paris: Gabriel Buon, 1575), 1–41, at 30–32.

[76] *Chyrurgerie*, 39.

make the heart expand or compress, moving spirits and natural heat in relation to the evaluated object. While broadly agreeing with Galen's (and the *Pantegni's*) physiological interpretations of the movements of the passions, he nonetheless moved away from the standard Galenic view of anger as one of the primary passions, focusing instead on the four basic passions distinguished by the Greek Stoics and by Cicero (*Tusculan Disputations*, 4: 13–21). He also followed Cicero's (and Augustine's) distinctions between the passions according to positive or negative cognitive evaluations of objects and their time frame: joy arises from the judgement or belief that the good is present, desire when the object judged as good is perceived as future, sadness when the object judged as evil is present, and fear when the object judged as evil is perceived as future. Like Cicero, he saw anger as a type of desire.[77]

In the *Art of Physick* (translated into English from the Latin edition of 1628), La Framboisière followed Cicero again in referring to shame as a form of fear, and to anger as "a burning Desire of Revenge." His new definition of the passions as "Motions of the Mind, violent and contrary to right Reason," established an opposition between passion and reason which was absent from *Le Gouvernement*.[78] This opposition was also a departure from medieval and Renaissance views, such as Villanova's and Maineri's suggestion that it is reasonable to display anger against unjust matters or unlawful actions, or Thomas Elyot's defence of a moderate type of anger which should be displayed by intelligent governors and masters in dealing with the negligence of their subjects or servants, just as it was displayed by Christ against those who were using the temple as a market.[79]

---

[77] "De là vient que nous sommes agitez de diuerses passions de l'ame, procedantes de l'opinion du bien ou du mal, present ou aduenir, lesquelles pour l'apprehension de l'object font dilater ou comprimer le coeur, l'esbranlant esmeuuent soudainement les esprits & la chaleur naturelle, de sorte que la couleur de la face en est incontinent changée. De l'opinion du bien present, vient, la ioye, & du future la cupidité, à laquelle se rapporte la cholere, qui est vn desir de vengeance: du mal present prouient la tristesse, & de l'aduenir la crainte." *Le Gouvernement* (Paris: Michel Sonnius, 1600), 156–57.

[78] La Framboisière, *The Art of Physick Made Plain and Easy* (London: Dorman Newman, 1684), 86–87.

[79] "et ideo cavende sunt eius occasiones, nisi quantum ex precepto racionis adversus illicita concitatur." Villanova, *Regimen sanitatis ad regem Aragonum*, in *Arnaldi de Villanova. Opera Medica Omnia*, X.1, pp. 423–70, at 436; hereafter, *Regimen ad regem*. "Igitur cauende sunt eius occasiones nisi quantum ratio precipit aduersus: illicita: iuxta illud. Irascimini & nolite peccare." Maineri, *Regimen*, 45v. The idea was conveyed in the various vernacular regimens attributed to Villanova. See, for instance: "ez ensy dan, daz man von rechtes wegen tzoernen muesse, alzo so man vnrecht digk horet." *Regel der Gesundheit*, 86. See also Thomas Elyot, *Castel of Helth* (London: Berthelet, 1539), 65.

Nonetheless, as in his previous work, La Framboisière continued to stress the physiological dimension of the passions, which could "cause an alteration in the Body, because of the extraordinary force of the Native Heat acting together with the Spirit and Bloud, both without and within." Despite this reference to the extraordinary force of the passions, he did distinguish different degrees of intensity when suggesting that gladness or joy and desire could be "wholesome" (healthful) if they were moderate, and pernicious if they were not.[80]

Like La Framboisière, the late-seventeenth-century German physician Jacob Joseph Joepser also drew on a mixture of ideas from Aristotelian faculty psychology and Stoicism when discussing the passions in his Latin regimen of health. While referring to them in Stoic terms as diseases of the soul (*morbus animi*), he stressed their force using a faculty psychology paradigm: "strong alterations of the sensitive appetite as regards the goodness or badness of an object perceived by the senses and the imagination." He noted that the bodily alterations brought about by the passions were sometimes significant, sometimes minor.[81]

In *Cerebri anatome* (1664), Willis suggested that the transmission onto the cerebellum of the impressions produced when strong passions were conceived in the brain caused a disturbance in the spirits, which affected the body's vital functions:

> the irregular motions of the Spirits, inhabiting the Cerebel, are wont also, by reason of the force of the affections, to be transmitted from thence to the Brain; for as often as a violent passion, such as Joy, Sadness, Anger, Fear, or of any kind, is conceived in the Brain, presently the impression of the same being brought through the by paths of the Prominences into the Cerebel, disturbs the Spirits destinated to the vital or merely natural function in their very fountain, and for that reason presently induces notable mutations in the Organs of those Functions.[82]

While in this early work he had referred specifically to joy, sadness, anger and fear (the main four passions discussed by Galenists), in his later

---

80 *The Art of Physick*, 86–87.

81 "vehemens appetitus sensitivi immutatio, circa bonum vel malum, sensu & imaginatione perceptum; jam majorem, jam verò minorem corporis alterationem inferens." Joepser uses the phrases "de animi affectibus," "animae affectionibus," "affecttibus, seu pathematibus animi," "excedentes animi passiones" and "morbus animi." *Isagoge, seu manuductio ad vitam longiorem: variis, de tuenda, reparandaque valetudine, dissertationibus illustrata: et selectis, tum veterum, tum recentiorum medicorum scitis placitisque stabilita* (Nuremberg: M. & J. F. Endter, 1680), 135–36.

82 *Anatomy of the Brain*, 95.

classification of the passions in *De anima brutorum* (*The Soul of Brutes*, ch. 8–9) Willis referred instead to the eleven passions distinguished by scholastic philosophers (concupiscible "Pleasure and Grief, Desire and Aversion, Love and Hatred," and irascible "Anger, Boldness, Fear, Hope, and Desperation"), arguing that this list was neither congruous nor sufficient, since it omitted shame, pity, emulation, envy and other affections. In this text he relied both on Aristotle and on a modified version of the Galenic notion of the spirits in describing the passions as perturbations of the corporeal soul:

> as soon as the Imagination conceives any thing that is to be embraced or shuned, presently the Appetite is formed by the spirits inhabiting the Brain, ordered into a Series; then by an impression sent to the *Praecordia*, as they are either dilated or contracted, the Blood is carried into various Motions of Fluctuations, and then by an instinct of the Appetite transmitted to the proper Nerves, the respective Motions are drawn forth: And upon these kind of Furnitures and Affection of the Spirits and Humors, and of the Solid Parts, the Affections or Passions of the Mind wholly depend, we have elsewhere shewed, after what manner, and by what Trajection or Irradiation of the Spirits, within the Nervous Processes, such quick Commerces are made, between the Brain and the *Praecordia*, and between both these and other Motive Parts.[83]

It is possible to establish continuities between Villanova's, Paré's and Willis's accounts of the passions as arising in the evaluations made by the imagination. In this respect, it can be argued that Willis only departed from medieval and Renaissance faculty psychology in ignoring the differentiation (found in Avicenna, Villanova and Paré) between the imagination and other internal senses (like the *vis estimativa* and *vis cogitativa* shown in Figures 5 and 6). His position is in line with that of the philosophers, who by 1600 had returned to a closer reading of Aristotle (purified from Arabic interpretations) by conflating all such embodied cognitive functions into the imagination.[84]

The above passage also shows how Willis maintained the Galenic distinction between spirits, humours, and solid parts of the body. Even though, in his view, the animal spirits were produced directly from the brain's blood (and not from the vital spirits distilled from blood in the heart, as was thought in medieval and Renaissance Galenism), he followed the Galenic tradition in seeing them as the "immediate instruments

83 *The Soul of Brutes*, 45–46.
84 See Park, "The Organic Soul," 480–81.

of thoughts." Like Villanova, he emphasized the role of animal spirits in transmitting the brain's evaluations and impressions to the heart, making it dilate or contract. Nonetheless, he provided a distinct explanation of the ensuing physiological processes. While Villanova and other Galenic authors described movements of natural heat and vital spirit (carried in the arterial blood) towards and away from the heart, Willis was able to draw on more accurate anatomical representations of the circulatory system, and thus simply referred to movements of disturbed blood.[85]

Where Willis clearly departed from Galenic knowledge was in his account of the anatomy of the brain and the cerebellum, in his dismissal of the explanatory model of the humours and also in his theory (based on Gassendi) of the intercostal nerve connecting the brain and the heart.[86] Nonetheless, like the Galenic authors examined in this section, he emphasized both the cognitive and physiological aspects of the passions. We will now see how this dual aspect was discussed in relation to anger.

The Physiological Basis of Anger: Individual Differences

In the *Pantegni*, anger (*ira*) was defined in Aristotelian terms as the boiling of the blood in the heart area with a rush of heat to the surface of the body in preparation for revenge.[87] In this short definition the readiness for revenge is not referred to as a mental state preceding or following the movement of bodily heat. Here mind and body are seen to act together, exemplifying the Galenic principle that the faculties of the soul depend on the temperature of the body.

Among the authors who provided a more nuanced account of anger, Arnald of Villanova noted both its physiological basis and the alterations

[85] "transmitted to the Breast, [the conception in our mind of good or evil things belonging to us] inordinately either Contracts or Dilates the Breast, and so pours forth the Affection, together with the disturbed Blood, on the whole Body." *The Soul of Brutes*, 48.

[86] Rina Knoeff focuses on the role Willis attributed to the intercostal nerve in enabling humans to control passion with reason; "The Reins of the Soul: The Centrality of the Intercostal Nerves to the Neurology of Thomas Willis and to Samuel Parker's Theology," *Journal of the History of Medicine and Allied Sciences* 59:3 (2004): 413–40. See also Jamie Kassler, "Restraining the Passions: Hydropneumatics and Hierarchy in the Philosophy of Thomas Willis," in *The Soft Underbelly of Reason: The Passions in the Seventeenth Century*, ed. Stephen Gaukroger (London: Routledge, 1998), 147–64; Noga Arikha, *Passions and Tempers: A History of the Humours* (New York: HarperCollins, 2007), 223–29.

[87] "Ira est ebullitio sanguinis qui in corde consistit et motus caloris subito extra corpus exeuntis ad vindicandum." *Pantegni*, Theorica, Bk 5, ch. 109, 25v.

it produces in the body.[88] In explaining the strong desire for revenge as being associated with choleric blood, he presupposed that only those whose blood was sufficiently warm and thin would be able to feel revengeful. Nonetheless, he did not make any explicit distinctions between different temperaments and did not refer to gender and age differences in bodily temperature. He simply stressed the physiological basis of moral disposition by providing a clear account of how choleric blood would build up the courage to attack by moving towards the heart together with spirit. He also sought to provide a rational explanation for the expansiveness usually associated with anger by suggesting that it was produced because its inward movement had the effect of kindling and heating the heart more than was needed, making it expand faster and more frequently than usual. This expansion of the heart would move the spirit towards the outer parts of the body, warming them up, thus preparing the body to fight. Anger could thus have a positive value in enabling action.

Maineri provided a similar explanation of the physiological basis of anger, though he made an explicit distinction between two movements: an initial sudden and impetuous inward movement of heat and spirits, which kindles the heart, and a subsequent outward movement.[89] His account differs from Villanova's both in its emphasis of the health risks entailed by the outward movement, which might leave the heart unprotected (*denudatum*), and in omitting any explicit references to how courage and the desire for revenge might be built up in the blood and its refined by-product, spirit.

Also in contrast with Villanova, Maineri noted individual differences in the external manifestations of anger, suggesting that they would depend on physiological differences such as the availability of bodily heat and spirits. He distinguished between the people who would become red when they were angry because their bodily heat was strong and their spirits abundant, and those who would become pale and shaky when they felt the desire for revenge because their bodily heat was too weak to reach the surface of their body. As we saw earlier, the distinction between red and

---

[88] "Nam in ipsa propter vehementem appetitum vindicte colericus sanguis movetur ad cor ut ipsum inflammet ac spiritus ad audaciam invadendi quo supercalefacto necesse est dilatari frequencius solito ac totum corpus maxime circa exteriora cum impetu calefieri, cum spiritus ad illas partes ex appetitu invadendi subito moveatur." Villanova, *Speculum medicine*, 25r.

[89] "In ira quidem movetur calor et spiritus subito et impetuose ad extra non totaliter relinquendo radicem sed accenditur in radice primo et postea movetur ad extra [...] et interdum totaliter radix: puta cor relinquitur denudatum." Maineri, *Regimen*, 45r.

pale angry faces was still seen as significant in the debates between Le Brun and his fellow members of the Académie Royale in the late seventeenth century. Maineri, however, had argued that paleness could not be seen as a straightforward sign of anger, and should be interpreted instead as being caused by the mixture of anger and fear.[90] Where Villanova explained how courage is built up by (hot) choleric blood together with spirit, Maineri suggested that without sufficient heat, there is no complete anger ("non est ira perfecta"). His interpretation "est quodammodo timor cum ira" tallied with the widespread pre-modern medical and natural philosophical belief that people whose natural heat was scarce (e.g., due to their innate temperament or due to illness) would tend to be fearful.

While we generally see courage as a character trait, independent of a person's physical constitution or physiological state, a number of medieval and early modern medical authors discussed it as a disposition which required abundant spirit or natural heat. For instance, Helkiah Crooke (d. 1635) drew attention to the physiological pre-disposition to courage as the basis for the differentiation between wrath and other types of anger. Citing Galen's reference (*Commentary on the Epidemics*, 1.2) to wrath as being associated with manly courage and distinct from the anger experienced by faint-hearted people like women and fearful men, Crooke described the latter as fretfulness and pettishness:

> The Temper of these two sorts is very different; for those that are angry, pettish, fretfull or wantle, chuse you which you will call them, are cold; but those that are wrathfull are hot. If therefore women are Nockthrown or easily mooued of the hindges, that they haue from their cold Temper, and from the impotencie and weaknes of their mind, because they are not able to lay a law vpon themselues.[91]

Drawing directly on Galen (rather than on medieval Galenists like Avicenna or Villanova) and endorsing widespread Aristotelian ideas, Crooke saw mental strength as being based on physiological disposition, and particularly on the proportion of natural heat, which was thought to be largely determined by factors such as age and gender.

---

[90] "et precipue in habentibus calorem fortem et multos spiritus. In habentibus enim calorem debilem irascuntur: et vindictam appetunt; calor non potest cum fervore dispergi ad extrema corporis et sic remanent exteriora membra albescentia et frigida non obstante quod calor sit ascensus in corde. Unde videmus multos iratos appetentes vindictam in actu ire livescere, et in talibus non est ira perfecta, sed est quodammodo timor cum ira." Maineri, *Regimen*, 45v.

[91] *Mikrokosmographia* (London: William Iaggard, 1615), 276.

Among the seventeenth-century medical authors who stressed the physiological basis of courage, La Framboisière simply noted that when spirits move outward at great speed, they impart strength to the outer parts of the body, thus facilitating courageous revenge.[92] He did not make any distinctions between temperament in the experience of anger in either *Le Gouvernement* or in *The Art of Physick*. Instead, he suggested that the movement of natural heat in anger is so vehement that if the anger endures, the heat "throws it self forth with violence into the outmost parts," causing redness in the face and warming up the whole body. He also stressed the causal link between physiological alterations and changes in attitude: "the whole Body being warm, becomes more bold, and ready to put it self forth into danger."[93] He thus maintained the traditional connections between anger and courage made by Aristotle (and reinforced through physiognomic accounts and through visual cues such as Ripa's and Peacham's inclusion of the lion in their emblem of the choleric type; see Figures 1 and 2), and by medical writers as far apart as Galen, Villanova and Crooke. Nonetheless, he also warned that being overconfident ("confidentius") might lead to unnecessary risks.

Moving away from Galen, though maintaining some continuity with the Aristotelian approach, Willis defined anger in *De anima brutorum* as being similar to boldness, though also involving simultaneous movements of sadness, characterized by contraction and heat, and readiness for revenge, characterized by expansion:

> Anger is of some Kin to Boldness, in which the sensitive soul, by reason of the evil unworthily brought to it, at the same time is made sad, and grows hot; wherefore, as she contracts her self by reason of Sadness, so presently girding her self for Revenge, she is dilated; therefore, as here divers Contractions come together, this Passion is performed with a mighty Perturbation of Spirits, and of the Blood.[94]

---

92 "la cupidite & la cholere font pareillement dilater le coeur: [...] celle-cy pour enuoyer vistement la chaleur naturelle auec le sang & les esprits du dedans au dehors, afin de fortifier tellement les membres, qu'ils puissent courageusement venger le tort qu'on nous a faict. C'est pourquoy elle les pousse avec vne grande vehemence & furie." *Le Gouvernement*, 157.

93 La Framboisière, *The Art of Physick*, 88. Note how the English "boldness" is used to translate the Latin term *confidens*: "Vbi corpus rubicundius, calentius, confidentius & ad omne facinus pattandum promptius redditur." *Schola Medicae*, in *Oeuvres* (Paris: Jean-Antoine Hvgvetan, 1644), 829–51, at 901.

94 *The Soul of Brutes*, 54.

Willis made no distinction between individual differences in the experience of anger based on temperament or physiological disposition. In line with Aristotle, he emphasized how the sadness caused by a perceived undeserved slight or evil would give rise to the desire for revenge.

While we might think of the passions or perturbations as mental states, Willis's understanding of anger as a perturbation did not separate the mind from the body. His view that thought, sadness and readiness for action involve an alteration of the spirits and the blood was indebted to the Aristotelo-Galenic approach promoted by medical writers like Avicenna, Villanova, and La Framboisière. Like them, Willis did not see strong passions as 'diseases of the soul', but as perturbations of the spirits, which could seriously affect the functioning of the vital organs.

The Harmful Effects of Anger

Medieval and early modern medical authors tended to agree that anger could have deleterious effects on health, though there was a huge disparity of opinions as to the specific diseases and impairments that it could lead to, and the processes this involved. For instance, Bernard de Gordon noted how paralysis (i.e. a softening of the nerves causing loss of movement and sensory loss) could result from excessive anger or great fear, just as it could be caused by a fall, a wound to the nerves, friction, a broken bone, a deep cut, a cold obstructing compression or a heat loss.[95] Villanova followed Avicenna in stressing that one of the main effects of anger is that it makes the heart dry (though to a lesser extent than in sadness), and that this happens through the process of frequent contraction and as a result of overheating.[96] Both Villanova and Maineri emphasized that anger could lead to mental confusion by heating the heart's blood, making it boil, and producing inflammation in all the parts of the body.[97]

By contrast, most of the medieval and early modern regimens of health tended to mention only the heating or drying effects of anger on the body. For instance, the *Regel der Gesundheit* (one of the fifteenth-century German regimens of health attributed to Villanova) explained that the heat

95 *Lilio*, I, 585–86.

96 "cor etiam exiccatur ex frequentia sui motus et supercalefactione, licet minus quam in tristitia." *Speculum medicine*, 25r.

97 "Quoniam ira supercalifacit omnia membra et propter fervorem cordis omnes actus racionis confundit." *Regimen ad regem*, 436. Maineri's wording is very similar; *Regimen*, 45r.

and the movement of the heart produced by anger would overheat all parts of the body.[98] The fifteenth-century French *Regime tres utile* (published under Villanova's name) referred to Avicenna's *Canon* in suggesting that anger warms up excessively all parts of the body, thus drying it up.[99] The various Salernitan regimens of health published in English between 1528 and 1650 simply cited Avicenna, mentioning succinctly that "heat dryeth up mans body."[100]

The English lawyer Thomas Elyot, in his very popular *Castel of Helth* (1539), warned against a wider range of physical effects, including trembling, fevers, apoplexy, palsy, sensory and mental numbness ("priuation of sencis"), restlessness ("vnquietnes of mynde"), lack of appetite, insomnia, "feeble digestion" and facial disfigurement ("deformitie of visage").[101] While in the later Renaissance it was typical for medical authors to draw on the newly available Latin translations of Greek medical texts, the regimens of health still tended to rely on Arabic Galenic sources rather than on Galen directly. For instance, the late-sixteenth-century Spanish physician and theologian Blas Álvarez Miraval (d. 1598) referred to the authority of Avicenna in noting that anger could cause heart palpitations and heart disease, and to Averroes in suggesting that it could make people spit or cough blood and produce ephemeral fever and epilepsy.[102] Relying both on medieval Galenism and on Galen directly, the late-seventeenth-century Latin regimen of health by the German physician Jacob Joseph

---

98 "Warumb tzorn verhitzet alle die gelider dez leibs von der hitz vnd der bewegunge dez hertzen vnd geschendet alle werck der bescheidenheit. Vnd darumb, waz von syne oede ist, daz sol sich hueten vor den sachen, die tzorn, druren brengen." *Regel der Gesundheit*, 86.

99 *Le regime tres utile et tres proufitable pour conserver et garder la sante du corps humain* (Lyons, 1491), 1r; for a critical edition, see *Le regime tres utile… With the commentary of Arnoul de Villeneuve*, ed. Patricia W. Cummins (Chaperl Hill: North Caroline studies in the Romance Languages and Literatures, 1976).

100 See, for instance, *Regimen sanitatis salerni or the Schoole of Salernes Regiment of Health* (London: B. Alsop, 1650 [1534]), 2. The extremely popular *Regimen sanitatis Salernitanum* circulated in over 100 manuscript versions from the thirteenth century onwards and was widely available in print in Latin and in a number of European languages in the sixteenth and seventeenth centuries in over 250 editions. For the English versions, see Paul Slack, "Mirrors of Health and Treasures of Poor Men: The Uses of the Vernacular Medical Literature of Tudor England," in *Health, Medicine, and Mortality in the Sixteenth Century*, ed. Charles Webster (Cambridge: Cambridge University Press, 1979), 237–73.

101 *Castel of Helth*, 65.

102 "la palpitación del corazon, como lo dize Avicena, y el sputo de la sangre, y la tosse, la calentura ephimera, y la epilepsia, como lo enseña Averroes en el tercero del colliget, en el capitulo 41 y juntamente con esto una passion grande del coraçon, que se llama cardiaca." Álvarez Miraval, *La conservación de la salud del cuerpo y del alma* (Medina del Campo: S. del Canto, 1597), 24r. See Averroes, *Colliget*, Bk 3, ch. 41.

Joepser suggested that, besides apoplexy and paralysis, anger could also produce acute pain in the male genitals.[103]

As regards the specific advice given by medieval and early modern physicians in their instructions or *consilia* to people suffering from a disease or medical condition, the most typical recommendation was that they needed to avoid anger, fear, worrying, and sad thoughts. For instance, people suffering from epilepsy were usually advised to eschew all accidents of the soul, such as anger, fear, worrying and any action which might move their spirits outward, or suddenly inward.[104]

The need to avoid anger was also stressed in all plague tracts. For instance, the late-fifteenth-century Latin, Spanish and Portuguese versions of the *Regimen contra pestilentiam* of Joannes Jacobi (a Catalan physician who became Chancellor of the University of Montpellier, d. 1384) noted the need to avoid anger because it produced excessive heat and thus would make people more susceptible to the plague.[105] A number of plague tracts referred to Galen and to Joannes Jacobi in emphasizing that wrath, excessive joy and sexual intercourse, were to be avoided because of their heating effects, while moderate joy and honest mirth could be very helpful.[106] Other authors, like the Licenciado Fores in the plague tract he wrote in Seville in 1481, warned about the dangerous impact of anger, sadness, fear and worrying in making people more susceptible to contagion, and recommended that pleasure and joy should be promoted through songs, tunes and instruments, and by telling pleasant stories.[107] The plague treatise published in 1516 by the royal physician Fernand Álvarez (d. 1526) mentioned the detrimental effect of sadnesss and worrying, and argued

103 Joepser, *Isagoge*, 135, 144.

104 Bernard de Gordon, *Lilio*, I, 569.

105 "et os homens que se muyto esqueentan con grande trabalho ou grande yra, teem os corpos mais dispostos para reçeber ha pestilencia." *Regimento proueytoso contra ha pestenencia*, trans. Luis de Raz (1496), facsimile edition (Lisbone: Tipografia Idea, 1961), a4r. Jacobi's brief treatise was first published in Latin 1476. It was also bound together with the Regimen attributed to Villanova, *Regimen sanitatis salernitanum cum expositione Arnoldi de Villanova* (Cologne: J. Guldenschaff, 1494), 76r–79v. A Spanish translation was included in Johannes de Ketham, *Epilogo de medicina* (Pamplona: Arnau Guillen de Brocar, 1495), tr. 7, ch. 8, fols 46v–47r.

106 See, for instance, Velasco de Taranta, *Tratado de la peste*, in Velasco de Taranta, Licenciado Fores, Fernando Álvarez, Diego Álvarez Chanca, *Tratados de la peste*, ed. María Nieves Sánchez (Madrid: Arco/Libros, 1993), 15–76, at 50.

107 *Tratado útil e muy prouechoso contra toda pestilencia y aire corrupto*, in *Tratados de la peste*, ed. Sánchez, 77–158, at 106. On this little-known work, see Randal P. Garza, *Understanding Plague: the Medical and Imaginative Texts of Medieval Spain* (New York: Peter Lang, 2008), 47–56.

that anger and anxiety (like walking too fast) were harmful because they made the breath (or spirit) move too quickly, though it suggested that honest pleasures should be cultivated as a way of counteracting the accumulation of moisture (and ensuing putrefaction) produced by a sedentary lifestyle.[108] Similarly, Thomas Lodge (d. 1625) also noted that honest pleasurable activities would induce a calm form of joy, as a way of preventing the unhealthful movements of spirit: "let them leade their life in peace, and quiet of minde, in ioy, disport and honest pleasure, auoyding all perturbations of the spirit, and especially sadnesse, melancholy, wrath, feare, and suspect, which are the most daungerous accedents that may encounter a man in such like times."[109] While all these authors agreed that the excessive heat produced by anger would make people more prone to contracting the plague, they also stressed the importance of maintaining the body's moderate heat.

The regulation of anger, fear and worry was seen as crucial in preventing premature death, as well as in particular situations such as pregnancy, when a woman's state of mind would affect not only her health, but also that of the baby she carried. Drawing on Rhazes's and Avicenna's regimental advice for pregnancy, medieval authors stressed the importance of avoiding anger and sadness because of their drying effect.[110] The summary of medical knowledge in verse published in the late fifteenth century by the Spanish royal physician Francisco de Villalobos (d. 1549) mentioned the need for pregnant women to avoid fear, anger and sadness, while the treatise for midwives published by Damián Carbón four decades later explains in greater detail how anger could cause miscarriage by heating up the spirits of the pregnant woman, leaving the fetus with inadequate air and rotten nourishment.[111]

---

108 *Regimiento contra la peste* (1501), in *Tratados de la peste*, ed. Sánchez, 159–75, at 166.

109 Thomas Lodge, *A Treatise of the Plague* (London: Edward White and N. L., 1603), ch. 6.

110 See, for instance, *Bartholomäus Scherrenmüllers Gesundheitsregimen* (1493) (Heidelberg: Institut für Geschichte der Medizin, 1970), ed. Wolfram Schmitt, 51; hereafter, *Gesundheitsregimen*. See Rhazes, "De regiminis pregnantis et conservatione fetus eius," *Liber de medicina ad Almansorem*, IV; Avicenna, "De regimine universali pregnantis" and "De abortu," in *Canon*, Bk 3, fen. 21, tr. 2, ch. 2 and 9.

111 Francisco López de Villalobos, *El sumario de la medicina con un tratado de las pestíferas bubas* (1498), ed. María Teresa Herrera (Salamanca: Instituto de Historia de la Medicina Española, 1973), 404; Damián Carbón, *Libro del arte de las comadres o madrinas y del regimiento de las preñadas y paridas y de los niños* (1541), ed. Daniel García Gutiérrez (Zaragoza: Anúbar, 2000), 20v.

Nonetheless, while warning against the dangers of anger to physical and mental health, and endorsing the general recommendation that it should be avoided, some medical authors made nuanced distinctions between different types of anger, depending on its intensity, and the presence or absence of the desire for revenge, as we shall now see.

The Therapeutic Uses of Anger

In his treatise on how to slow down the effects of old age, *De retardatione accidentium senectutis*, the Franciscan Friar Roger Bacon (d. 1294) suggested that anger, a typical "accident" associated with the aging body, can also have a healthful impact. Drawing on a wide range of medical authors (including Galen, Rhazes, Avicenna and Isaac Israeli) and on the *Secret of Secrets* attributed to Aristotle, Bacon emphasized the strengthening effects of wrath and anger, moderate exercise or wrestling, joy, mirth and "whatever provokes laughter," conversations with friends, listening to instrumental music or songs, and obtaining victory over one's enemies, thereby filling up with self-confidence.[112] He explained that all such operations and movements of the soul are strengthening and conducive to good health because they spread the blood around the body. Similarly, in the late-seventeenth-century English version of this text, its translator, Richard Browne, noted that "choler" could be beneficial to health because its heat could help prevent the putrefaction of the humours.[113]

At first sight, the suggestion that anger could have a positive impact on health appears to be at odds with the frequent remarks made by medical authors about the need to avoid anger, fear or sadness. For instance, Bernard de Gordon advised that one should not be angry, afraid or saddened (*nec irascaris, nec timeas, nec doleas*) by any loss, death of friends,

---

[112] "alius modus fit in operationibus et actionibus anime et motibus, sicut iracundia et ira et alteratio et exercitium temperatum et luctatio; et iterum sicut gaudium et letitia et que faciunt mouere risum, et musica instrumenta audire cum cantinelis et absque cantinelis et sedere cum sociis animum delectantibus, [...], et de inimicis consequi victoria et suam fiduciam complere, et cum dilectis ratiocinare, ut dicit Aristoreles in epistola ad Alexandrum." *De retardatione accidentium senectutis, cum aliis opusculis de rebus medicinalibus*, ed. A. G. Little and E. Withington (London: Clarendon, 1928), 71. The seventeenth-century English translation omits reference to exercise and wrestling and does not translate "et suam fiduciam complere." See *The Cure of Old Age and Preservation of Youth*, trans. Richard Browne (London: Thomas Flesher and Edward Evetts, 1683), 128.

[113] "Choler is by some reckoned the Salt of the Microcosm, which helps to keep the Flood of Humors from Putrefaction," *The Cure of Old Age*, 133.

imprisonment or banishment, and that one should not feel indignant in the face of disgrace or abuse (*pro aliquo vituperio non indigneris*). Despite the apparent contrast between his position on anger and Bacon's, it can be argued that de Gordon placed the emphasis on moderation, rather than complete avoidance of the accidents of the soul.[114] Like de Gordon, Bacon also noted the importance of moderation in emphasizing that the six non-naturals, a necessary part of human existence, had such a great impact in preserving and altering the body, that their intensity and frequency needed to be regulated (*administrantur in qualitatibus et quantitatibus*) so as to promote good health.[115] Yet the fact that Bacon mentioned the strengthening effect of both wrath and anger is consistent with the medieval Galenic view that health could be maintained by counterbalancing one non-natural factor of health with another, one passion with another.

The idea that anger could be beneficial to some people, depending on their complexion and state of health was a widespread one in the medieval and early modern regimens of health. For instance, the richly illuminated abridged versions of Ibn Boṭlān's eleventh-century health handbook produced in Latin in the late fourteenth and early fifteenth centuries, known as *Theatrum sanitatis* or *Tacuinum sanitatis*, suggest that in making the heart's blood boil, anger could restore the body's heat ("calorem transmutantes restituens").[116] This brief reference is part of the three-line text which accompanies the visual representation of "Ira" as a woman with furrowed brows, wearing no headdress, exposing part of her breasts and, as it seems, being admonished by a learned man (see Figure 7). Like the Liege and Paris *Tacuinua sanitatis*, the *Theatrum* notes that anger could also help those who suffer from paralysis or from pain in the mouth.[117]

---

[114] He adds the qualification "sine rationabili causa," as well as stressing moderation or temperance: "in omnibus actibus suis homo sciat temperare se in accidentibus animae." Bernard de Gordon, *De conservatione vitae*, ed. Joachimus Baudisius (Leipzig: Rhamba for E. Vogelin, 1570), 79.

[115] "Nam doctrina regiminis precipit obuiare causis senectutis cum mensuratione sex generum causarum necessarium que conseruant corpus et mutant, et sic iste cause sunt completiue sanitatis et infirmitatis: quia, quando adminstrantur in qualitatibus et quantitatibus secundum quod oportet, et partibus, usus erorum conseruant sanitatem. Et quando non administrantur secundum quod oportet, transeunt in illo et faciunt accidere egritudinem, quando perseuerat transitus et multiplicatur. Collige in *Tegni* G. cum expositio Haly ibi tractat de regimine sanitatis." *De retardatione*, 13. See *The Cure of Old Age*, 12–13.

[116] *Theatrum sanitatis*, ed. Manuel Moleiro Rodríguez (Barcelona: Moleiro, 1998). This is a facsimile edition of Ms. 4182 of the Biblioteca Casanatense in Rome.

[117] See *The Medieval Health Handbook: Tacuinum sanitatis*, ed. Luisa Cogliati Arano, trans. Oscar Ratti and Adele Westbrook (London: Barrie & Jenkins, 1976), plate 67 shows fol. 66 of the Liege codex and plate 174 shows fol. 66 of the Paris codex.

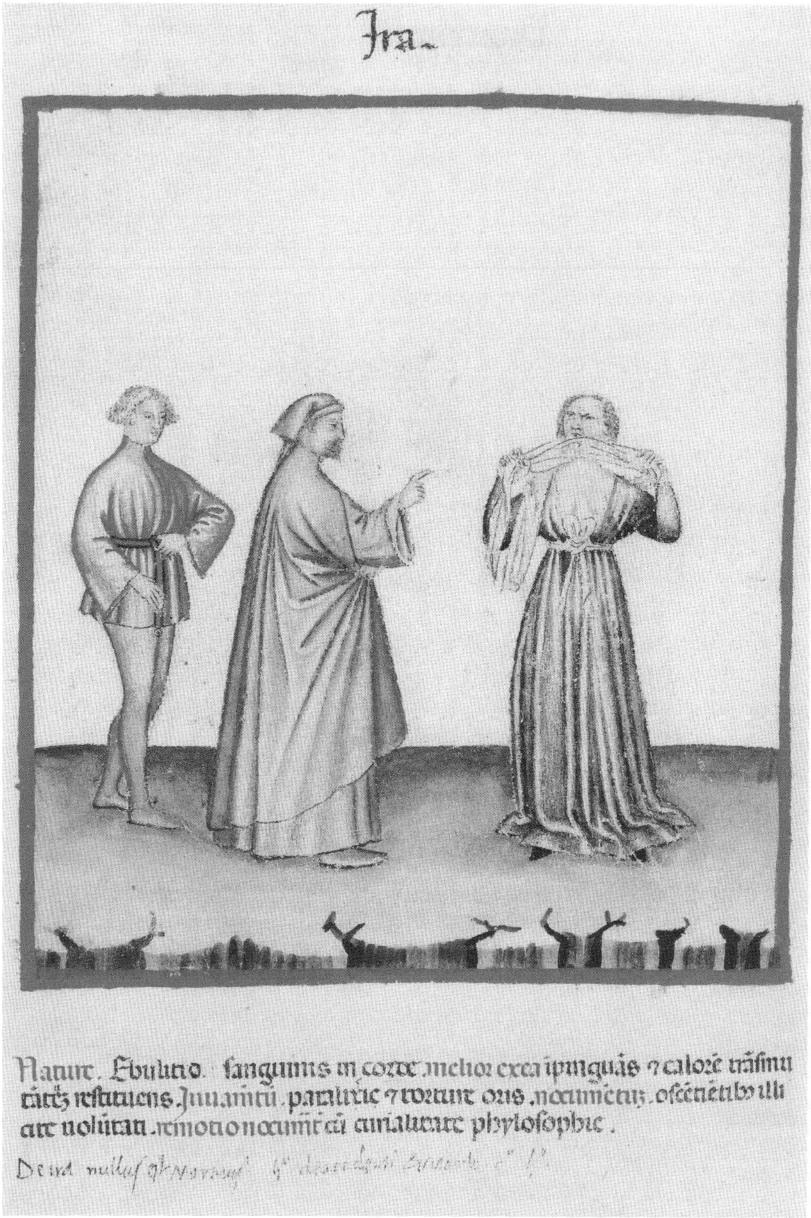

Fig. 7. "Ira." *Theatrum sanitatis*, facsimile of Ms. 4182 of the Biblioteca Casanatense in Rome, ed. Manuel Moleiro Rodríguez (Barcelona, 1998), cxc. Courtesy: Wellcome Library, London.

The Vienna *Tacuinum* also mentions that the kind of anger which moves the blood outward and fills the veins would be a good antidote against paralysis, though it warns that if the anger was too strong or prolonged, it would make the skin yellow, and cause trembling, fever and anxiety.[118] All four versions of the text point out that anger can be beneficial, and that philosophical education can prevent its potentially harmful effects. They thus emphasize both the physiological dimension of anger and its cognitive component. More importantly, the text and the illustration accompanying it also show a social context in which anger might manifest and be managed.

The belief that anger is not always harmful, and might sometimes be healthful, also appears in the therapeutic instructions given by Taddeo Alderotti (d. 1296) in his *Consilia*, which include a reference to each of the non-naturals. For instance, a patient with pain in the kidneys caused by a build-up of phlegm (a cold condition) could get angry without this having a negative impact on his health.[119] For patients suffering from "weak nerves," who would shake every time they experienced an accident of the soul, the drying heat of anger could even be beneficial in the longer term.[120] We can follow the logic of this advice by bearing in mind that "weak nerves" were seen as a cold and moist condition and that anger was believed to have a drying and warming effect on the body.

The suggestion made by Alderotti that a patient suffering from inflammation of the liver and the spleen should avoid excessive anger seems to indicate that moderate anger was sometimes acceptable, perhaps because the patient could not easily avoid being angry, or because his anger was not thought to be damaging in view of his overall physiological condition.[121] Here one should bear in mind the social context of the type of advice

118 *L'Art de vivre au Moyen Age: Codex vindobonensis serie nova 2644 conservé à la Bibliothèque nationale d'Autriche*, ed. Daniel Poirion and Claude Thomasset (Paris: Editions du Félin, 1995), 98v.

119 "caveat a tristitia superflua, sollicitudine et a coitu; gaudeat tamen et letetur, et si aliquando ad aliquam iram commotus fuerit, non nocebit." Alderotti, *Consilia*, ed. Piero P. Giorgi and Gian F. Pasini (Bologna: University of Bologna, 1997), 458.

120 "Dico igitur quod omnia accidentia ante tremorem eccitant in presenti cum fiunt, sed quia desiccant corpora omnia preter gaudium, ideo in processu non ledunt, sed iuvant aliqualiter potius, et maxime ira cuius [est] humiusmodi desiccatio et calefactio; sed timor et tristitia, licet desiccant, quia infrigidant, nocent cum pauco iuvamento." *Consilia*, 290–92.

121 "De accidentibus anime: abstineat ergo a coitu et ab omni solicitudine, tristitia, timore et ira superflua; inducatur sibi gaudium et letitia temperate. Et hec est eius cura per dietam." *Consilia*, 226.

given in the *Consilia*. The recommendation that anger or sadness should be avoided did not simply put the onus on the patient to control his or her reactions. Caregivers were expected to ensure that the sick person was not given bad news or any reason to be sad or angry, in much the same way as they were expected to give him or her the type of foods prescribed by the physician.

In the best Galenic practice, the treatment suggested for each patient was personalized and took into account his or her physiological make-up, age and circumstances, rather than the disease *per se*. This can perhaps explain why moderate anger might have been considered harmless for a patient with an inflamed liver and spleen, while the advice for another patient suffering from a similar disease (an inflamed liver) was to avoid all anger.[122] This differing advice can also help us understand Galenic views on how the impact of anger would depend on each person's particular mixture of primary qualities. In a conceptual framework in which inflammation of the spleen (diagnosed in one of Alderotti's patients suffering from an inflamed liver but not in the other) could be interpreted as the effect of the retention of (cold, dry) black bile, it was also possible to assume that the gentle heat of moderate anger would make the black bile less dense, helping it flow better.

While Alderotti did not distinguish between different types of anger in his *consilia*, other medieval authors stressed the correlation between the intensity of anger and its effects on health. For instance, Benedictus de Nursia argued that, by making the blood boil in the heart, temperate anger could be conducive to health because it could strengthen the body's natural heat if it was weak or sluggish.[123] He nonetheless also argued that the alterations produced by wrath were dangerous because their excessive movement of bodily heat outwards (in preparation for revenge) could lead to the dissolution of the body's natural heat. The distinction between unhealthful and healthful forms of anger was also emphasized in the manual for physicians of Estéfano de Sevilla (d. 1387), which explicitly referred to Galen's views (in *De morbo et accidente* 5.6 and in *De causis* 3) that while wrath might be detrimental both for people with a good temperament and for those whose body was cold, the type of anger which involved no desire for revenge ("saña sin enojo de ninguna persona") could help the

122 "abstineat ab omni sollicitudine et tristitia, ira." *Consilia*, 92.

123 "sua ebullitione & accidente caliditate, calorem naturalem debilitatum aut sopitum confortat & expergefacit, & ad bonam sanitatem iuuamentum prebet." *Pulcherrimum*, ch. 96 [262].

body to maintain its natural heat in a moderate effervescence, thus ensuring that the blood reached and vivified all the bodily organs.[124]

As regards individual differences, the *Regimina sanitatis* often mentioned that anger could be conducive to health in people lacking warmth. For instance, the fourteenth-century regimen attributed to Joannes de Burgundia suggested that "thy wrath profyteth to flewmatyk men and hit harmeth coleryk."[125] Similarly, Bartholomäus Scherrenmüller's *Gesundheitsregimen* (1493) noted that anger can be healthful for people with a cold heart.[126] The regimen of health published in French in 1491 indicated that, in producing and maintaining bodily heat, anger can also be beneficial to people who had been made cold by poisoning.[127]

When Ambroise Paré wrote for surgeons in the late sixteenth century, he noted that anger caused an effusion of heat, like joy, but only far speedier, thus making the spirits and humours so inflamed that it could cause putrid fevers. Knowing, however, that the heat of anger would have a different impact on different people, he suggested that it might be beneficial to people who lacked heat and had too much phlegm due to their sedentary lifestyle: "anger is profitable to none, unlesse by chance to some dull by reason of idlenesse, or opprest with some cold, clammy and phlegmaticke humor."[128]

Following the Hippocratic and Galenic principle of *contraria contrariis curantur*, it was possible to suggest that the heat of anger could help to counteract the excess of cold in the body, whether it was innate, or due to lifestyle, sickness or environmental conditions. Thus, the Vienna *Tacuinum sanitatis* notes that anger is more suitable to very old and infirm people and to those with a cold temperament, as well as in the winter and in cold regions.[129] This advice is a great example of how the non-natural factors of health and disease could be orchestrated to ensure an overall healthful

[124] Estéfano de Sevilla, *Visita y consejo médicos*, Madrid, BN MSS 18052, ed. Enrica J. Ardemagni, Rebecca Montague, Carmen Sáez, María Jesús Sánchez, Beth Markowitz, Cynthia M. Wasick and John Zemke, in CD-ROM *Textos y Concordancias Electrónicos del Corpus Médico Español*, ed. María Teresa Herrera and María Estela González de Fauve (Madison, 1997), 13r.

[125] *Gouernayle of Helthe*, 3r.

[126] *Gesundheitsregimen*, 87.

[127] "Et est a noter quels sont aucunes gens qui sont frois naturellement: ou par accident daucun maleficier poison auquels est utile et prouffitable pour la santé corporelle destre marris et courouez a ce que par ce moyen la chaleur naturelle en euls soit melee acquise et conservee." *Regime tres utile*, 1r.

[128] *Chyrurgerie*, 40. See *Introduction a la Chirurgie*, 32.

[129] See *L'Art de vivre au Moyen Age*, 98v.

balance: the cold weather (air, the first non-natural) and the coldness created by sedentariness (the third non-natural) could be counteracted by certain states of mind, such as anger (the sixth non-natural), which have a warming effect.

The principle that bodily coldness could be counteracted with the warmth produced by some of the alterations of the mind also underpinned the pre-modern medical belief that anger could be used as a means to cure cold diseases. For instance, Lluís Alcanyís referred in his plague tract (1490) to a famous physician who cured the extreme weakness of a patient by constantly reminding him of events from his past which provoked his anger, thus strengthening his natural heat.[130] In attributing a positive value to the warmth created in the patient by the negatively evaluated images from his past held in his memory and evoked through external auditory stimuli, this anecdote stresses the unity of mind and body. It also shows an implicit awareness of anger as both a 'cognitive' and a 'physiological' event.

The Renaissance belief in the effect of certain types of memories and mental evaluations on the body is also illustrated by a passage by the English physician William Bullein (d. 1576) on the potentially positive impact of anger. Referring to Galen's view that anger could keep the body moderately warm, Bullein suggested in the *Bulwarke of Defence* (1562 and 1579) that anger could be particularly beneficial for idle bodies with little natural heat, and that it could also help to counteract the effects of cold weather. In emphasizing (jokingly, perhaps) the advantages of anger over artificial ways of warming up the body, such as massaging it with oil, bathing in warm water or going into the stove (a heated room), he used a compelling argument, based on personal experience, which would be recognized by most of his readers. He simply invited them to try to recall the warmth they might have felt at times when they were being criticized or reprimanded:

> wee feele by our selues in colde weather, let our Enemy sodaynely appeere before us, or if we heare our selues shamefully rebuked, we neede no fyre, to kindle the flame of our choler, forthwyth we are in the house top, the holiest of vs all.[131]

---

[130] Lluís Alcanyís, *Regiment preservatiu et curatiu de la pestilencia*, ed Jon Arrizabalaga (Barcelona: Barcino, 2008), 94.

[131] "The Booke of the Vse of Sicke Men, and Medicines," 24v, in *Bulleins Bulwarke of Defence against all Sicknesse, Soarenesse, and Woundes that Doe Dayly Assaulte Mankinde* (London: Thomas Marshe, 1579 [1562]). For a study of this work in its cultural context, see

Bullein thus stressed how bodily heat could be produced when perceiving oneself being slighted, though he made no reference to any anger being expressed externally. This shows how anger was believed to originate in the cognitive process of judging an object or action as undeservedly harmful, and to manifest internally in the body, altering it before any action was taken.[132] It also emphasizes how the various non-natural factors of health and disease (air, rest and movement, and the accidents of the soul) could counterbalance one another.

The belief in the therapeutic use of anger in dealing with cold diseases seems to have survived into the late eighteenth century, when the popular medical author William Corp acknowledged the benefits of anger in conditions such as palsy and intermittent fevers. Corp, nonetheless, also criticized the then widespread view that anger could cure all kinds of diseases, including (hot) eruptive ones, like small pox or measles. In view of such mistaken views, he opted for the simple solution of denying that anger had any therapeutic value: "the employment of anger in the cure of diseases will be either hazardous, or useless."[133]

Conclusion

Judging from the evidence examined in this essay, pre-modern anger was not always seen as entirely distinct in its physiological manifestations from other emotional states. It could sometimes be mixed with fear (as suggested in Maineri's fourteenth-century Galenic regimen of health). It was conceptualized as a sequence of sadness and pleasure (in the Aristotelian view put forward in Montaña's sixteenth-century advice manual) or of sadness and the desire for revenge (in Willis's seventeenth-century Aristotelian interpretation). It was also understood as a form of desire (in the Ciceronian view propounded by La Framboisière in seventeenth-century France). Yet, beyond the disparity of the pre-modern medical definitions of anger, what emerges from the medical discussions is that (contrary to what modern scholars like Dirk Geeraerts have suggested) anger was not thought to be simply 'caused' by choler.

R. W. Maslen, "The Healing Dialogues of Doctor Bullein," *The Yearbook of English Studies* 38:1/2, Tudor Literature (2008): 119–35.

[132] For those who might feel moved by anger or any sudden 'affection' but might not wish to give it full rein, Bullein recommended the old remedy of reciting the alphabet.

[133] *Essay on the Changes Produced in the Body by Operations of the Mind* (London: Ridgway, 1791), 56–63.

The brief accounts of the passions found in the earlier medieval texts, like the *Pantegni* and the *Isagoge*, referred to them as movements of spirit and natural heat. Some medical authors, like Maineri in the fourteenth century and Crooke three centuries later, put forward seemingly deterministic views in suggesting that anger was highly dependent on the individual's physiological make-up: while hot-blooded, spirited men might experience wrath, colder individuals (like women, the elderly or the sick) would experience a less intense form of anger. More generally, however, the regimens of health stressed the role of the will as they urged people to moderate their anger. The medieval and early modern medical authors who discussed anger tended to see it in Aristotelian terms as involving a physiological response to an evaluative representation (impressed in spirit) of a perceived, remembered or anticipated object or situation. In their view, anger was neither caused by choleric humour, nor by the objects or situations themselves, but by the particular ways an individual evaluated them, which in turn were dependent on prior experience and physiological disposition.

The importance pre-modern medical authors attached to physiological disposition in the experience of anger, fear, sadness and joy makes it difficult to conceptualize such states as readily identifiable categories. It does suggest, however, that they should be thought of as both cognitive and physiological states. Even though the pre-modern explanations in terms of the Galenic theory of spirits (acting as material instruments of the soul in its mental operations) are no longer valid, modern neuroscientists continue to emphasize the material basis of the mind-body connection by looking for visible signs of brain activity, trying to establish neural correlates of cognitive and affective function. Nonetheless, one area in which modern scientific research is still lagging behind is the study of the differing impact of emotions on people's health. There are few modern scientific answers to the question posed by Damasio in 1994 of why excessive emotion seems to be damaging to health only in some circumstances. This contrasts with the repeated warnings found in medieval and early modern medical texts about the dangers of excessive anger, fear, sadness or worrying in situations such as epidemics and conditions such as pregnancy.

Medieval and early modern regimens of health and plague tracts stressed the importance of maintaining a balanced proportion of heat and moisture in the body through a balanced lifestyle. Rather than seeing the passions as "forces of nature" (to use Paster's phrase) to which people were subject, they promoted the idea that individuals had some agency in moderating their passions, and that this was achievable with the help of other people (think, for instance, of the 'social interaction' shown in Figure 7). One way of doing this was by actively seeking to counter one passion with another. As we have seen, plague tracts such as that of Licenciado Fores in the late fifteenth century or that of Thomas Lodge in the seventeenth suggested that the best way to counteract or prevent unhealthful movements of spirit such as anger, fear or sadness was through the 'honest' joy and pleasure produced by music and by telling pleasant stories (i.e., usually social activities), which had the beneficial effect of maintaining the body's moderate warmth and moisture. In contrast with modern experimental research into the impact of depression or anxiety on health, which tends to isolate one particular mood state as a variable condition, the pre-modern regimens tended to see anger, fear, sadness and joy as events interacting with (and counteracting) one another in their longer-term effects on bodily and mental health.

Seeing anger as a cognitive-physiological event which stimulated the production and movement of heat within the body in preparation for action allowed pre-modern medical authors to suggest ways in which it could be managed according to the Hippocratic-Galenic principle of *contraria contrariis curantur*. This principle informed the medical practice of influential thirteenth-century physicians like Alderotti (who adapted his advice on the 'accidents of the soul' to the particular conditions of the patients he discussed in his *Consilia*), and was still propounded in the Salernitan regimens of health published in the mid-seventeenth century. Even though prolonged anger was generally considered to have deleterious effects on health, it was thought that the non-natural (non-organic) heat of anger could be therapeutic in helping to counteract natural factors such as cold temperament or in restoring to balance the contra-natural cold produced by infirmity (e.g., 'weak nerves') or by poisoning. In the wider context of preventive medicine, anger and joy were also believed to counteract the effects of other 'non-natural' factors of disease, such as a cooling diet, insufficient food intake, or lack of exercise. Thus, to prevent the putrefaction allegedly caused by the accumulation of moisture produced by a sedentary lifestyle, some authors, like Álvarez in his 1501 plague tract, recommended the cultivation of joy, while others, like Paré in 1564, suggested that anger could be useful. Bullein, writing in 1562, noted that anger (one of the sixth non-naturals) could counteract the cold produced in the body by the weather (the first non-natural) or by sedentariness (the third non-natural).

At a time when psychologists cannot agree on whether the 'emotions' are primarily biological or cognitive events, it is best to move away from dualist paradigms (and from trying to establish unidirectional causative links between mind and body) by considering the wider patterns of a person's diet, lifestyle and environment. Looking back at approaches from the distant past, we see a multiplicity of co-existing ways of conceptualizing anger as an event. The late-fourteenth-century illumination of *ira* in the *Theatrum sanitatis* presents extreme anger within a framework of social interaction which might help to moderate it: philosophical advice. In the late seventeenth century, Le Brun sought to capture the experience of anger visually by focusing on its facial expressions, and explained these as the visible signs of the movements of invisible material spirit between the brain, the heart and the surface of the body. While medical authors might have interpreted the label 'anger' (or related pre-modern terms like *ira, cholère, tzorn, yra* or *saña*) as referring to sadness mixed with pleasure, as the desire for revenge, as a sign of courage, or as evidence of excessive heat or choleric humour in the body, their contemporaries would have used the same words with meanings more directly related to the particular social interactions in which their experiences of anger were embedded, perhaps focusing more on whether the expression of their anger was beneficial in achieving their shorter-term goals than on the longer-term impact it might have on their health.

Finally, given the recent proliferation of cognitive therapies and cognitive behavioural therapies which place the emphasis on changing or eradicating emotions through cognitive readjustments, it seems increasingly relevant to consider the Aristotelian view (taken by influential medieval Galenists like Villanova and Renaissance humanists like Elyot) that anger can be compatible with reason. In recognizing that there are many forms of anger, we can see beyond the existing ways of conceptualizing it as caused by temperament (or, in modern terms, by enduring personality traits), by humoral (or hormonal) imbalances, or by the 'forces of nature' (Paster's phrase for the pre-modern passions, still applicable to some modern biological arguments). We can also question the Stoic and Neostoic views of anger as a disease of the soul, and think of the more productive ways in which individuals, in their specific circumstances and their particular physiological states, can judge whether it is beneficial, feasible or reasonable to suppress, to moderate or to redirect the heat of anger.

NON-NATURAL LOVE: COITUS, DESIRE AND HYGIENE IN MEDIEVAL AND EARLY MODERN SPAIN

Michael R. Solomon

Lurking in the shadows of every western manifestation of heterosexual love is the prospect of penetrating bodily members and the exchange of fluids known as coitus. Be it expressed forthrightly such as William IX of Aquitaine who bluntly exhorts us to hear how many times he "fucked" two courtly ladies—a hundred and eighty-eight times—or shrouded in deep melancholy and intense yearning for a faraway love (*amor de lonh*), as Jaufre Rudel would have it, coitus appears to be the destination of, or at least a frequent or tempting rest stop on the road to fulfilling, amorous desire.[1] Medical writers in the late middle ages acknowledged the need for patients to regulate coitus and amorous affect as a means of keeping the body healthy. But working within the Galenic non-natural paradigm, these writers treated coitus and love as distinct phenomena with separate hygienic imperatives. In vernacular medical treatises designed to instruct lay people on how to keep healthy by controlling their diet, daily activities, environment, and emotions, they categorized coitus among the non-natural category of evacuation that required the regular expulsion of superfluous bodily matter through bowel movements, bathing, and sexual intercourse. Love, however, fell into the movements of soul or the emotions, and was grouped with other affective conditions such as sadness, worry, and anger. This essay explores the representation of love and coitus in the vernacular medical writing from late medieval and early modern Spain and points to the way nonprofessionals exploited, conflated, or ignored conflicting hygienic imperatives that emerged from medical works on love and coitus.

Starting in the early fourteenth century and gaining momentum in the fifteenth and sixteenth centuries, the Iberian Peninsula experienced an explosion of concise and simplified vernacular medical treatises. Spanish physicians and medical theorists attempted to disseminate information

---

[1] For examples see William's song "Farai un vers pos mi sonelh" and and Jaufre Rudel's poem "Lanquan li jorn son lonc en may" in Frede Jensen, *Troubadour Lyrics: a Bilingual Anthology* (New York: P. Lang, 1998), 70, 122.

on health and hygiene in ways that could be readily understood by non-professionals.[2] Typical is court physician Alfonso Chirino's popular *Menor daño de la medicina (Least Damage from Medicine).* Printed twenty-five times in the sixteenth century, Chirino's work tells readers explicitly that "everything you find written herein will not be in medical jargon or obscure words; rather I will speak in a way that anybody can understand."[3] The author then proceeds to promise that he includes only the useful information that can be readily used by a non-specialized public. Throughout the sixteenth century, writers of vernacular medical treatises presented their works as highly useful artifacts in which medical information was reorganized, indexed, and reduced to provide only the most effective and proven hygienic and therapeutic imperatives. These works—cast as plague tracts and *regimina santitatis* or as vernacular translations of works on surgery, pharmacology, anatomy, and pathology encouraged readers to believe that information bound in manuscripts or books could provide remedies, relief, and some sense of control over the bewildering conditions of their bodies.

For many medieval and sixteenth-century physicians, the vernacular dissemination of medical information to the general public could be dangerous, encouraging lay people to make a diagnosis or embrace a cure based on limited knowledge.[4] The "New Galenism" that emerged from the medical school in Montpellier in the late thirteenth century and quickly spread to Spain posited a radical individualism in which the ailments of each patient had to be considered in relation to many internal and exogenous factors.[5] As the fourteenth-century Galenist Juan de Aviñón pointed out in his gloss on Hippocrates' first aphorism, "this art is long ... because it

[2] See my *Fictions of Well-Being: Sickly Readers and Vernacular Medical Writing in Late Medieval and Early Modern Spain* (Philadelphia: University of Pennsylvania Press, 2010) for a complete overview of the rhetorical strategies used in vernacular medical writing to convince readers that these works would be easy to use and useful in helping them preserve their health.

[3] "Todo lo que aquj fallardes escripto non será por vocablos de medeçina nin por palabras escuras salvo fablando vulgarmente que qualquier omne puede entender." Chirino, *Menor daño de la medicina*, Escorial MS b.IV.34, fol. 3r.

[4] Solomon, *Fictions*, 22.

[5] For an overview of " 'New Galenism' or 'Medieval Galenism' and its dissemination in Spain see Luis García-Ballester, *Galen and Galenism: Theory and Medical Practice from Antiquity to the European Renaissance* (Aldershot: Ashgate, 2002); "Arnau de Vilanova (c. 1240–1311) y la reforma de los estudios médicos en Montpellier (1309): el Hipócrates latino y la introducción del nuevo Galeno," *Dynamis* 2 (1982): 97–158.

is divided into seven parts, and each part requires a long time to acquire."[6] Medical training was complicated and time-consuming, a process that no patient could be expected to acquire without many years of training and least of all while in the throes of illness.

As a compromise, medical writers established a distinction between therapeutics ("a regimen of cure"), which should fall into the hands of a trained physician, and hygiene ("a regimen of preservation"), which helped patients organize their daily activities so as to maintain a state of well-being and avoid the onset of disease.[7] The works that best served a hygienic reader were *regimina sanitatis* (health guides) and plague treatises, each based on the Galenic non-natural paradigm and each designed to instruct lay people on how to stay healthy by controlling their diet, daily activities, environment, and emotions. Non-natural hygiene required individuals to control six exogenous phenomena: air and environment, food and drink, motion and rest, sleep and vigilance, the excretion of superfluous matter, and control of the emotions.[8] Each of these categories focused on one type of hygiene, and writers offered health guidelines or regimens specific to each non-natural. In an ideal setting, a competent physician using a process of testing through trial and error could help a patient determine how much of each of these substances and activities the patient needed to preserve his or her health, but when physicians were not available, medical writers assured their readers that the more

[6] "Ypocras que dijo, la vida es breve: el arte es luenga, el juicio grave, el tiempo angosto, y la prueba dudosa. E la razón porque esta arte es muy luenga, según dijo Boecio, es por razón que ella es departida en siete partes y en cada parte ha menester luengo tiempo para alcanzarla" (Hippocrates said that life is short, art is long, judgment grave, time brief, and proof doubtful. The reason that this art [the art of medicine] is long, according to Boethius, is because it is divided into seven parts, and each part requires a long time to acquire). *Sevillana medicina*, 5r. See Solomon, *Fictions* 21.

[7] Jacme d'Agramont, for example, argued at the beginning of his treatise on the plague: "E de regiment de preservació pot tot hom usar ab aquest present tractat sens de metge, sens tot periyll. Mas lo regiment de curació és apropriat al metge en lo qual cascú sens de la art de medicina porie leugerament errar"(Any man can use this treatise with confidence as a regimen for preserving his health, without the aid of a physician. But the regimen for curing is reserved for the physician, because anyone who does not know the art of medicine could easily err). *Regiment de preservació a epidèmia o pestilència e mortaldats*, ed. Enrich Ardeiu and Joseph M. Roca (Biblioteca Virtual Joan Lluís Vives, 2000): http://www.lluisvives.com/servlet/SirveObras/jlv/12920522027817162321435/index.htm. See also Solomon, *Fictions*, 22.

[8] For an overview of the concept and the development of the non-naturals see García-Ballester, "On the Origin of the 'Six Non-Natural Things' in Galen," in *Galen und das hellenistische Erbe*, ed. Jutta Kollesch and Diethard Nickel (Stuttgart: Steiner, 1993), 105–15.

general concepts found in vernacular medical works built on the non-naturals could serve them well.

As I mentioned above, coitus fell into the category of excretion of superfluous matter, along with bathing and bowel movements. Love, however was a completely different hygienic concern and pertained to the more elusive category of movements of the soul, phenomena that we traditionally associate with the emotions. I will examine each of these in their non-natural context followed by a discussion of the way these distinct hygienic imperatives converged in popular thinking about amorous desire.

Coitus

By and large, vernacular medical writers treated coital hygiene as a necessary excretion or expulsion that allowed men and women, according to their temperaments and other factors, to rid themselves of excess semen as a preventive measure against illnesses related to the retention of seminal fluids.[9] Although writers often included caveats and provisions for men with religious obligations, they generally spoke about coitus, candidly in a manner similar to their treatment of diet, bathing, exercise, sleep, and bowel movements. Discussions on coitus generally began by comparing the benefits and dangers of insufficient or excessive coition.

On the positive side, writers offer a long list of health-preserving benefits including the way coitus in moderation lightens the body, pacifies anger, eliminates disturbing thoughts, lifts men's spirits, cures kidney pain, sharpens vision, and cures all types of gout; in women, it reduces the possibility of developing suffocation of the womb. Coitus helps men avoid the retention of seminal fluids that can turn to poison in the body and cause sudden and unexpected death. According to some authors, excess semen left in the body leads to fevers or dangerous heat in the genitalia that can spread to the heart and brain causing terrible afflictions.[10] Physicians warn that sudden deprivation of coitus for those accustomed to it leads to

[9] For a more extensive overview of medieval treatises on coitus, see Danielle Jacquart and Claude Alexandre Thomasset, *Sexuality and Medicine in the Middle Ages* (Princeton, N.J.: Princeton University Press, 1988), 116–38.

[10] "la tal superfluydad detenida se escalentara mucho dentro en sus vasos, y se causara fiebre o calentura, porque los miembros genitales y sus cercanos se encenderan o excalentaran continuamente hasta que el calor allegue al coraçon, y algunas vezes el vapor de la tal superfluydad, sube hasta el celebro adonde engendra muy malas enfermedades." Francisco Núñez de Coria, *Tratado del uso de las mujeres* (Madrid: Pierres Cusin, 1572), 289r–320r, at 292r.

headaches, loss of sight and appetite, and to mental incapacity; excessive seminal vapors in the brain can cause melancholia, madness, involuntary trembling, and scotoma (loss of vision). We frequently find anecdotes from antiquity describing men who copulated regularly and then stopped only to start suffering from many of the ailments listed above.

If insufficient coitus threatens well-being, excessive or immoderate coition also has it dangers. Vernacular medical writers warn that this leads to fatigue, memory loss, a weakening of the five senses, the development of coughs, bad breath, appetite loss, indigestion, deteriorating of the heart and liver, the onset of dropsy, kidney stones, gout, all types of fevers, sores on the penis, hernias, shortness of breath and sudden death. The hygienic imperative that emerges from these vernacular discussions is for patients to engage in thoughtful deliberation, preferably in consultation with their physician, on the proper amount of—and best times for—the expelling of excess semen.

When translating the Latin *coitus* into Spanish or Catalan, medical authors employ a variety of words or expressions including a direct translation (*coyto* or *coito*) or "venereal act" (*acto venéreo*) and more euphemistic renderings such as "laying with women" (*jaer ab mujer*) and "conversing," or "communicating with women" or "venereal coupling" (*conversación con mugers, comunicación con mugeres, ayuntamiento venéreo*), venereal affairs (*negocios venéreos*), and venereal use (*uso venéreo*). Francisco Nuñez de Coria translates coitus broadly as "the use of women," as seen in the title of his treatise, *El tractado del uso de las mugeres*.

Announcing that he will write in a way that all men can understand, avoiding medical jargon, the author of the fifteenth century *Speculum al foderi* attempted to translate the term as *foder* (Lat. *futuere*). In the mind of the author and in spite of its crude connotations—very close to the modern English "fuck"—"foder" offered the most forthright way to express the highly corporeal act of bodies entwined in sexual intercourse. Curiously, in all these attempts to render an understandable translation for the term coitus, none of the authors I have examined use the term love (*amor*) or any variation thereof to describe the act of sexual intercourse and we find no expressions that approach the more modern euphemism "to make love." For the most part, authors who describe the hygienic implications of coitus are completely indifferent to questions of amorous affect or emotion and to the possible relation between being in love and moderating the body through sexual intercourse.

If coitus is necessary on occasion, or even with certain regularity to stay healthy—as vernacular medical writers insist—how do men and women go about complying with this hygienic imperative when no willing or convenient sexual partner is available? For the most part medical writers are silent on this matter. In fact, there is a general tendency to suppose that coition is as casual and uncomplicated as having a bowel movement. Given that the salutary objective is the expulsion or retention of semen, we might assume that masturbation would offer a convenient method of regulating bodily fluids; yet, there are almost no references whatsoever to this alternative form of treatment. Rather some writers offer men who need to avoid coitus for religious or ascetic reasons a series of dietary regimens designed to moderate or eliminate the production of semen in the body. But these remedies seem to be tenuous at best, and most writers appear eager to list the health-producing benefits that moderate coitus will produce. Still, although the underlying assumption is that coitus will take place in a heterosexual context, there is little discussion in vernacular medical treatises on the relation between the hygienic subject and his or her partner. One notable exception is the previously mentioned short treatise known as *Speculum al foderi* or "The Mirror for Fuckers," as some modern historians have suggested the work should be translated.[11]

Written in the kingdom of Aragon probably during the early fifteenth century, the *Speculum al foderi* is by and large a Catalan translation of the Latin *Liber minor de coitu*.[12] Perhaps the most remarkable aspect of this translation, in addition to the expressed desire to make information on coitus available to all men (*tot hom*), is the insertion of three chapters, most likely from Arabic sources, that address the question of securing a willing partner for the presumed health-preserving benefits of coitus. These chapters attempt to teach men how to seduce a sexual partner and how to stimulate and prepare women for sexual intercourse, and offer a description of twenty-six coital positions. Part *ars amandi* and part *Kama Sutra*, these inserted chapters offer a remarkable departure from Latin

---

[11] Jacquart and Thomasset, *Sexuality and Medicine*, 135.

[12] See Enrique Montero Cartelle, "Sobre el origen árabe del *Speculum al foderi* catalán y su relación con el *Liber minor de coito* salernitano," *Anuari de Filologia* 14 (1991): 71–80. There have been several modern attempts to edit the *Speculum al foderi*; the most recent and most reliable to date is *Speculum al foder*, ed. Ana Alberni (Bellcaire d'Empordà: Vitel·la, 2007). See also *Speculum al joder: tratado de recetas y consejos sobre el coito*, ed. and trans. Teresa Vicens (Barcelona: Hesperus, 1978); *The Mirror of Coitus: A Translation and Edition of the Fifteenth-Century* Speculum al foderi (Madison, Wis.: Hispanic Seminary of Medieval Studies, 1990); Pere Vallribera Puig, *Literatura médica medieval catalana. "Speculum al foderi." Transcripció i estudis medics d'un text del segle xv sobre sexología* (Barcelona: Universidad de Barcelona, 1993); *El kamasutra català: mirall del fotre, anónim del segle XIV*, ed. Patrick Gifreu (Barcelona: Columna, 1996), a modernized Catalan edition.

and vernacular treatises on hygienic intercourse. Of particular interest is chapter eight, which treats the "the manners and customs of women." Here, unlike most vernacular writing on the non-naturals, the author links coital hygiene to amorous desire and provides observations and strategies for obtaining a sexual partner, including making use of a go-between. The author describes the type of men whom women find desirable and lists the bodily and facial gestures that indicate a woman's amorous interest. He describes in detail the way women fall in love and advises men who would seek the love of women (*amor de les fembres*) to recognize that women experience great desire and take great pleasure in coitus; even the most noble, gallant, and wealthy man, we are told, will fail to win a woman's love if he does not acknowledge this.

By conflating coitus, desire and love in a hygienic context, the *Speculum al foderi* created an innovative departure from previous treatments of the non-naturals. This work, however, was an anomaly, and future vernacular treatments of coitus failed to develop or even include discussions on desire and love. Rather, throughout the sixteenth century we see a movement towards a more cautious approach to hygienic coition, with greater concern over dangers or negative effects of intercourse. In his plague treatise *Preservative and Curative Remedies in Times of Pestilence* (1597) Miguel Martínez de Leiva, for example, briefly acknowledges that coitus has some health-preserving properties, but spends several pages denouncing the ills of excessive coitus. He reminds readers of the longstanding idea that excessive and habitual coitus expends life itself and he offers the example of how plants and flowers that have lost their seeds immediately begin to wither and die.[13] There is a decidedly moral tone to these arguments, and medical authorities such as Galen and Avicenna are exploited to remind readers that the venal act debilitates the heart, brain, and stomach and makes men more receptive to pestilent fevers. As increasingly is the case, Martínez ends his treatment on evacuation by coitus by offering alternative suggestions for avoiding or eliminating superfluous bodily matter, such as regular bowel movements, moderation in eating and drinking and pharmaceutical remedies. Other writers, such as Andrés Laguna, simply warn men to avoid coitus altogether; he suggests that there are much

[13] "Y que este vicio carnal consuma la vida, veese por exemplo de la plantas, como dezia un Filosofo, que quando echan de si su siemente se consumen y secan." Miguel Martínez de Leiva, *Remedios preservativos y curativos para el tiempo de la peste* (Madrid, 1597), 106.

better alternatives for reducing seminal fluids than yielding to what he calls the "dirty and abominable" practice of coitus.[14]

Amor

As a hygienic concern, love (*amor*) appears in the category of the six non-naturals dedicated to movements or accidents of the soul. In his *Sevillana medicina*, Aviñón identifies these as follows:

> It is necessary that men who want to preserve their health do not become angry, full of rage, or worried if they can avoid these [emotions] as they will learn that they cause great harm to the body. Therefore, men should be tempered in all the movements of the soul such as rage, fear, love, disaffection, pity, cruelty, generosity, avarice, wisdom, ignorance, and in cunning, cowardliness, pleasure, and sadness.[15]

The term "movements of the soul" corresponds awkwardly with the modern notion of emotions. While there is little trouble identifying rage, fear, and sadness as emotional states, other medieval movements of the soul such as pity, generosity, avarice, and cunning would seem to be better categorized as moral virtues or defects, rather than straightforward emotions. Clearly, if we are to think of the sixth non-natural as a hygienic regulation of emotive states, we must do so by accepting the most capacious definition possible of the term "emotion."

Movements of the soul were perhaps the most complicated of the non-naturals from a physiological standpoint, requiring a rather extensive explanation of the way pneuma or spirits (air) and organs such as the heart affect the various ventricles of the brain.[16] Of all the non-naturals these are most closely linked with or at least marked by strong pathological implications.

---

[14] "Nosotros no debemos tener en tanto, que nos haga imitarle en un caso tan suzio e abominable, mayormente pudiendo por otros medios mas licitos librarnos de aquel insolente humor." Andrés de Laguna, *Discurso breve sobre la cura y preservación de la pestilencia* (Salamanca, 1566), 28r–29r.

[15] "Es menester que se guarde el ome que quiere conseruar su salud que non tome saña ni enojo ni cuydado en quanto pudiere despues quel ome vee que faze tan gran daño en el cuerpo. Y por ende debe ser el ome templado a todos movimientos animales: assí como saña & miedo y amor y desamor y piedad y crueldad y largueza y avaricia y saber y non trassaber. Y en ardidez y en cobardía o en plazer o en tristeza." *Sevillana medicina*, 123v.

[16] For a complete overview of the sixth non-natural and the underlining physiology, see Pedro Gil-Sotres, "La higiene de las emociones," in Arnaldus Villanova, *Regimen sanitatis ad regem Aragonum*, ed. Luis García-Ballester and Michael McVaugh (Barcelona: Edicions Universitat Barcelona, 1996), 803–27.

In fact, there is a tendency among some authors to call these "passions or accidents of the soul," stressing their status as diseases. As pathologically oriented, often demanding therapeutic or curative intervention, the sixth non-natural does not lend itself to extensive hygienic imperatives. Although patients were told to avoid violent emotions such as rage or extreme anger, the primary exhortation regarding the sixth non-natural was simply to moderate affects and emotions such as sadness, love, fear, and joy, and to control the propensity to be generous, feel pity, or seek pleasure. Thus, in vernacular medical treatises on the non-naturals, the movements of the soul are given a highly cursory overview. When writers provide more elaborate discussions, they tend to focus almost entirely on one of two emotions, most commonly happiness (*alegria*) and sadness (*tristeza*). Alfonso Chirino, for example, begins his section on the "passions of the soul" by warning men that the lack of happiness or heartfelt joy is one of the greatest impediments to enjoying good health.[17] He continues to warn against the ill effects of anger, envy, and avarice on the body, but he fails to include any discussion on love or amorous affection. This is very common. Although love properly fits into the category of the sixth non-natural, there are very few vernacular medical works that treat this emotion at any length or even list it among the passions or movements of the soul. This is not to say that physicians ignored the biomedical implications of love; rather they discussed amorous affect most frequently as a disease or ailment rather than a hygienic concern.

Well known are the extensive medieval and early modern treatments of lovesickness, which physicians usually identified as *amor hereos* or heroic love. In vernacular medical writing from Spain we find discussions on excessive love with its corresponding summary of symptoms, diagnostic techniques, and cure in treatises on pathology such as the fifteenth-century Spanish translation of Ibn al-Khatib's *Tratado de patología* (15v) or the Spanish translation of Bernard of Gordon's *Lilio de medicina*.[18] Love in these treatises is defined as an excess and an obsession, caused by the visual fascination with the image or figure of the beloved that leads to obsessive fixation on the pleasure that the patient believes there is to find in the

[17] "De las cosas que guardan la salut y fortefican las potençias naturales para que fagan conplidamente sus naturales obras en el cuerpo humanal es el alegria o gozo del coraçon o la verdadera paçiençia en estas cosas: terrestes quando non andan a nuestra voluntat." *Menor daño de la medicina*, 29r.

[18] *Lilio de medicina*, 60r–61r. See Ibn al-Khatib, *Tratado de patología general*, ms 10.051, Biblioteca Nacional, Madrid, 15v; see also the Spanish translation of Bernard of Gordon's *Lilium medicinae: Lilio de medicina*, ms I-315, Biblioteca Nacional, Madrid, 60r–61r.

object of his desire. The condition, often linked to melancholy, leaves the patient depressed, despondent, and listless, often lost in deep penetrating thoughts that lead to madness and ultimately death if not cured. Treatment is generally a process of distracting so as to break this obsessive fixation on the beloved. For mild cases physicians recommend that the patient be taken on a trip, surrounded by good friends, and encouraged to see other women. When the condition is more severe, the patient should be given a good beating and subjected to abject demonstrations in which an old woman denigrates the beloved, often comparing her to excrement and even showing her menses-soaked rags. In the treatment of pathological love, medical writers offer little prophylactic or hygienic advice for avoiding the disease. The fifteenth-century physician Francisco López de Villalobos simply suggests that the stricken man flee from the beloved "like the way men flee from harmful air in times of pestilence."[19]

Couched in general works on pathology or in specific treatises such as Arnau de Villanova's Latin *Tractatus de amore heroico*, medical writers treated love as an ailment or disease rather than an emotion that could be moderated as part of a hygienic regimen.[20] Although there are many treatises that prescribe coitus as a possible cure for lovesickness, medical writers do not recommend amorous affection as part of successful hygienic coitus, with the exception of the previously mentioned *Speculum al foderi*. It is clear that physicians were concerned with the disease of love, as manifested in Constantine the African's gloss on the *Viaticum*, Arnau de Villanova's *Tractatus de amore heroico* and Jacques Ferrand's *Traité de l'essence et guérison de l'amour (Treatise on Lovesickness)*, but these concerns almost never appear in *regimina sanitatis* and plague treatises that were organized according to non-natural hygiene.[21] Advice related to love in vernacular medical treatises is very seldom hygienic and almost always points to the idea that love is a disease that must be cured by a physician rather than managed by the patient. Simply stated, the concept of

[19] "aparten con gran diligencia/ d'aquella señora como en pestilencia/ se apartan los hombres del ayre dañado." Francisco López de Villalobos, *Sumario de la medicina con un tratado sobre las pestíferas bubas* (Salamanca: Antonio Nebrija, 1498), 4r.

[20] See *Tractatus de amore heroico; Epistola de dosi tyriacalium medicinarum*, in *Arnaldi de Villanova Opera medica omnia*, III (Barcelona: Edicions Universitat de Barcelona, 1985).

[21] See Jacques Ferrand, Donald A. Beecher, and Massimo Ciavolella, *A Treatise on Lovesickness* (Syracuse University Press, 1994). For an overview of the history and the development of lovesickness, see Mary Frances Wack, *Lovesickness in the Middle Ages: the Viaticum and its Commentaries* (Philadelphia: University of Pennsylvania Press, 1990).

non-natural love does not emerge in the medical guides designed to help lay people preserve their health.

Disease and Desire

Late medieval non-natural hygiene, while offering patients basic guidelines on controlling their consumption of food and drink, and on the proper amount of rest, exercise, sleep, waking, bathing and bowel movement, failed to provide any advice on managing the emotion of love. Rather, there is evidence suggesting that the imperatives related to coitus and the treatment of love as a non-hygienic pathological condition created new vehicles for fulfilling amorous desire. The dissemination of vernacular medical treatises offered laymen new ways to "disease" themselves. As I have argued elsewhere, the ability to identify an individual—or to declare oneself—as being diseased not only gave meaning to bodily phenomena, including the itch of sexual desire and the fascination with the figure of the beloved, but it also conferred certain rights and privileges (and, conversely limitations) on those identified as suffering from a particular ailment.[22]

To cast one's desires as a disease or as a concern requiring hygienic intervention allowed patients to manipulate medical knowledge gleaned from vernacular sources in ways that would allow them to fulfill amorous longings and sexual impulses. For example, the fourteenth-century *Libro de buen amor* was written by Juan Ruiz, Archipreste de Hita, from the point of view of a lecherous clergyman, who tells readers that he, like all men, has experienced the great love of women and that this practice of "trying out women" is justified on the grounds that "testing" is valuable because it allows him to determine what is best for him. Here the Arcipreste makes a tongue-in-cheek allusion to a basic Galenic procedure for determining the correct amount of non-natural substances and practices (including coitus) that a patient needs to stay healthy. He is suggesting that the trial and error involved in testing and determining the right type and amount of food that a patient needs applies likewise to ascertaining the type and amount of sexual intercourse that is needed for him to

[22] See my discussion on the "power to disease," in "Women, the power to disease, and the fictions of the Counter-Clinic," in *The Literature of Misogyny in Medieval Spain: the "Arcipreste de Talavera" and the "Spill"* (Cambridge: Cambridge University Press, 1997), 149–79.

remain healthy according to the hygienic guidelines related to non-natural coitus.[23] Later, at the end of the fifteenth century, Calixto, a young upper-class man in Fernando de Rojas' work *Tragicomedia de Celestina and Melibea* becomes lust-stricken when by chance he meets Melibea, a beautiful young woman. He immediately pathologizes his desires and begins to feign the symptoms of lovesickness. But when he realizes that the cure his servants offer for treating this disease will not lead to the quick sexual act he desires, he encourages them to treat him according to the hygienic need to regularly expel excess semen as a health-preserving necessity.[24]

In the popular and literary mind, concepts of hygienic coitus and pathological love became conflated and confused. Among the morass of beliefs, counsels, perceptions, seductive ruses, and plaintive sighs that have come to dominate the western expression of love from Ovid to Andreas Capellanus to Petrarch and beyond, medical knowledge disseminated in the vernacular only continued to complicate the ideas surrounding amorous affection. If literature does indeed represent the sexual practices and attitudes of late medieval and early modern Spaniards, we can see how individuals harnessed selective hygienic and therapeutic principles as a way to fulfill desire. Thus when we read the familiar complaints of a courtly lady, for example, who beckons her lover to come to her bedside to cure her of an ailment—as we often find in late medieval courtly literature—we should remember that this suffering might not be merely emotional or based on some other bodily malady; rather we should acknowledge that she might be couching her desire to see her beloved in an allusion to superfluous seminal fluids that have suffocated her womb. The only cure according to treatises such as the *Speculum al foderi* and other works on non-natural coitus is sexual intercourse, thus allowing desire, disease, and coital hygiene to coalesce in the pleasure of the amorous embrace.

---

23 Following a discussion explaining that men live, according to Aristotle, to copulate and consume food, the Arcipreste tells: "E yo, como só omne como otro, pecador,/ ove de las mugeres a vezes grand amor;/ provar omne las cosas non es por ende peor,/ e saber bien e mal, e usar lo mejor." *Libro de buen amor*, strophe 76.

24 See my article "Calisto's Ailment: Bitextual Diagnostics and Parody in Celestina," *Revista de Estudios Hispánicos* 23:1 (1989): 41–64.

A DISEASE UNTO DEATH: SADNESS IN THE TIME OF SHAKESPEARE*

Erin Sullivan

There are many factors that make William Shakespeare's *Antony and Cleopatra* (c. 1606) a difficult play to stage. There's the fact that it contains close to double the typical number of scenes found in Shakespeare's other plays, the fact that the action takes place on two different continents with more or less two discreet casts of characters, the fact that Cleopatra has to hoist up the dying Antony with a rope from a lower level to her placement in her monument, the fact that woven throughout the tragedy and pathos of this play are unexpectedly comic lines ("How heavy weighs my lord!," Cleopatra remarks as she pulls her dying lover up (4.16.33)).[1] As if these issues weren't challenging enough, there is also the fact that one of the play's central characters, a follower of Antony named Enobarbus, has an onstage death scene in which he dies of a grief-stricken, broken heart. Having betrayed Antony to his enemy Octavius Caesar, Enobarbus swiftly regrets this decision and falls into a debilitating slump towards death, which he narrates to the audience: "Throw my heart/ Against the flint and hardness of my fault," he laments, "Which, being dried with grief, will break to powder,/ And finish all foul thoughts" (4.10.14–17). Just five lines later, Enobarbus does in fact die, with no other cause being indicated than the sadness he feels for his unfaithfulness to his leader and friend.

For modern audiences, this can be a strange moment to take in; like the death of Mr Krook from spontaneous human combustion in Charles Dickens's *Bleak House* (1852), the death of a relatively young, strapping soldier from excessive sadness does not fit with the model of human physiology many of us have come to expect. Unlike Dickens, however, who after the

* Many thanks are due to Andrew Wear and Elena Carrera, both of whom read early drafts of this chapter and improved it significantly with their observant and insightful comments. Thanks also to the students and staff at the Shakespeare Institute, who through friendly conversation helped add to my tally of characters in Renaissance drama that suffer from deadly grief, and also to the Wellcome Trust, which generously funded the period of study in which the bulk of this research took place.

[1] All references to Shakespeare's plays are to *The Complete Works*, ed. Stanley Wells, Gary Taylor, John Jowett, and William Montgomery, 2nd edn (Oxford: Oxford University Press, 2005). Dating of the plays also follows this edition.

publication of this episode wrote in vigorous defence of the possibility of spontaneous combustion, which many of his readers doubted, Shakespeare did not need to launch a justification for the manner in which Enobarbus died.[2] Although deaths from overwhelming sorrow were not considered commonplace in Shakespeare's England, neither were they thought impossible or fantastical. As this chapter will show, many different people in sixteenth and early seventeenth-century England understood all excessive emotion (or passion, as it was then known) to be physiologically dangerous, but none so much as sadness, which not only damaged the body but was also known to kill. This belief was firmly entrenched in the learned medical teachings of the time and its acceptance among a wider audience can be seen in medico-philosophical treatises, mortality records, and popular dramas from the period. Such evidence illustrates how strong mind-body sympathy was perceived to be within the Galenic humoral system dominant in Shakespeare's time, and accordingly how important it was to moderate sorrowful passions before detrimental physiological changes could take hold. Treatment for such passionate 'dis-ease' covered a broad range of therapies, but most important, we will see, was the expression and genuine communication of sadness from the sufferer to a sympathetic listener, who not only offered thoughtful advice but also a willingness to share in the sufferer's sorrows and by doing so help dissipate them.

The Vocabulary of Sadness

As recent scholarship on emotions and passions has shown, there is no simple answer as to what an 'emotion' or 'passion' is, much less what a particular passion such as sadness might be. Although today sadness is regularly categorized as one of the 'basic' emotions, suggesting that it is common among humans regardless of culture, considerable research from anthropology and cultural psychology complicates any simple assertion of essential or universal emotion categories.[3] In early modern England,

---

[2] For the Krook episode, see chapter 32, "The Appointed Time," in Charles Dickens, *Bleak House* (Oxford: Oxford University Press, 1966), 443–56, as well as Daniel Hack, "'Sublimation Strange': Allegory and Authority in *Bleak House*," *ELH* 66:1 (1999): 132–34.

[3] Paul Ekman's work on facial expression and emotion across culture has been highly influential in making the case for basic or core emotions; for a review of his work and other studies in this field see Ekman, "Cross-Cultural Studies of Facial Expression," in *Dar-*

passionate states described as 'sadness' could involve a range of different influencing factors and associations, and what it meant to be sad could vary significantly depending on whether writers were drawing on medical, moral, or religious contexts to frame the experience of passion (or some combination of the three).[4] For the purposes of this chapter I will be focusing specifically on medically oriented discussions of sadness, acknowledging of course that such discussions never divorced themselves altogether from moral or religious issues. The important distinction, however, is that such discussions framed the understanding of sadness centrally through the workings of the humoral body, as opposed to, for instance, the relationship between man and God in a postlapsarian world. Although such discussions often invoked God, they based their explanations of the aetiology and effects of sadness in a system of natural philosophy that stretched back to Hippocratic times.

It is important to note early on that while the word 'sadness' features frequently in sixteenth and seventeenth-century English writings on the passions, it is often used more or less interchangeably with a set of other words, most notably 'sorrow' and 'grief.' For modern readers this can seem strange, first and foremost because as scholars of emotions research we have become accustomed to taking a strongly nominalist approach to the study of emotional states, meaning that we understand the specific names of abstract concepts to play a major part in how they take on significance and meaning. Such an approach has become particularly prevalent in light of the influential findings of anthropologists and linguists, who have shown that many emotions words and concepts are not easily translated across languages and cultures.[5] The second reason is that, in modern

win and Facial Expression: A Century of Research in Review, ed. Paul Ekman (New York: Academic Press, 1972), 169–222. Key anthropological work, largely undertaken in the 1970s and 80s, sought to challenge this view; see for instance Catherine A. Lutz's helpful review article, Lutz and Geoffrey M. White, "The Anthropology of Emotions," *Annual Review of Anthropology* 15 (1986): 405–36. More recently work in cognitive linguistics and 'semantic metalanguage' has begun to suggest a middle way; see Anna Wierzbicka, *Emotions across Languages and Cultures* (Cambridge: Cambridge University Press, 1999).

[4] This complex cultural negotiation is the subject of my current project, available at present as Erin Sullivan, "Secret Contagions: Sadness and the Self in Early Modern England" (unpublished PhD thesis, University of London, 2010).

[5] See for instance Michelle Z. Rosaldo's work on the Ilongot people of the Philippines and the emotion *liget*, which has no clear translation in English; Rosaldo, *Knowledge and Passion: Ilongot Notions of Self and Social Life* (Cambridge: Cambridge University Press, 1980). Catherine A. Lutz's work offers similar evidence and conclusions; see Lutz, *Unnatural*

English parlance, the words 'sadness,' 'sorrow,' and especially 'grief' are often taken to have very distinct meanings, with 'grief' frequently being related to the experience of severe loss or bereavement.[6] In the early modern context the word 'grief' was certainly also used to describe bereavement—in Shakespeare's *King John* (c. 1596), for instance, Lady Constance describes how "Grief fills the room up of my absent child" (3.4.93) following the death of her son Arthur—but it also had a much broader field of meaning, signifying any form of pain, be it inward or outward. In the dictionary of Sir Thomas Elyot (c. 1490–1546), first published in 1538, we find grief equated with the Latin *dolor*, which Elyot defines as "griefe or paine of body or mynd, also sorowe," an entry illustrating the wide range of physiological and mental pains the word might describe. Such openness might in fact leave us wondering if the word 'grief' could signify anything more specific than a general sense of pain, but if we turn our attention to early modern definitions of *aegritudo* we begin to get an idea of its particular meaning within the context of the passions. In his entry for *aegritudo* Elyot offers the gloss, "grief of mynde, or sorow," a definition that is followed word for word by Richard Huloet in his 1552 dictionary, Thomas Cooper in his 1584 thesaurus, and Thomas Thomas in his 1587 dictionary.[7] The preacher Thomas Rogers (c. 1553–1616) again reiterates the semantic links between 'grief,' 'sorrow,' and *aegritudo* in his 1576 treatise on the passions, writing that "This Sorrowe, the *Stoikes* call griefe, and dolor, & they saye it is an unmeasurable contraction of the minde . . . In Latin it is called *Aegritudo*."[8] The word 'sadness' also appears alongside 'grief' and 'sorrow' in such writings, suggesting its acceptance as a near synonym: in Randall Cotgrave's 1611 *Dictionary of the French and English Tongues*, for instance, *doleur* is glossed as "Griefe, sorrow, anguish, woe, sadnesse."[9]

Such texts suggest that we cannot differentiate too strictly between terms like 'grief,' 'sorrow,' or 'sadness,' despite particular resonances they

---

Emotion: Everyday Sentiments on a Micronesian Atol and Their Challenge to Western Theory (Chicago: Chicago University Press, 1988).

[6] See for instance the work of Elizabeth Kübler-Ross, such as *On Grief and Grieving: Finding the Meaning of Grief through the Five Stages of Loss* (New York: Simon and Schuster, 2007).

[7] These dictionary quotations come from the results for 'grief' in the *Lexicons of Early Modern English* (*LEME*), ed. Ian Lancashire (Toronto: University of Toronto Press): http://leme.library.utoronto.ca/ [accessed 1 March 2011]. Birth and death dates follow those given in the *Oxford Dictionary of National Biography* (Oxford: Oxford University Press, 2004 (online edition 2007)): http://www.oxforddnb.com/.

[8] Thomas Rogers, *The Anatomie of the Minde* (London, 1576), 39v.

[9] *LEME*, "grief."

may have today. Although in some contexts it can be argued that writers intended specific meanings, resonances, and experiences according to their chosen terminology—there is some evidence, I think, that references to 'grief' emphasize the acute painfulness of sadness—it is not possible to delineate specific connotations in a uniform manner. Within the context of the passions words like 'sadness,' 'sorrow,' and 'grief' were seen as broadly synonymous, occupying a similar space in the same semantic field. This linguistic proximity is important to bear in mind as we begin to explore the ways in which discussions of sadness appear in different kinds of evidence from the period, as I will be drawing on examples that use all three of these terms as well as variations on them.

Medical Theory and Dramatic Literature

Medical knowledge and practice in sixteenth and early seventeenth-century England was composed of many different ideas, products, and approaches, resulting in an eclectic range of services that has been described as a "medical marketplace."[10] Despite this variety, however, the fundamental knowledge system underlying such ideas and practices was more or less a unified one, based on the ancient tradition of humoral medicine. Composed of four liquid humors—blood, yellow bile, black bile, and phlegm—the humoral body was a holistic system that stressed correspondences and sympathies across physical, mental, and spiritual functioning, as well as connections between the internal and external world.[11] The body's humors and the soul's passions were particularly interconnected, and most writers on the subject indicated that each humor was linked to a particular passion (in the case of sadness, black bile or melancholy was the related humor), and also that the passions depended on both movements in the soul and changes in the body (such as blushing, weeping, a quickened heartbeat, or sensations like leadenness) in order to be fully experienced. "[P]assions are drowned in corporall organs and instruments," wrote the English Jesuit Thomas Wright (c. 1561–1623) in his book *The Passions of the Minde in Generall* (1601), adding elsewhere that

[10] Patrick Wallis and Mark S. R. Jenner, "Introduction: The Medical Marketplace," in *Medicine and the Market in England and its Colonies, c. 1450–c. 1850*, ed. Wallis and Jenner (Basingstoke: Palgrave Macmillan, 2007), 1–23, Andrew Wear, *Knowledge and Practice in English Medicine, 1550–1680* (Cambridge: Cambridge University Press, 2000), 28–29.

[11] Wear, *Knowledge and Practice*, 37–40.

this sympathy worked both ways: "there is no Passion very vehement, but that it alters extreamly some of the foure humors of the body."[12]

In this model, what occurred in the body influenced the soul, and what occurred in the soul influenced the body, sometimes to the point that such links seem to be understood less as cause and effect and more as simultaneous happening. How entirely the body and soul were seen as intertwined did vary according to writer, but for the purposes of this chapter it is enough that there was a general consensus that body and soul were highly linked. Any intense passion could lead to disorder in the body and consequently illness, prompting writers like the doctor Stephen Bradwell (b. 1590/1) to advise that "*Passions* must (by a wise watching over our selves) be beaten off, whensoever they but offer to set upon us," for if they grew too strong disease would follow. This was nowhere more true than in the case of sadness or sorrow, which according to Bradwell "afflicts the Heart, disturbes the Faculties, melts the Braine, vitiates the humours, and so weakens all the principall parts; yea, sometimes sinkes the Body into the grave." Like the humoral system itself, such ideas about the dangers of sadness stretched back to the Romans and Greeks; Galen produced a text sometimes translated as "On the Avoidance of Grief," and ancient myths and histories included characters like Adrastus, King of the Argives, who reputedly died of sorrow upon receiving news of the death of his son, or Julia, daughter of Julius Caesar, who did the same following the death of her husband.[13]

But what exactly was it about sadness that had such a devastating effect on the body? Bradwell's description suggests that the passion sent all the vital organs of the body into severe disorder, but he does not say much about the specific physiological processes involved. Most writers in and around Shakespeare's time who addressed this issue focused on the intense strain sadness placed on the heart, which Thomas Wright, along with many other writers, thought to be "the peculiar place where that Passions allodge." According to Wright, when the brain perceived sensory information that might give rise to passion, it transmitted this information down to the heart, initiating a very physical response that occurred alongside the generation of feeling:

---

[12] Thomas Wright, *The Passions of the Minde in Generall: A Reprint Based on the 1604 Edition*, ed. Thomas O. Sloan (Urbana, IL: University of Illinois Press, 1971), 8, 4.

[13] Stephen Bradwell, *Physick for the Sicknesse, Commonly Called the Plague* (London, 1636), 37, 34. Many thanks to Vivian Nutton for bringing Galen's text to my attention.

> the purer spirits, flocke from the brayne, by certaine secret channels to the heart, where they pitch at the dore, signifying what an object was presented, convenient or disconvenient for it. The heart immediately bendeth, either to prosecute it, or to eschew it: and the better to effect that affection, draweth other humours to helpe him.[14]

In the case of sadness, this process was particularly damaging, as the humor involved was melancholy, characterized by its cold and dry qualities that were capable of chilling the body's vital spirits: "when he [a man] grieveth, the vitall spirits are contracted and stifled," wrote the theologian Samuel Hoard (1599–1658/9) in his book on "the grieving of the spirit," and Wright similarly noted that sadness caused "the gathering together of much melancholy blood about the heart, which collection extinguisheth the good spirits, or at least dulleth them ... the which humour being cold and drie, dryeth the whole body, and maketh it wither away."[15] Medical books were not the only sources of information advocating this view, and the Bible itself emphasized the damaging effects of sorrow, as in Proverbs 17.22: "A joyful heart causeth good health: but a sorowful minde dryeth the bones."[16]

Aspects of such theories can be seen very clearly in literary works from the period, including Shakespeare's plays. Returning to the case of Enobarbus, we can see how Shakespeare emphasizes the dryness of sorrow or grief, which has so desiccated Enobarbus's heart that he feels it "will break to powder" and put an end to his life. Other characters in Shakespeare's works that reportedly die from sorrow include Lady Montague, from *Romeo and Juliet* (c. 1595), whose husband says to the Prince in the final scene, "Alas, my liege, my wife is dead tonight./ Grief of my son's exile hath stopped her breath" (5.3.209–10); Brabantio, father of Desdemona in *Othello* (c. 1603/4), who dies from sorrow over Desdemona's elopement—"Thy match was mortal to him," says Graziano, "and pure grief/ Shore his old thread in twain" (5.2.212–13); Gloucester in *King Lear* (c. 1605/6), whose "flawed heart ... Burst[s] smilingly ... 'Twixt two extremes of passion, joy and grief" (24.193–96 (5.3)), as well as Lear himself, who, following his daughter Cordelia's death, bids his heart "Break ... prithee break," a line

---

14 Wright, *Passions of the Minde*, 32, 45.

15 Samuel Hoard, *The Soules Miserie and Recoverie: Or, the Grieving of the Spirit How It Is Caused, and How Redressed* (London, 1636), 11; Wright, *Passions of the Minde*, 61.

16 *The Geneva Bible: A Facsimile of the 1560 Edition* (Peabody, MA: Hendrickson, 2007), 272v.

that turns out to be his last (24.306 (5.3)).[17] If we include characters who are *said* to have died of sorrow, but for reasons of plot secretly survive, the list grows considerably longer: Juliet from *Romeo and Juliet* ("with which grief/ It is supposèd the fair creature died" (5.3.50–51)), Helena from *All's Well That Ends Well* (c. 1606/7) ("the tenderness of her nature became as a prey to her grief... now she sings in heaven" (4.3.54–56)), Hero from *Much Ado about Nothing* (c. 1598/9) ("Hero was in this manner accused, in this very manner refused, and upon the grief of this suddenly died" (4.2.59–61)), and Hermione from *The Winter's Tale* (c. 1609/10) ("This news [of her young son's death] is mortal to the Queen. Look down/ And see what death is doing" (3.2.147–48)). These lists include only the characters clearly stated to have died from some form of sorrowful passion, leaving out those whose deaths are linked to sorrowful events (Lady Macbeth, Lady Constance in *King John*, Ophelia in *Hamlet*, Falstaff in *2 Henry IV / Henry V*, the Duchess of Gloucester in *Richard II*) or who are said to be physically weakened by sadness and care (Henry IV, Titus Andronicus, Richard II, the Nurse in *Romeo and Juliet*, Cesario's imaginary sister in *Twelfth Night*, Antonio in *The Merchant of Venice*, to name only a few). Were we to take into account all the instances in which sorrow and grief are said to mar or age characters, our tally would become even longer.

Although the idea of a broken heart may conjure up a sense of sudden, acute pain that places great stress on the organ and quickly damages it, medical and literary writings emphasized that illnesses from sorrow often took hold gradually, slowly drying up the body's moisture and causing it to wither away, which speeded up the natural process of aging. According to Elyot, in his extremely popular medical regimen, *The Castell of Health* (reprinted sixteen times between 1536–1595),[18] sorrow "exhausteth both naturall heate and moysture of the bodie," much as a lamp uses up its oil or a candle its wax, a metaphor that was itself frequently linked in ancient and early modern times to the process of growing old.[19] Shakespeare's plays echo this sentiment, suggesting that sorrow, like age, saps the body

---

17 References to *King Lear* are to the quarto version, printed in the Oxford *Complete Works* as *The History of King Lear* and split into scenes as opposed to acts and then scenes. The equivalent Folio act and scene numbers are given in parentheses and follow the notation of the Oxford editors.

18 Paul Slack, "Mirrors of Health and Treasures of Poor Men: The Uses of the Vernacular Medical Literature of Tudor England," in *Health, Medicine, and Mortality in the Sixteenth Century*, ed. Charles Webster (Cambridge: Cambridge University Press, 1979), 248.

19 Thomas Elyot, *The Castell of Health* (London, 1595), 98. For the lamp metaphor and aging see Peter H. Niebyl, "Old Age, Fever, and the Lamp Metaphor," *Journal of the History of Medicine* 26:4 (1971): 351–68.

of its moisture, leading a person towards death. In *Richard II* (c. 1595), for instance, John of Gaunt describes his aging body as an "oil-dried lamp," adding that the "sudden sorrow" of his son's exile "Shorten[s] my days" and "help[s] time to furrow me with age" (1.3.214, 220–22) (two scenes later, he does in fact die). Such dangers were not limited to older characters; in *Romeo and Juliet*, for example, Romeo highlights the drying (and by extension damaging) properties of sorrow as he leaves Juliet's balcony for the second and final time. Juliet, noting her lover's palor, tells him, "now thou art so low,/ As one dead in the bottom of a tomb," to which he responds, "trust me, love, in my eye so do you./ Dry sorrow drinks our blood" (3.5.55–59).

This emphasis on the dryness of both sorrow and aging leads to a strong correlation between the process of growing old and that of grieving in many of Shakespeare's works. Once again, in *Romeo and Juliet*, we see the Nurse argue with Juliet over Romeo's killing of her cousin Tybalt, crying, "Give me some aqua vitae./ These griefs, these woes, these sorrows make me old" (3.2.88–89), and likewise in *Richard III* (c. 1592/3) the Duchess of York tells Richard, "Either thou wilt die by God's just ordinance… Or I with grief and extreme age shall perish" (4.4.184, 86). Throughout the plays grief is characterized as "beauty's canker" (*The Tempest* (c. 1610/11), 1.2.418), a deteriorating illness that makes you "sick and pale" (*Romeo and Juliet*, 2.1.47), "set[s] the jaundice on your cheeks" (*Troilus and Cressida* (c. 1602), 1.3.1), and forms "trenches"—more commonly known as wrinkles—in your face (*Titus Andronicus* (c. 1592), 5.2.23). In *The Comedy of Errors* (c. 1594), Egeon forgives his son Antipholus of Ephesus for not recognizing him, explaining that "grief hath changed me since you saw me last,/ And careful hours with time's deformèd hand/ Have written strange defeatures in my face" (5.1.298–300). In many ways, sorrow, time, and by extension age can be seen as roughly synonymous in these plays, since with added years come new losses, disappointments, and causes for grief. For the most unlucky characters, such misfortunes arrive all at once, causing age and the physical deterioration it inevitably brings to take hold before their natural time.

Medical Practice: Doctors' Case Notes and the London Bills

Taken together, such quotations and examples show us not only that Shakespeare corroborated ideas found in works of medical theory on the dangerous nature of sadness, but also that he did so consistently throughout his career as a playwright, which spanned from the early 1590s to the late

1600s. While these plays are of course works of imaginative fiction, they are also very much linked to the understanding of the body found in popular medical works from the period, suggesting significant uniformity of belief when it came to the damaging powers of sadness. Some question might remain, however, as to whether or not such theoretical and fictional accounts had much bearing on actual, day to day experience. After all, plays like those of Shakespeare were written first and foremost with drama in mind, aiming in many ways to exceed the confines of normal human life, and it could be argued that they exaggerate and hyperbolize many aspects of human experience, especially those relating to the passions and their effects. To die of a broken heart might have been believable on the stage, an arena in which tragedy and romance prevail, or even in a work of medical theory, which focuses on what *could* happen to the body in the most extreme of circumstances, but can we see any sign of this belief system in typical medical practice in the period?

The short answer is yes, although the evidence becomes much slimmer when we turn our attention from books of medical theory and dramatic fiction and towards accounts that help us explore the social historical side of this question. This is partly because the sources themselves are scarcer; doctors' casebooks, for instance, do not survive in great numbers, nor do written accounts of patient experience. Among the Cecil Papers at Hat field House is one account that gives brief, yet vivid insight into what doctors and patients made of sadness and its effects on the body and mind. Dated June 20, 1601, it is a letter addressed to Sir Robert Cecil, Secretary of State (1563–1612), who had instructed a group of physicians to visit an ailing London merchant named Rowland Lee and see if he was able to carry on with the running of his business. In the letter the physicians explain that they have "spent longe time in Conference both with himselfe and suche as have attended him in his sicknes" and have determined that "the infirmitie of his sicknes and other greefes ... [is due to] the late losse of his wief," which has "made his bodie weake and easelye stirred to lamentinge he beinge of a very tender feelinge in that behalfe."[20] Among the physicians present was William Gilbert (1544?–1603), physician to Queen Elizabeth and James I, reflecting the fact that belief in the physical dangers of excessive sorrow was not just the province of popular stage plays or printed texts. Those involved in medical practice also acknowledged the

[20] In Richard Hunter and Ida Macalpine, eds, *Three Hundred Years of Psychiatry, 1535–1860* (London: Oxford University Press, 1964), 64–65.

painful disruptions it could cause in the mind and body, leaving sufferers like Lee enfeebled, exhausted, and unable to look after themselves.

The physiological agonies of sorrow also appear in the medical notes of the astrological physician Richard Napier (1559–1634), who saw over 40,000 patients during his thirty-seven years as a practitioner in Great Linford, Buckinghamshire. According to historian Michael MacDonald, who has analysed all of Napier's cases relating to mental disturbance,

> many of Napier's patients became ill after they experienced grief or fright. They blamed a wide range of physical ailments on their emotional distress, including, for example, consumption, rheumatism, lameness, bloated faces, swollen limbs, amenorrhea, greensickness, and all manner of fevers.

MacDonald further notes that in a few extreme cases, cause of death was attributed to the sorrow of a broken heart, including two maidens jilted by their lovers and a woman who "died of a consumption taken by grief of her husband's debts."[21] In the far shorter published casebook of the physician John Hall (1574/5–1635), who was Shakespeare's son-in-law, illness and sorrow likewise appear side-by-side. In an entry for Lady Elizabeth Browne, for instance, a list of troubling afflictions, including "binding of the Belly, Melancholy, Watchfulness, troublesom sleep, Obstruction of the Courses," and a sense that "some live thing [was] leaping in her Belly," appear alongside the note that "All these happened from the death of her Daughter, dying in Child-bed." As is the case with the vast majority of the patient entries that appear in Hall's book, Lady Browne recovered fully and "came to enjoy perfect health," though not without some lingering concern during her course of treatment about "Scorbutic Pain of the Belly," an entry that helps remind modern readers how deeply intertwined emotional, mental, and physical ailments were often believed to be.[22]

The medical reality of the damaging effects of sadness can be seen even more starkly in surviving copies of the London Bills of Mortality, which were printed broadsides that tallied the total number of births and deaths in the city and its suburbs each week (yearly bills were also produced later in the seventeenth century). Such documents are unusual for their time; London was the first city in Europe to collect, print, and distribute

---

[21] Michael MacDonald, *Mystical Bedlam: Madness, Anxiety, and Healing in Seventeenth-Century England* (Cambridge: Cambridge University Press, 1981), 181–82.

[22] John Hall, *John Hall and His Patients: The Medical Practice of Shakespeare's Son-in-Law*, ed. Joan Lane and Melvin Earles (Stratford-upon-Avon: Shakespeare Birthplace Trust, 2001), 192–94.

this sort of demographic information to a wide readership with any regularity.[23] The system originated in manuscript form in the late sixteenth century as a way of keeping track of plague deaths (both in terms of number and location), moved into print in the early part of the seventeenth century, and then from 1629 onwards included tallies of all causes of death, including categories such as fever, bleeding, drowned, palsy, lunacy, and—particularly interesting for our purposes—fright and grief (see Figure 1 for an example of a yearly bill featuring many of these categories). As I have argued elsewhere, the bills were a familiar feature of London life, with citizens paying careful attention to the broadsides, particularly during times of plague, and their contents reflect widely acknowledged disease and illness categories in the period.[24] The presence of fright and grief in these documents therefore illustrates the extent to which passion, particularly sadness, was seen as a dangerous and even deadly force at this time. It should be noted as well that it is unlikely that deaths from grief in the bills were understood to be suicides, as there are separate categories that cover suicide, mental instability, and more mysterious misfortunes, including "Made away themselves," "Hanged themselves," "Drowned," "Dead in the street," and "Lunatique."

Although the exact number of deaths from grief listed in the bills is difficult to calculate, mainly due to the fact that these ephemeral documents do not survive in great numbers, extant weekly and yearly bills from the years 1629–1660 show that at least 357 deaths in London were attributed to the pains of grief and sadness (see Table 1).[25] Of course, in

---

[23] Some cities in Italy (most notably Florence and Milan) kept detailed municipal mortality records from as early as the fourteenth century, but they were not printed and distributed among the citizenship as the London Bills were. For more on these Italian "Books of the Dead," see Ann G. Carmichael, *Plague and the Poor in Renaissance Florence* (Cambridge: Cambridge University Press, 1986), 27–35, Carlo M. Cipolla, *Public Health and the Medical Profession in the Renaissance* (Cambridge: Cambridge University Press, 1976), 30–31.

[24] There is considerable evidence to suggest that the bills were produced for and circulated among a large readership; for further discussion see Erin Sullivan, "Physical and Spiritual Illness: Narrative Appropriations of the London Bills of Mortality," in *Representing the Plague in Early Modern England*, ed. Rebecca Totaro and Ernest B. Gilman (New York: Routledge, 2010), 79–84.

[25] Most scholars interested in the seventeenth-century bills rely on the data provided in John Graunt, *Natural and Political Observations, Mentioned in a Following Index, and Made upon the Bills of Mortality*, 2nd edn (London, 1662), fold-out table between 70–71. Graunt's table offers a helpful summary of the bills, but it is not entirely accurate and is missing information for several years. My calculations are based on the yearly and weekly bills that are held in the Guildhall Library's printed collections St. 42.9, Broadsides 23.70, and Granger 1.3.3 and the Bodleian Library's rare books collection G. A. Lond. 4° 95–7. For

comparison to the major killers in seventeenth-century London, this number was admittedly small: of the 281,352 people recorded as dying in the city and its outlying parishes in the bills, grief amounted to 0.1109 percent of deaths, which meant that for every 1,000 Londoners, just over 1 might expect to die of grief, as compared to the nearly 200 who would die of consumption, 130 of problems during infancy, 105 of ague and fever, and 70 of plague.[26] Still, deaths from grief are significant in their very existence, illustrating that the passion was considered harmful both in theory and in practice, and they also outstrip several other causes of death, including murder and suicide, which according to the bills were responsible for 113 and 283 deaths respectively.[27] Certainly no other passion proved more fatal: though medico-philosophical treatises suggested that any passion could kill if it grew too intense, a look through the long list of causes of death in the bills shows that only two other categories explicitly allude to the passions, with the more obvious being "fright" and the more ambiguous being "lethargy."[28] Over the same period of time, a total of 30 deaths resulted from fright and 79 from lethargy, which combined still fall short of half of the deaths from grief. Furthermore, as opposed to some of the other afflictions in the bills, which might vary from year to year or be called one thing in the early part of the century and something else towards the end, deaths from grief remained consistent and reliable over time, with at least one person dying from the malady every year from 1629 until 1818.[29] Indeed, John Graunt (1620–1676), a merchant and statistician who wrote

more information on the extant bills see Sullivan, "Physical and Spiritual Illness," 81–83, especially n. 21–22.

[26] By consumption I mean all given deaths for "consumption," "consumption and cough," and "consumption and tissick" (55,669); by problems in infancy I mean all given deaths for "christomes and infants" (35,984); by ague and fever I mean all given deaths for "ague," "ague and fever," and "fevers" (29,623); and by plague I mean all given deaths for "plague" (19,501). These figures are based on the numbers printed in extant yearly bills from 1629–1660.

[27] By murdered I mean all given deaths for "murdered" and "murdered, slain, and shot;" by suicides I mean all given deaths for "hanged and made away with themselves."

[28] While it is certainly possible that other causes of death, such as suicide, the "mother" (commonly understood as an early modern version of hysteria), spleen (the organ along with the liver responsible for the production of bile in the body), and perhaps "apoplex" (a form of heart attack), involved emotional turmoil, I am talking about categories in which the passions themselves are identified as the primary agent causing death.

[29] Even after 1818 deaths from grief appear sporadically in the bills; see Paul Laxton, *London Bills of Mortality* (Cambridge: Chadwyck-Healy, 1984), 1818 slide, 2, J. Marshall, *Mortality of the Metropolis* (London, 1832), fold-out tables following 82. As far as I am aware Laxton's microfiche collection is at present only available in England at Oxford's Bodleian Library.

a book about the bills in 1662, described grief as "*Chronical*" since it bore "a constant proportion unto the whole number of *Burials*" throughout the years.[30] Though Graunt queried some of the causes of death listed in the bills, he did not question grief's validity, a point that further suggests that dying from the passion remained a natural, uncontroversial idea in London over the course of the seventeenth century.

While the simplicity and absolutism of the data in the bills is in some ways highly appealing, getting to the more personal case histories behind such statistics is a considerable challenge. The data in the bills was based on the records kept in each parish's register book, a system that had begun in 1538 when city magistrates instructed all London parishes to maintain birth, marriage, and death records of all the people living within their limits.[31] Parishes were expected to employ clerks to look after these records, as well as local 'searchers,' most often elderly women, to declare the official cause of death for any person dying within the parish limits. When the bells of the parish church tolled to announce the passing of one of its inhabitants, the searchers would go to see the body to 'search out' the cause of death. This would be done both by observing the 'signs and tokens' visible on the body and by gaining information about the deceased person's final days from any family members, friends, or attending physicians that might have been present.[32] In this way cause of death would often be determined collectively, reflecting both the authority of lay knowledge (a doctor did not have to be there to determine a cause of death) and the widespread acknowledgement among London citizens that prolonged grief could cause serious physiological harm.

By the end of the century all parishes had some form of register book, but they were by no means uniform in their method of record-keeping. Causes of death are rarely recorded in these books aside from during plague years, when a 'p' sometimes appears beside death entries to indicate those who died in the epidemic. Such record-keeping would have been critical

30 Graunt, *Natural and Political Observations*, 16–17. Graunt later highlights how certain categories, such as rickets, changed considerably during the seventeenth century (23–24).

31 For more detailed descriptions of the history of the institution of the bills, see Stephen Greenberg, "Plague, the Printing Press, and Public Health in Seventeenth-Century London," *Huntington Library Quarterly* 67:4 (2004): 512–22, J. C. Robertson, "Reckoning with London: Interpreting the Bills of Mortality before John Graunt," *Urban History* 23 (1996): 328–334, Sullivan, "Physical and Spiritual Illness," 77–79.

32 For an excellent discussion of the searchers and their role in the parish, see Richelle Munkhoff, "Searchers of the Dead: Authority, Marginality, and the Interpretation of Plague in England, 1574–1665," *Gender & History* 11:1 (1999): 1–29.

to the creation of each week's bill, an enterprise that was overseen by London's Worshipful Company of Parish Clerks.[33] What is less clear, however, is how such information was managed from 1629 onwards, when all causes of death were listed in the bills. We might expect these causes to be recorded in the parish records alongside death entries, but in practice such notation was very rare. In a few parish records we can find some indication of causes of death and a handful of cases that were attributed to grief. In the parish records of St. Giles without Cripplegate, for instance, the clerk recorded the death of "Suzan daughter of Tho:[mas] Jaupper" on December 17, 1653, simply adding the word "Greife" next to the entry. He also noted that she had been admitted to Bethlem Hospital, more commonly known as 'Bedlam' asylum, London's municipal mental institution, suggesting perhaps that she died there. Madness was not always present in cases of grief, but as can be seen in many of the literary sources already discussed it was not an uncommon side effect of prolonged and intense passion.[34]

Other records of people dying from sadness and anxiety can be found in the unusually discursive parish records for St. Botolph without Aldgate. In his detailed study of the parish, Thomas Rogers Forbes has uncovered various burial entries for those dying of a kind of affliction commonly described as "grief of mind" or "thought," a term that takes us back to Shakespeare's Enobarbus, who in his sadness says that "swift thought... blows my heart" (4.6.34–5).[35] The physician William Bullein (c. 1515–1576) likewise acknowledged the pernicious nature of excessive rumination and its connection to sadness, noting in a passage on the passions in his *The Governement of Healthe* that "many men have bene caste awaye by thoughte, and moste for losse of estimacion."[36] Though the deaths in the Aldgate records pre-date the grief deaths in the bills by roughly thirty years, they provide some insight into the kinds of situations that families, searchers, and parish clerks might have later set down as deaths from grief. The records are brief, but one common feature that emerges is the role that anxiety and worry played in the onset of such

33 Greenberg, "Plague," 516.

34 Guildhall Library Manuscript 6419, vol. 5 (Baptisms, marriages, and burials in St. Giles Cripplegate, 1653–7), 6v.

35 Forbes writes that such grief is the "stated or implied" cause of death in twenty-one entries, eleven of which are men and ten women. See Thomas R. Forbes, *Chronicle from Aldgate: Life and Death in Shakespeare's London* (New Haven, CT: Yale University Press, 1971), 117–18.

36 William Bullein, *The Governement of Healthe* (London, 1558), 52v.

deaths. In July 1597, for instance, the parish clerk himself, who earlier in the year had been temporarily excommunicated, "dyed of inward griefe of mind or of a thowght," and in 1598 a female parishioner died on Christmas Eve under similar emotional duress, "hir husband being in prison."[37] Unresolved suits at court, or "the law's delay," as Hamlet called them in his "To be or not to be" speech (3.1.74), seem to have been particularly pernicious.[38] In June 1597 a forty-year-old man died "of a thowght having had long sute in Lawe," and five years earlier a carpenter from Buckinghamshire had come to the city to pursue a lawsuit, which caused him to fall ill from "inward griefe" of mind and eventually die at the home of his kinsman, who lived in the parish (thinking back to Dickens's *Bleak House*, mentioned in the introduction to this chapter, we might imagine a sixteenth-century Jarndyce vs. Jarndyce scenario).[39] In each case these records offer a brief glimpse into the lives and stories of those who died from maladies associated with sadness and worry, showing how the hardships of life might provoke an illness that proved unmanageable. Though most of the victims of grief tallied in the bills remain anonymous, it is likely that the circumstances surrounding their deaths were of a similar nature, arising from worldly misfortune and ending in personal tragedy.

Coping with Sadness

Given this widespread belief in the physiological dangers of sadness, we may well ask what doctors advised people to do to protect their health when the passion did strike. As with almost all approaches towards illness in this period, moderation and regimen were key. Passions were one of the six non-natural factors believed to affect health (the other five being diet, environment, sleep, exercise, and excretion) and like their counterparts they required careful regulation if body and mind were to be kept in healthful balance.[40] One way to attempt to balance any of the non-naturals was to adjust the levels of the other five, such as prescribing

---

[37] Forbes, *Chronicle from Aldgate*, 26, 118.

[38] In his critical edition of *Hamlet* T. J. B. Spencer describes such prolonged suits as a "typically Elizabethan misfortune"; see Spencer, ed., *Hamlet* (London: Penguin, 2005), 233.

[39] Forbes, *Chronicle from Aldgate*, 117–18.

[40] For more on non-naturals and regimen see Wear, *Knowledge and Practice*, 155–58, Heikki Mikkeli, *Hygiene in the Early Modern Medical Tradition* (Helsinki: Finnish Academy of Science and Letters, 1999), 19–23, 54–58.

lighter foods (to counter the cold, heavy, and dry qualities of sorrow and melancholy), a trip to the countryside to enjoy fresh air, more (or less) sleep, increased activity such as dancing or horseback riding, or a host of clysters intended to clear away any blockages in the intestines.[41] In the eyes of many doctors, however, such treatments could only go so far, since they did not get at the root of the problem. "[W]ee can but talke of *Topicall remedies*," wrote Bradwell, "as to apply *Mirth, Musicke, delightfull businesse, good Company, and lawfull Recreations*; such as may take up all time from carefull thoughts and passionate affections: Then have wee done." Further treatment, he suggested, had to come from religious men, since passions were at their root "diseases of the *Soule*" and required wise and holy counsel if they were truly to be cured.[42]

This emphasis on wisdom and counsel is widespread in books addressing the problem of sadness: "The syckenes of the body muste have medicine, the passions of the mynde, must have good counsel," wrote Bullein, and Elyot similarly suggested that disorders of passion required "the connsaile of a man wise and well learned in morall Philosophie."[43] In his essay on the subject, Francis Bacon (1561–1626) stressed the necessity and virtue of accepting counsel, writing that "The wisest princes need not think it any diminution to their greatness, or derogation to their sufficiency, to rely upon counsel. God himself is not without [it]" (along these lines Bacon subtitled his own book *Counsels Civil and Moral*).[44] The efficacy of counsel when it came to easing sadness, however, could sometimes be brought into question. Shakespeare depicts this struggle between painful passion and rational counsel multiple times in his plays, highlighting the difficulty, even hypocrisy of rationalizing away a debilitating sorrow. *Much Ado about Nothing* explores this problem in some detail, with Benedick noting early on that "everyone can master a grief but he that has it" (3.2.26). In this early scene the tone is comic—Benedick is trying to hide the fact that he is in love, passing off his mopish behaviour as the effect of a toothache—but towards the end of the play the issue surfaces again, albeit in a much darker way. Following Claudio's rejection and shaming of his bride Hero, whom he accuses of adultery, Hero's father

---

41 See for example Elyot, *Castell of Health*, 102–3, Wright, *Passions of the Minde*, 63–65, Nicolas Coeffeteau, *A Table of Human Passions*, trans. Edward Grimeston (London, 1621), 346–48.

42 Bradwell, *Physick for the Sicknesse*, 37–38.

43 Bullein, *Governement of Health*, 52v, Elyot, *Castell of Health*, 95.

44 Francis Bacon, *The Essays, Or Counsels Civil and Moral*, ed. Brian Vickers (Oxford: Oxford University Press, 1999), 46–47.

Leonato violently disowns her for the shame and sadness she has brought to their family, bidding her to die from this grief:

> Do not live, Hero, do not ope thine eyes,
> For did I think thou wouldst not quickly die,
> Thought I thy spirits were stronger than thy shames,
> Myself would on the rearward of reproaches
> Strike at thy life. (4.1.124–28)

The truth is that Hero is innocent, but even after agreeing to a plan to pretend that Hero has indeed died from grief (a strategy intended to provoke public pity for her), Leonato struggles to moderate his own sorrow. At the start of Act 5 he enters with his brother Antonio, who warns him, "If you go on thus [in great sadness], you will kill yourself" (5.1.1), to which Leonato responds, "I pray thee cease thy counsel,/ Which falls into mine ears as profitless/ As water in a sieve" (3–5). In the long speech that follows, Leonato questions the benefit that learned counsel can offer grieving men, for while it does attempt to stimulate the reasoning faculties, which in turn can temper passion, it is too academic, cerebral, and detached to connect with the minds of those who are truly sick with sadness. Leonato derides men who will "Patch grief with proverbs" (17), offering pithy maxims for overcoming passion, for no one, he asserts, can actually abide by such casual advice when "the load of sorrow" bears down on him (28). "I will be flesh and blood," he concludes,

> For there was never yet philosopher
> That could endure the toothache patiently,
> However they have writ the style of gods,
> And made a pish at chance and sufferance. (34–38)

Leonato's reference to the toothache harkens back to his earlier scene with Benedick, a move that shows how this one-time joke has now become all too serious. Likening the pain of passion to pain in the body, he suggests that neither can be willed away by philosophy or reason; all pain, his lines emphasize, has a vital, real presence that mocks lazy platitudes and patronizing counsel. Although the exact nature of Leonato's sorrow in this scene is unclear—the fact that he is complicit in the plan to recover Hero's honor could suggest that he is no longer so upset about her alleged unchastity, meaning that his grief in this scene is entirely feigned (it is certainly put on to the extent that he knows that Hero has not actually died)—there is also reason to take his comments on the inefficacy of counsel as authentic. His extreme reaction to Claudio's allegations in the wedding scene establish a strength of passion that could credibly carry over into this later scene, despite the twists in plot, suggesting to readers and audiences a character that is genuinely distraught over what will become of his daughter, chaste or unchaste, living or deceased. Either way, the sentiments he expresses concerning the intensity and urgency of sorrow highlight the inescapably embodied nature of the passion, as well as the shallowness of moral counsel that seeks to instruct without stopping to consider what it is like to feel. Such passion, Leonato suggests, is not only unavoidable, but also desirable, as it possesses an honesty about what it means to be human that is absent in the cool, disinterested logic of stoical counsel.

In several other plays by Shakespeare we similarly encounter grieving characters who emphasize the importance of actively expressing sorrow, whether in the form of words, actions, tears, or all three. Rather than attempt to use reason to mitigate and control one's grief, these characters suggest that it must be "expressed," not only in the sense of articulated, but also in the sense of pressed out, in order for mental and bodily health to be preserved. In *Macbeth* (c. 1606), for instance, when news arrives of the murder of Macduff's wife and children, Malcolm urges Macduff to say something rather than suffer quietly in silence: "Give sorrow words. The grief that does not speak/ Whispers the o'erfraught heart and bids it break" (4.3.210–11). Such lines are reminiscent of Hamlet's anguish early in his eponymous tragedy (c. 1600/1) about the pain of not being able to discuss one's sadness and discontent with others: "But break, my heart, for I must hold my tongue" (1.2.159). In *Macbeth*, Malcolm insists that Macduff's "deadly grief" must be eased through verbal expression and also through action, which he calls the "medicines of our great revenge" (something that we might also consider with regard to Hamlet's situation), and accordingly he encourages Macduff to "Dispute it [i.e. act on his grief] like a man" by turning his attention to overthrowing the man responsible for murdering his family, Macbeth (215–16, 221). While Macduff eventually agrees, he insists that he "must also feel it as a man," a point that emphasizes the need to acknowledge and engage with sorrow, despite its potential physiological harms or its perceived feminizing effects (largely due to the fact that it leads to weeping) (223). Likewise, in *Titus Andronicus*, Titus's brother Marcus finds that grief must be expressed rather than expunged; looking at his niece Lavinia, who has been brutally raped and mutilated, and her tongue cut out so that she can no longer speak, he says,

> O that I knew thy heart, and knew the beast,
> That I might rail at him to ease my mind!
> Sorrow concealèd, like an oven stopped,
> Doth burn the heart to cinders where it is. (2.4.34–37)

Bottled sorrow, these lines indicate, only aggravates the already pernicious effects of the passion, stifling the heart and pushing it towards breaking point. According to Marcus, words must have vent, and in the following scene he suggests that tears must be shed too if health is to be at all preserved. Bringing Lavinia to her father, he warns, "Titus, prepare thy agèd eyes to weep,/ Or if not so, thy noble heart to break./ I bring consuming sorrow to thine age" (3.1.58–60).

Marcus's characterization of sorrow suggests that it is both a canker that eats away at the body ("consuming" and aging it), as well as a kind of pressure cooker, in which the heart violently contracts and the spirits are suffocated ("like an oven stopped"). The emphasis on heat in this second model is somewhat at odds with the medical explanations of sorrow outlined above, a difference that might be explained by the suddenness of sorrow in these instances (with heat resulting from the intense clenching of the heart) or the fact that anger, a hot and surging passion, is also present. In both cases, writers suggested that words and especially tears could act as the body's natural defences against the damages of sorrow, as they offered a physical and mental release that could help alleviate some of the strain placed on the heart. According to the French Catholic preacher Jean-François Senault (c. 1601–1672), sorrow "drops away by Tears; and abandons the Heart, when it gets up into the Face," and his countryman Nicolas Coeffeteau (1574–1623) likewise wrote that "Teares are also proper to disperse heavinesse... when wee powre forth teares, we cast out that which afflicts us, & emptying the humor which oppresseth us, and smothers us within, by this meanes we free our selves from a heavy burthen which lay upon our hearts."[45] In Shakespeare's early history play, *King Henry VI, Part 2* (c. 1590/1), the distressed King echoes this idea, claiming that his tears are his body's way of draining excess liquid from his heart:

> ... my heart is drowned with grief,
> Whose flood begins to flow within mine eyes,
> My body round engirt with misery;
> For what's more miserable than discontent? (3.1.198–201)

---

[45] Jean-Francois Senault, *The Use of the Passions*, trans. Henry Earl of Monmouth (London, 1649), 485, Coeffeteau, *Table of Humane Passions*, 348–49.

Through crying the body has a means of regulating the imbalances caused by sorrow, though this method of release is not always strong enough to offset entirely the passion's malign effects. Furthermore, some individuals, particularly men, might attempt to stifle tears because of their association with womanish behaviour, noted briefly above. Claudius, for instance, chastises Hamlet for his "unmanly grief" in the wake of his father's death (1.2.94), and although Lear sheds tears early in his story when his first daughter challenges his authority, saying, "I am ashamed/ That thou hast power to shake my manhood thus" (4.290–1 (1.4)), when he experiences the same rejection at his second daughter's hands he vows to stifle this physiological impulse, whatever the consequences: "I have full cause of weeping, but this heart/ Shall break into a hundred thousand flaws/ Or ere I'll weep.—O fool, I shall go mad!" (7.443–5 (2.2)).[46] In the end, both of these predictions prove true: the King descends into distraction, experiencing a sorrow that ultimately breaks his heart. His story, as well as many others from the period, illustrates the deep physiological impact the passions were believed to have when they overwhelmed the mind and body, weakening the control of the reasoning faculties and burning, drowning, stretching, and straining the heart past endurance.

This urgent need for physical and verbal expression to some extent draws into question the high value writers in the period placed on the patient acceptance and internalization of moral counsel. If we open up the idea of moral counsel to a two way exchange, however—that is, a conversation that involves both expression and advice, as opposed to the passive acceptance of a learned lecture—the efficacy of counsel becomes more convincing. In his essay on the subject, Bacon suggests that personal disclosure is a natural and necessary part of counsel, meaning that trust and a sense of mutuality between the counselled and the counsellor is important: "The greatest trust between man and man is the trust of giving counsel," adding that "in other confidences men commit the parts of life ... but to such as they make their counsellors, they commit the whole."[47] This emphasis on the exchange of trust, secrets, and indeed

---

[46] In her analysis of male expressions of emotion, Jennifer C. Vaught suggests that while common conceptions of masculinity in the period argued that crying was emasculating (an idea Lear echoes in his own lines), many literary and cultural representations suggested that "men who ally themselves with women by adopting conventionally feminine forms of expression such as weeping and wailing are often strengthened rather than weakened as a result." Vaught, *Masculinity and Emotion in Early Modern English Literature* (Aldershot: Ashgate, 2008), 2.

[47] Bacon, *The Essays*, 46.

oneself suggests that the best counsel is predicated on friendship and mutual feeling, an idea that Bacon explores in greater detail in his essay "Of Friendship." Here he explains that the cornerstone of friendship is the ability to express feelings and unburden oneself of the physiological and mental pains they will cause if left uncommunicated:

> A principal fruit of friendship is the ease and discharge of the fullness and swellings of the heart, which passions of all kinds do cause and induce. We know diseases of stoppings and suffocations are the most dangerous in the body; and it is not much otherwise in the mind ... no receipt openeth the heart, but a true friend; to whom you may impart griefs, joys, fears, hopes, suspicions, counsels, and whatsoever lieth upon the heart to oppress it, in a kind of civil shrift or confession.[48]

Friendship and community facilitate the healthy regulation and flow of passion in a way much more natural than enforced rationalization, which can be "too piercing and corrosive" to do any good. "Reading good books of morality is a little flat and dead," Bacon explains, noting elsewhere that "a man were better relate himself to a statua or picture, than to suffer his thoughts to pass in smother."[49] Sorrows must have expression, in some cases immoderate or even unmanly, in order for health to be preserved, and furthermore this expression must be acknowledged and valued by some form of friend or confidant. The theologian Edward Reynolds (1599–1676) indicated as much in his *A Treatise of the Passions* (1640) when he noted that "in matter of Griefe, the *Mind* doth receive ... some lightnesse and comfort, when it finds it selfe *generative* unto others, and produces *sympathie* in them."[50] True relief came not simply from extracting sorrow from one's heart, but from communicating it to others and seeing some sign of recognition, compassion, and sympathy in them. It is notable in Shakespeare's plays that the characters who suffer most from grief do so in isolation; Enobarbus, Lear, Lady Constance, and Ophelia, for instance, are all estranged from their friends and family in some way, meaning that when they do attempt to communicate their sorrow they find that it often falls on deaf, or at least unsympathetic, ears. Their examples suggest that sorrows must not only be acknowledged and expressed in order for the sufferer to find relief, but also heard and validated within a community of sympathetic listeners.

---

[48] Ibid., 60.
[49] Ibid., 63.
[50] Edward Reynolds, *A Treatise of the Passions* (London, 1640), 54–55.

Conclusion

This chapter has sought to illustrate how strongly many people living in and around the time of Shakespeare believed sadness to be a damaging, debilitating, and even deadly force. Although writings on sadness and friendship suggest to some extent that the experience of sorrows could have some positive effects (for instance, the coming together of friends or the realization of who might be considered a true friend), such benefits were not enough to ease writers' concerns about the steep physiological costs the passion could exact. Most writers in this period criticized a strictly stoical approach to dealing with the passions, arguing that such an approach "woulde cut of, and as it were gelde men of those thinges which are grafted and planted in them by nature."[51] Passions were a natural and intrinsic part of the human experience, meaning that they could and should never be completely eradicated. Writers like Wright suggested that the passions could be "stirred up for the service of vertue," but nevertheless they wondered whether a passion as harmful as sadness could in fact be marshalled positively. Though Wright gave instructions in his book as to how one might provoke different passions in oneself and also in others, he omitted sadness from this discussion, implying through his silence that this particular passion was too dangerous and its effects too negative to warrant any reason for encouraging it.[52] An examination of the effects of intense sadness in the plays of Shakespeare suggests as much, for while it is true that in many of these plays characters gain knowledge or wisdom through their sorrows (think of Lear, for instance), it cannot be denied that they suffer immensely in their bodies, minds, and souls because of it. Of all the passions, sadness was by far considered the most hazardous, resulting in a widespread acknowledgement that if left unaddressed it could indeed prove to be a disease unto death.

---

51 Rogers, *Anatomie of the Minde*, B1v.
52 Wright, *Passions of the Minde*, 17, 260–93.

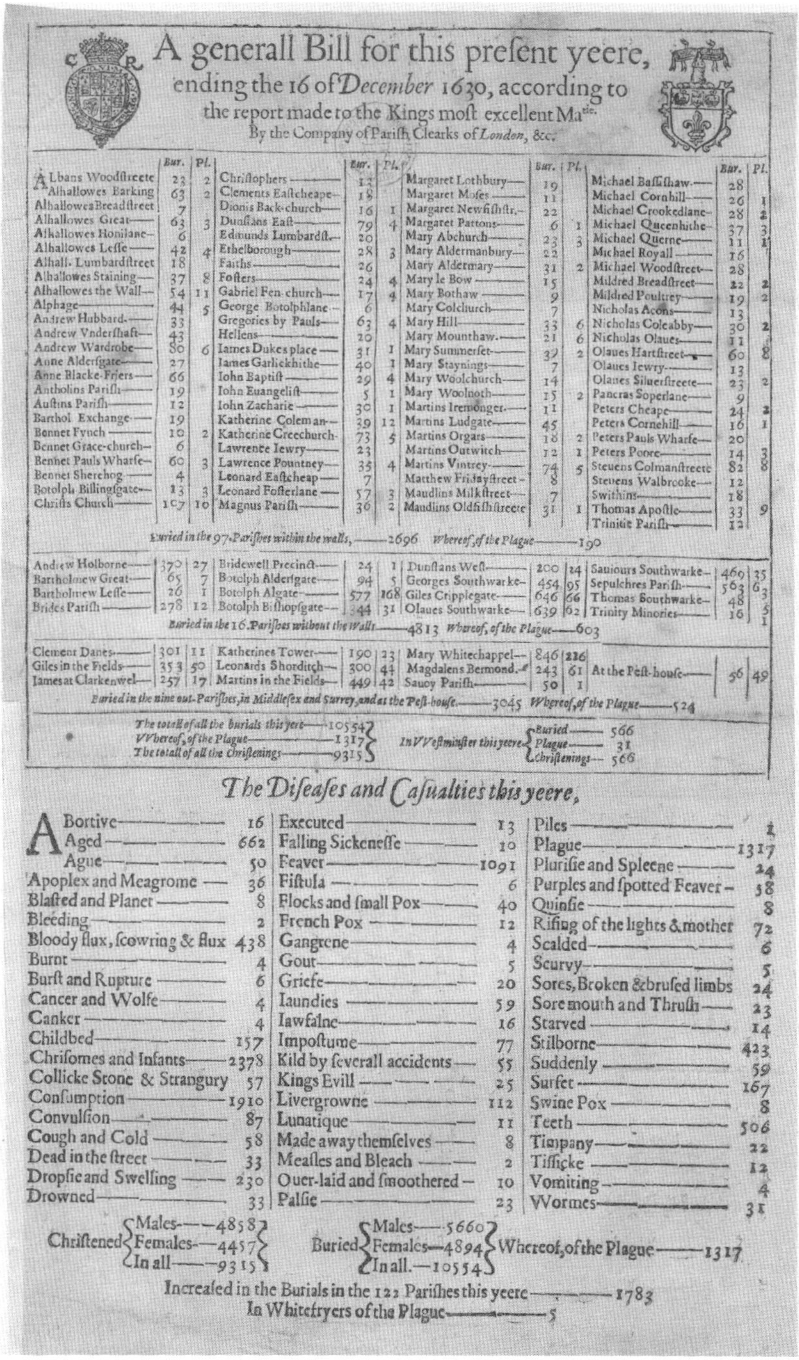

A generall Bill for this preſent yeere, ending the 16 of *December* 1630, according to the report made to the Kings moſt excellent Ma[tie.] By the Company of Pariſh Clearks of *London*, &c.

	Bur.	Pl.		Bur.	Pl.		Bur.	Pl.		Bur.	Pl.
Albans Woodſtreete	23	2	Chriſtophers	13		Margaret Lothbury	19		Michael Baſſiſhaw	28	
Alhallowes Barking	63	2	Clements Eaſtcheape	18		Margaret Moſes	11		Michael Cornhill	26	1
Alhallowes Breadſtreet	7		Dionis Back-church	16	1	Margaret Newfiſhſtr.	22		Michael Crookedlane	28	2
Alhallowes Great	63	3	Dunſtans Eaſt	79	4	Margaret Pattons	6	1	Michael Queenhithe	37	3
Alhallowes Honilane	6		Edmunds Lumbardſt.	20		Mary Abchurch	23	3	Michael Querne	11	1
Alhallowes Leſſe	42	4	Ethelborough	28	3	Mary Aldermanbury	22		Michael Royall	16	
Alhall. Lumbardſtreet	18		Faiths	26		Mary Aldermary	31	2	Michael Woodſtreet	28	
Alhallowes Staining	37	8	Foſters	24	4	Mary le Bow	15		Mildred Breadſtreet	22	2
Alhallowes the Wall	54	11	Gabriel Fen-church	17	4	Mary Bothaw	9		Mildred Poultrey	19	2
Alphage	44	5	George Botolphlane	6		Mary Colchurch	7		Nicholas Acons	13	
Andrew Hubbard	33		Gregories by Pauls	63	4	Mary Hill	33	6	Nicholas Coleabby	30	2
Andrew Vnderſhaft	43		Hellens	20		Mary Mounthaw	21	6	Nicholas Olaues	11	
Andrew Wardrobe	80	6	Iames Dukes place	31	1	Mary Summerſet	32	2	Olaues Hartſtreet	60	8
Anne Alderſgate	27		Iames Garlickhithe	40	1	Mary Staynings	7		Olaues Iewry	13	
Anne Blacke-Friers	66		Iohn Baptiſt	29	4	Mary Woolchurch	14		Olaues Siluerſtreete	23	2
Antholins Pariſh	19		Iohn Euangeliſt	5	1	Mary Woolnoth	15	2	Pancras Soperlane	9	
Auſtins Pariſh	12		Iohn Zacharie	30	1	Martins Iremonger	11		Peters Cheape	24	2
Barthol Exchange	19		Katherine Coleman	39	12	Martins Ludgate	45		Peters Cornehill	16	1
Bennet Fynch	10	2	Katherine Creechurch	73	5	Martins Orgars	18	2	Peters Pauls Wharfe	20	
Bennet Grace-church	6		Lawrence Iewry	23		Martins Outwitch	12	1	Peters Poore	14	3
Bennet Pauls Wharfe	60	3	Lawrence Pountney	35	4	Martins Vintrey	74	5	Steuens Colmanſtreete	82	8
Bennet Sherehog	4		Leonard Eaſtcheap	7		Matthew Fridayſtreet	8		Steuens Walbrooke	12	
Botolph Billingſgate	13	3	Leonard Foſterlane	57	3	Maudlins Milkſtreet	7		Swithins	18	
Chriſts Church	107	10	Magnus Pariſh	36	2	Maudlins Oldfiſhſtreete	31	1	Thomas Apoſtle	33	9
									Trinitie Pariſh	12	

Buried in the 97. Pariſhes within the walls,—2696 *Whereof, of the Plague*—190

Andrew Holborne	370	27	Bridewell Precinct	24	1	Dunſtans Weſt	200	24	Sauiours Southwarke	469	35
Bartholmew Great	65	7	Botolph Alderſgate	94	5	Georges Southwarke	454	95	Sepulchres Pariſh	563	63
Bartholmew Leſſe	26	1	Botolph Algate	577	168	Giles Cripplegate	646	66	Thomas Southwarke	48	3
Brides Pariſh	278	12	Botolph Biſhopſgate	344	31	Olaues Southwarke	639	62	Trinity Minories	16	5

Buried in the 16. Pariſhes without the Walls—4813 *Whereof, of the Plague*—603

Clement Danes	301	11	Katherines Tower	190	23	Mary Whitechappel	846	216	At the Peſt-houſe	56	49
Giles in the Fields	353	50	Leonards Shorditch	300	44	Magdalens Bermond.	243	61			
Iames at Clarkenwel	257	17	Martins in the Fields	449	42	Sauoy Pariſh	50	1			

Buried in the nine out-Pariſhes, in Middleſex and Surrey, and at the Peſt-houſe.—3045 *Whereof, of the Plague*—524

The totall of all the burials this yere—10554
VVhereof, of the Plague—1317
The totall of all the chriſtenings—9315

In VVeſtminſter this yeere *Buried*—566 *Plague*—31 *Chriſtenings*—566

The Diſeaſes and Caſualties this yeere,

Abortive	16	Executed	13	Piles	1
Aged	662	Falling Sickeneſſe	10	Plague	1317
Ague	50	Feaver	1091	Pluriſie and Spleene	24
Apoplex and Meagrome	36	Fiſtula	6	Purples and ſpotted Feaver	58
Blaſted and Planet	8	Flocks and ſmall Pox	40	Quinſie	8
Bleeding	2	French Pox	12	Riſing of the lights & mother	72
Bloody flux, ſcowring & flux	438	Gangrene	4	Scalded	6
Burnt	4	Gout	5	Scurvy	5
Burſt and Rupture	6	Griefe	20	Sores, Broken & bruſed limbs	24
Cancer and Wolfe	4	Iaundies	59	Sore mouth and Thruſh	23
Canker	4	Iawfalne	16	Starved	14
Childbed	157	Impoſtume	77	Stilborne	423
Chriſomes and Infants	2378	Kild by ſeverall accidents	55	Suddenly	59
Collicke Stone & Strangury	57	Kings Evill	25	Surfet	167
Conſumption	1910	Livergrowne	112	Swine Pox	8
Convulſion	87	Lunatique	11	Teeth	506
Cough and Cold	58	Made away themſelves	8	Timpany	22
Dead in the ſtreet	33	Meaſles and Bleach	2	Tiſſicke	12
Dropſie and Swelſing	230	Ouer-laid and ſmoothered	10	Vomiting	4
Drowned	33	Palſie	23	VVormes	31

Chriſtened { Males—4858, Females—4457, In all—9315 }

Buried { Males—5660, Females—4894, In all.—10554 } Whereof, of the Plague—1317

Increaſed in the Burials in the 122 Pariſhes this yeere—1783

In Whitefryers of the Plague—5

Fig. 1. The annual Bill of Mortality for 1630. Image courtesy of the Guildhall Library, City of London.

Table 1. Deaths from grief in the London Bills, 1629–1660.

Year	Deaths	Source
1629	18	GH, St. 424.9
1630	20	GH, St. 424.9
1631	22	GH, St. 424.9
1632	11	GH, St. 424.9
1633	14	GH, St. 424.9
1634	15	GH, St. 424.9
1635	5	GH, St. 424.9
1636	20	GH, St. 424.9
1637	No record	N/A
1638	4	Bod., G.A. Lond. 4° 95–7
1639	5	Bod., G.A. Lond. 4° 95–7
1640	No record	N/A
1641	18	GH, Broadsides 23.70
1642	12	Bod., G.A. Lond. 4° 95–7
1643	5	Bod., G.A. Lond. 4° 95–7
1644	8	Bod., G.A. Lond. 4° 95–7
1645	1	Bod., G.A. Lond. 4° 95–7
1646	10	Bod., G.A. Lond. 4° 95–7
1647	12	Graunt, *Observations*
1648	13	Graunt, *Observations*
1649	16	GH, Granger 1.3.3
1650	7	GH, Granger 1.3.3
1651	17	GH, Granger 1.3.3
1652	14	GH, Granger 1.3.3
1653	11	GH, St. 424.9
1654	17	GH, Granger 1.3.3
1655	10	GH, Granger 1.3.3
1656	13	GH, Granger 1.3.3
1657	10	Birch, *A Collection*
1658	12	GH, Granger 1.3.3
1659	13	GH, Granger 1.3.3
1660	4	GH, Granger 1.3.3
TOTAL	357	

Source key: GH = Guildhall Library, Bod. = Bodleian Library, Graunt = John Graunt's *Natural and Political Observations*, 2nd edn (London, 1662), Birch = Thomas Birch's *A Collection of the Yearly Bills of Mortality, 1657–1758* (London, 1759).

MEDICINE, PSYCHOLOGY, AND THE MELANCHOLIC SUBJECT IN THE RENAISSANCE

Angus Gowland

The corrupt nature of man after the Fall, according to the *Discours des maladies mélancoliques* (1597) by André du Laurens, physician to Henri IV and renowned professor of anatomy at the university of Montpellier, is to be seen in two kinds of 'alteration.' The first occurs in the soul, which contains (as du Laurens's English translator puts it) the "ingraven forme" of God but which "becommeth more outragious then a lyon, more fierce then a tyger, and more filthie and contemptible then a swine" when man gives way to his unruly appetites and passions. The second takes place when the body, the "vessell of the soule," is "so greatly altered and corrupted" that the soul's faculties are "likewise corrupted," a process that arises "most sharply" in three diseases: "the frensie, madnes, and melancholie." Just as the actions of frenetics and the mad are in no way "worthie of a man," so "melancholike men" are "so cast downe" and abased "that they become companions to the brute beasts." In such cases, from being "the best furnished and most perfect of all other living creatures," a man can thereby become

> most caitife and miserable creature that is in the world, spoyled of all his graces, deprived of iudgement, reason and counsaile, enemie of men and of the Sun, straying and wandring in solitarie places: to be briefe, so altered and chaunged, as that he is no more a man, as not retaining any thing more then the very name.[1]

Just over twenty years later the Oxford divine and amateur medical enthusiast Robert Burton wrote similarly of the postlapsarian deformation of the human being in his *Anatomy of Melancholy* (1621). "Man," according to Burton, once "the most excellent, and noble creature of the World," has become "*miserabilis homuncio*, a cast-away, a catiffe, one of the most miserable creatures of the World, if he be considered in his owne nature, and

[1] André Du Laurens, *A Discourse of the Preservation of the Sight: of Melancholike Diseases; Of Rheumes, and of Old Age*, trans. Richard Surphlet (London, 1599), 80–81 (Du Laurens, *Discours de la conservation de la veue, des maladies melancholiques, des catarrhes, et de la vieillesse* (Paris, 1597), 108r–110v).

so much obscured by his fall that (some few reliques excepted) he is inferiour to a beast." When we yield to our "lusts" and give way to "every passion and perturbation of the minde," we "metamorphosize our selves, and degenerate into beasts," provoking God to anger and bringing upon ourselves "this [disease] of *Melancholy*, and all kindes of incurable diseases."[2] For Burton as for du Laurens, melancholy could reveal and incarnate postlapsarian misery in its quintessence, as a condition in which man was subject to disturbing emotions and irrational impulses, and thereby came to resemble "bruit Beasts... void of all reason."[3]

These works suggest that to be melancholic in this period was to be—or at least, be perceived to be—in some sense sub- or inhuman. In part, this perception originated in long-standing commonplaces concerning extreme emotions or psychic perturbations that associated passions with irrational animals.[4] But as I hope to show here, the notion that the melancholic was somehow not fully human had implications for the sufferer's selfhood that went beyond his or her simple resemblance to "bruit Beasts." This notion was also a product of a complex and wide-ranging nexus of medical, psychological, moral and spiritual ideas about human nature, and more specifically about human subjectivity and the self. In this essay, then, I shall be investigating the relationship between ideas about melancholy and those about the self in the Renaissance, with a view to outlining the contours of the specifically 'melancholic subject.'

I

There has been much interesting work done in the past thirty years on expressions of selfhood in early modern literature. The pioneering study in English literary studies was Stephen Greenblatt's *Renaissance Self-Fashioning* of 1980, which initiated the 'new-historicist' project of treating early modern texts as cultural artifacts to reveal contemporary subjectivities and senses of self. These were typically shown to be of a markedly

---

[2] Robert Burton, *The Anatomy of Melancholy*, ed. R. Blair, T. Faulkner, and N. Kiessling, 6 vols (Oxford: Clarendon, 1989–2000), 1.1.1.1, vol. 1, pp. 121–22, 128.

[3] Burton, *Anatomy*, vol. 1, pp. 61–62. For descriptions of the 'beastly' attributes of melancholics see, for some examples, vol. 1, pp. 36, 42–43, 52; 1.2.3.4, vol. 1, p. 258; 3.1.3.1, vol. 3, p. 33.

[4] See Gail Kern Paster, *Humoring the Body: Emotions and the Shakespearean Stage* (Chicago: University of Chicago Press, 2004), 135–88 for some illustrations of this association.

paradoxical character: fluid and malleable, and the product of complex and subtle authorial artifices, but simultaneously constituted by social, political and economic discourses external to the self, and perhaps above all, products of the historically constituted power-relations that structured those discourses.[5] However, intellectual historians of the early modern era have—with some notable exceptions—been comparatively reticent about entering into this diverse and complex territory.[6] Instead, Greenblatt's quasi-Foucauldian project has been developed by a series of literary-historical studies that have mined the dramatic and poetic texts of

---

[5] Stephen Greenblatt, *Renaissance Self-Fashioning from More to Shakespeare* (Chicago and London: Chicago University Press, 1980). For some important precursors, now often overlooked, see Hardin Craig, *The Enchanted Glass: The Elizabethan Mind in Literature* (Oxford and New York: Oxford University Press, 1936); J. B. Bamborough, *The Little World of Man* (London and New York: Longmans, Green & Co., 1952); and Thomas Green, "The Flexibility of the Self in Renaissance Literature," in *The Disciplines of Criticism: Essays in Literary Theory, Interpretation, and History*, ed. Peter Demetz, Thomas M. Greene, and Lowry Nelson (New Haven: Yale University Press, 1968).

[6] For an introductory survey, emphasizing the variety of conceptions of selfhood in his era, see Peter Burke, "Representations of the Self from Petrarch to Descartes," in *Rewriting the Self: Histories from the Middle Ages to the Present*, ed. Roy Porter (London and New York: Routledge, 1997), 17–28. For a selection of historical studies see Karl Joachim Weintraub, *The Value of the Individual: Self and Circumstance in Autobiography* (Chicago: University of Chicago Press, 1978); Vittor Ivo Comparato, "A Case of Modern Individualism: Politics and the Uneasiness of Intellectuals in the Baroque Age," in *The Individual in Political Theory and Practice*, ed. Janet Coleman (Oxford: Oxford University Press, 1996), 149–70; Martin Euringer, *Zuschauer des Welttheaters: Lebensrolle, Theatermetaphor und gelingendes Selbst in der frühen Neuzeit* (Darmstadt: Wissenschaftliche Buchgesellschaft, 2000); Geoff Baldwin, "Individual and Self in the Later Renaissance," *The Historical Journal* 44 (2001): 341–64; Timothy J. Reiss, *Mirages of the Selfe: Patterns of Personhood in Ancient and Early Modern Europe* (Stanford: Stanford University press, 2003); John Jeffries Martin, *Myths of Renaissance Individualism* (Basingstoke: Palgrave Macmillan, 2004); M. T. Jones-Davies, ed., *L'intériorité au temps de la Renaissance: Actes du colloque de Paris 2003–2004* (Paris: Honoré Champion, 2005); Raymond Martin and John Barresi, *The Rise and Fall of Soul and Self: An Intellectual History of Personal Identity* (New York: Columbia University Press, 2006), 109–22. Three important studies of theories of human nature more generally are Ernst Cassirer, *The Individual and the Cosmos in Renaissance Philosophy*, trans. Mario Damandi (Oxford: Basil Blackwell, 1963); Charles Trinkaus, *In Our Image and Likeness: Humanity and Divinity in Italian Humanist Thought*, 2 vols (London: Constable, 1970); and Paul Oskar Kristeller, *Renaissance Concepts of Man, and Other Essays* (New York: Harper & Row, 1972). For some important art-historical studies see John Pope-Hennessy, *The Portrait in the Renaissance* (London: Phaidon, 1966); Joseph Leo Koerner, *The Moment of Self-Portraiture in German Renaissance Art* (Chicago and London: University of Chicago Press, 1997); Gunter Schweikhart, *Autobiographie und Selbstportrait in der Renaissance* (Köln: W. König, 1998); Joanna Woods-Marsden, *Renaissance Self-Portraiture: The Visual Construction of Identity and the Social Status of the Artist* (New Haven and London: Yale University Press, 1998). For a collection of texts, see *Personal Disclosures: An Anthology of Self-writings from the Seventeenth Century*, ed. David Booy (Aldershot and Burlington: Ashgate, 2002).

the Renaissance, often in conjunction with vernacular works of medicine, psychology, moral philosophy and spiritual writing.[7]

Here I shall be approaching this territory with a similar, loosely Foucauldian concern with the elaboration of subjectivity in medical and psychological works, but adopting a slightly different perspective. In one sense, my approach will be broader. It takes a number of European as well as English texts into account, from the conviction that generally speaking for the questions with which I am concerned these works tend to agree more than they disagree. But in other senses the approach here is more specific. It will be focusing principally on the learned discourse of orthodox Galenic medicine and Aristotelian psychology; and as indicated above, it will address the relationships between the Galenic medical conceptions of the human subject, more general philosophical concepts of subjectivity and selfhood, and theories of melancholy in the Renaissance. It is important to emphasize that I shall not be addressing several areas of early modern discourse, both learned and popular, that would be important to any comprehensive understanding of ideas about the self in this period—particularly social conceptions of status and gender.[8] Instead, I shall be concentrating on those parts of intellectual production where a clear or significant relationship can be discerned between the medical psychology of melancholy and conceptions of what it is to be a human subject or self.

[7] A comprehensive bibliography of this territory, now vast, is not possible here, but amongst the more notable studies that are relevant to this essay are Katharine Eisaman Maus, *Inwardness and Theater in the English Renaissance* (Chicago, 1995); Michael C. Schoenfeldt, *Bodies and Selves in Early Modern England: Physiology and Inwardness in Spenser, Shakespeare, Herbert, and Milton* (Cambridge: Cambridge University Press, 1999); and Douglas Trevor, *The Poetics of Melancholy in Early Modern England* (Cambridge: Cambridge University Press, 2004). See also Joan Webber, *The Eloquent 'I': Style and Self in Seventeenth-Century Prose* (Madison: University of Wisconsin Press, 1968); Bridget Gellert Lyons, *Voices of Melancholy: Studies in Literary Treatments of Melancholy in Renaissance England* (London: Routledge & Kegan Paul, 1971); Louis van Delft, *Littérature et anthropologie: Nature humaine et caractère à l'âge classique* (Paris: PUF, 1993).

[8] On the gendering of melancholy in English writing of this era see Helen Hackett, "'A Book, and Solitariness': Melancholia, Gender and Literary Subjectivity in Mary Wroth's *Urania*," in *Renaissance Configurations: Voices/Bodies/Spaces 1580–1690*, ed. G. McMullan (Basingstoke: Macmillan, 1998), 64–88; Katherine Hodgkin, "Dionys Fitzherbert and the Anatomy of Madness," in *Voicing Women: Gender and Sexuality in Early Modern Writing*, ed. Kate Chedgzoy, Melanie Hansen, and Suzanne Trill (Keele: Keele University Press, 1996), 69–92.

II

One way of starting historical inquiry into subjectivity is to ask about the means by which different authors identified something called the 'self.' And one answer to this question, forming the basis for many rich literary explorations of early-modern subjectivity, is that self-awareness was frequently identified with a sense of inwardness. This has, unsurprisingly perhaps, been found to have been expressed most clearly in literary-poetic and dramatic works of all different kinds. These do not directly concern me here, though it can be noted in passing that the debate, begun in the 1980s, as to whether early modern texts express senses of interiority, or whether such interiority is an anachronistic imposition by the modern reader, has been more or less decisively settled in favour of the former position. The challenge now is to identify the historically contingent formations of interiority.[9] Other answers to the question of how conceptions of selfhood were expressed in this era, which I shall be touching upon here at different stages, rest on the notion that such conceptions were articulated in relation to various external others. In general terms, these included discussions of the relationships between individuals (as well as their internal motives and actions) in moral philosophy, between the self and the community in political thought, and between the self, nature, and God in natural philosophy and theology. In the works of some authors, such as Girolamo Cardano and Michel de Montaigne, such concerns were interwoven with an understanding of the role of narrative in the construction of selfhood.[10] My concern here, however, will be conceptions of self and subjectivity that are expressed in works of early modern medicine and psychology, conceptions which are fundamentally the product of a range of diverse and complex negotiations of an evolving relationship

---

9 See Maus, *Inwardness and Theater*, esp. 1–7.

10 On Cardano, see Anne C. E. Van Galen, "Body and Self-Image in the Autobiography of Girolamo Cardano," in *Modelling the Individual: Biography and Portrait in the Renaissance*, ed. Karl Enenkel, Betsy de Jong-Crane, and Peter Liebregts (Amsterdam: Editions Rodopi, 1998); Guido Giglioni, "Autobiography as Self-mastery. Writing, Madness, and Method in Girolamo Cardano," in *Bruniana and Campanelliana: Ricerche filosofiche e materiali storico testuali*, Vols 1–2, ed. Eugenio Canone and Elisa Germana Ernst (Rome: Istituti Editoriali e Poligrafici Internazionali, 2002), 331–62. The literature on Montaigne is immense, but see, for example, Richard L. Regosin, *The Matter of My Book: Mongtaigne's 'Essais' as the Book of the Self* (Berkeley and London: University of California Press, 1977); Craig B. Brush, *From the Perspective of the Self: Montaigne's Self-Portrait* (New York: Fordham University Press, 1994); and Allan Levine, *Sensual Philosophy: Toleration, Skepticism and Montaigne's Politics of the Self* (Lanham, MD: Lexington Books, 2001).

between Christian doctrine and classical philosophy. There is sometimes great variation between the precise formulations found in particular texts, but I shall be presenting a schematic outline of the territory, hopefully without distorting that variation too violently.

Before beginning, some points should be made about the terms 'self' and 'subject' (or 'subjectivity') as they will be employed here. It is hardly controversial to observe that since ideas about selfhood, and forms of subjectivity, are historically determined and have fluctuated wildly across the centuries, it would be self-defeating in an historical inquiry to be referring to an essential or transhistorical conception of the self or subject. On the other hand, however, in order to organize our analysis it seems that we must posit a conception of selfhood or subjectivity with some more or less stable characteristics—for example, to settle doubts about whether the texts we are dealing with are elaborating a conception of self or in fact something else. It will be a fundamental conviction of this paper that although there are many striking differences between premodern and modern conceptions of the self, and indeed that there were a variety of early modern conceptions of self, there is nevertheless enough common ground between the meanings of the term 'self' (and its various cognates) in the sixteenth and twenty-first centuries for us to make sense of this territory. If there were not significant family resemblances between our vocabulary and those employed in early modern texts, we simply would not be able to make sense of them. Here, then, I shall be using the term 'self' heuristically, to denote an aspect of an individual human being, that is to say, an individuated human person who experiences (and following Richard Sorabji) "owns" psychological states and actions, and therefore also is capable of expressing an 'I'-perspective that is truly his or her "own."[11] The individual self in this sense is distinct from the human being or person, as it refers to what is intrinsic to an individual person as opposed to what is adventitious. This approach to the concept of self has the advantage of being detectable in ancient as well as early modern and modern philosophy and literature.[12] Although it is common to use the

[11] Richard Sorabji, *Self: Ancient and Modern Insights about Individuality, Life, and Death* (Oxford and Oxford: Clarendon, 2006), 20–30, 32–33, 48–53. As will become clear, this essay is heavily indebted to Sorabji's work on classical conceptions of selfhood.

[12] See Sorabji, *Self, passim*. For other useful works on ancient conceptions of selfhood see Klaus Oehler, *Subjectktivität und Selbstbewusstsein in der Antike* (Würzburg: Köbigshausen & Neumann, 1997); Paulina Remes and Julia Sihvola, eds., *Ancient Philosophy of the Self* (Dordrecht: Springer, 2008).

terms 'self' and 'subject' more or less interchangeably, by the latter term, I shall be referring to a conception of the human being that is not individuated in this way, but to which characteristics, potentialities, operations, and actions are attributed. The 'subject' in this quasi-grammatical sense is the human being of which sets of things are predicated. This, it seems to me, is broadly in line with a Foucauldian conception of subjectivity, according to which the 'subject' is produced within discourse, or is constituted as an effect of power/knowledge.[13]

III

In the Galenic tradition that constituted the dominant orthodoxy within European medical circles from the middle ages to well into the seventeenth century, there were two modes of analysis of human nature pulling in opposite directions. In the first place, the status of the individual was sometimes clarified in Renaissance learned medicine by referral to the 'tree' of Porphyry, a tool of logical division which was used to distinguish genera from species, and which stipulates that individual human beings are the most specific kind of species, belonging to the genus human, and that they can be differentiated by their distinctive characteristics.[14] The nature of these characteristics is determined by the particularizing theory of idiosyncrasy, to which Galenic physicians were fully committed. As elaborated by Galen in the *Mixtures* (known in the Renaissance as the *De temperamentis libri III*), the nature of individual human beings is primarily a matter of their unique blend of humours and elements,[15]

[13] For Foucault's discussion of the relationship between the care of the self, self-knowledge, and truth (or the 'knowing subject'), see Michel Foucault, *The Hermeneutics of the Subject: Lectures at the Collège de France, 1981–1982*, ed. Frédéric Gros and trans. Graham Burchell (New York and Basingstoke: Palgrave Macmillan, 2005). The terms 'subject' and 'self' are differentiated along slightly different lines in Robert M. Strozier, *Foucault, Subjectivity, and Identity: Historical Constructions of Subject and Self* (Detroit: Wayne State University Press, 2002), 10–11.

[14] Ian Maclean, *Logic, Signs and Nature in the Renaissance: The Case of Learned Medicine* (Cambridge: Cambridge University Press, 2002), 121–23.

[15] "Constare animalium corpora ex calidi, frigidi, sicci, humidique mixtura, nec esse horum omnium parem intemperatura portionem, demonstratum antiquis abunde est, tum philosophorum, tum medicorum praecipuis." "Cum namque ex calidi, frigidi, sicci, & humidi temperatura conflari corpora dicunt, de ijs, quae summo gradu sic se habent, ipsis scilicet elementis, aere, igni, aqua, terra, intelligendum aiunt." Galen, *De temperamentis libri tres*, trans. Thomas Linacre (Paris, 1527), 1 and 3.

namely their peculiar bodily 'mixture' or *krasis* (hence ἰδιοσυγκρασία)—what would come to be called the 'complexion' (*complexio*) or 'temperament' (*temperamentum*).[16] Idiosyncrasies were considered to account for a wide variety of individual characteristics and capabilities: not just susceptibility to particular diseases, but also particular modes of perception, and extraordinary kinds of physical and mental ability. This permits us to say—somewhat speculatively, since Galen's theorization of the individuated self is relatively inchoate[17]—that there was a concept of 'self' in Galenic medical discourse. The physician was able to gain knowledge of this self through conjecture from sensory experience, but because it concerned infinite particulars, such 'artistic' knowledge could only ever be probable.[18]

On the other hand, Galenic medicine also contained a generalizing tendency to explain the attributes and capabilities of the human species within a comprehensive physiological theory. In the *Methodus medendi* (II.7), Galen contrasted the "special form" of the individual with the "unitary form" of man, and he was later associated with the view that medicine is concerned with the knowledge of species, not individuals.[19] In medieval and Renaissance Galenism, this generalizing tendency gave rise to the popular subfield of characterology, which located individuals schematically within complexionate categories according to dominant humoral mixture, and which attributed physical and mental characteristics that were considered to emanate from the qualities of the humour (or humours) in question.[20] In Thomas Walkington's *Optick Glasse of Humors*,

---

[16] On idiosyncrasy in the *Methodus medendi* see Galen, *Opera omnia*, ed. C. G. Kühn (1821–1833), vol. 10, p. 209.

[17] See, for example, the discussion of individual beings in Galen, *De temperamentis* I, in *Selected Works*, trans. P. N. Singer (Oxford: Oxford University Press, 1997), 218–21.

[18] On the logical issues involved here see James Allen, "Failure and Expertise in the Ancient Conception of an Art," in *Scientific Failure*, ed. Tamara Horowitz and Ira Allen Ira Janis (Lanham, Rowman & Littlefield, 1994), 81–108, at 96–97; id., *Inference from Signs: Ancient Debates about the Nature of Evidence* (Oxford: Clarendon, 2001), 89–97; and Maclean, *Logic, Signs and Nature*, 167–70.

[19] Galen, *On the Therapeutic Method Books I and II*, trans. and comment. R. J. Hankinson (Oxford: Clarendon, 1991), II.7.6–32, 65–75; Maclean, *Logic, Signs and Nature*, 169. On the importance of this text within the medical curriculum of Renaissance universities see Jeromy Bylebyl, "Teaching *Methodus Medendi* in the Renaissance," in *Galen's Method of Healing: Proceedings of the 1982 Galen Symposium*, ed. Fridolf Kudlien and Richard J. Durling (Leiden: Brill, 1991), 157–89.

[20] A useful overview of English Renaissance characterology and its influence on contemporary literature and drama can be found in Lawrence Babb, *The Elizabethan Malady: A Study of Melancholia in English Literature from 1580 to 1642* (East Lansing: Michigan State University Press, 1965).

a fairly typical English instance of this kind of writing first published in 1607, the Galenic doctrine that "the soule simpathizeth with the body and followeth her crasis and temperature" provided the foundational principle for the scheme of the "nine temperatures" (ideally well-balanced; cold; hot; moist; dry; hot and moist; cold and moist; hot and dry; cold and dry) that "are blazond out among the phisicions." Walkington's contention—commonplace in this genre—was that knowledge of humoral complexions was an essential component of self-knowledge, without which we put "all the faculties both of soule and body" at risk. The reader was encouraged to identify the position of his or her idiosyncrasy within these general complexionate schemes, in order to adopt a prescribed somatic and psychic regimen that would avoid unhealthy extremes: "Who keepes a golden meane is sure to finde, A healthfull body and a chearefull minde." The individual self is thereby related to a subjectivity that was centrally constituted in humoral terms.[21]

A generalizing theoretical tendency is also conspicuous in Galenic pathology and therapeutics. Despite the commonplace acknowledgement that treatment was always to be directed at and adapted to the mixture of the particular individual,[22] diseases were routinely treated by Galenic physicians as having basically stable sets of characteristics (causes, symptoms, prognostics, and cures) that applied to different degrees in each case. Here, again, we encounter the constitution of a subject, or a process of 'subjectivization,' that involves the construction of forms of subjectivity by Galenic discourse through the assignation of generic clusters of

[21] Thomas Walkington, *The optick glasse of humors. Or, The touchstone of a golden temperature, or the Philosophers stone to make a golden temper wherein the foure complections sanguine, cholericke, phlegmaticke, melancholicke are succinctly painted forth, and their externall intimates laide open to the purblind eye of ignorance it selfe, by which euery one may iudge of what complection he is, and answerably learne what is most sutable to his nature* (London, 1639), 8, 18, 78, 167. For an important predecessor to this work, which exerted considerable influence on Walkington, see Levinus Lemnius, *De habitu et constitutione corporis, quam Graeci κρασιν, triviales complexionem vocant, libri duo* (Antwerp, 1561), which appeared in English as *The Touchstone of Complexions*, trans. Thomas Newton (London, 1576).

[22] See Galen, *Methodus medendi* III.7.11, trans. Thomas Gale: "He is the best Phisition of everie particular patient, which hath gotten the method, wherby he may discerne natures, and also conjecture which are the proper remiedies of everie one. For it is an extreame madness, to judge that there is a common curation of all man." *Certaine workes of Galens, called Methodus medendi, with a briefe declaration of the worthie art of medicine, the office of a chirurgion, and an epitome of the third booke of Galen, of naturall faculties* (London, 1586), 54r.

capabilities and susceptibilities—as opposed to an individuated 'self' with characteristics that are entirely its own.

Another important characteristic of Galenic physiology is its functionalism. For Galen, the health or sickness of the human being was to be measured by the manner and extent to which the various parts of the organism—each of which has its own particular mixture that affects its functioning—were active. As we are told in the *De temperamentis*, a healthy organism is one in which each of its parts is performing its natural function,[23] and a diseased organism is one in which one or more of its parts' natural activities is impaired. Conversely, the essence of a disease is the disposition that impedes the activity of a bodily part.[24] To measure the extent to which any individual organism exhibits the characteristics that are to be expected of the species to which it belongs, then, is to assess the extent to which its bodily parts perform the functions which are appropriate to their nature: "This matter of "partaking most of the nature proper to the species" is evaluated in terms of the activities. The optimal state of any plant or animal is regarded as corresponding to the best performance of its activities."[25]

We can turn now to the Galenic understanding of the constituent parts of the human being, whether considered as a particularized idiosyncratic self or as a generically classifiable humoral subject, and the interlinked concepts of body and soul. For Galen and his followers, the human being was a body-soul composite, which was presented in physical terms as an entity whose workings were to be explained primarily (if not always exclusively) by means of factors that are located within the domain of nature.[26] Hence, the bulk of the discourse of learned medicine consists of a materialistic mode of analysis in which the principal explanatory tools were the concepts of elements, qualities, humours, and subtle 'spirits.' Similarly, the central principle of Galenic psychology, that the operations of the faculties of the soul depend in various ways upon the mixtures of the body,[27] was widely accepted by orthodox physicians. Nevertheless, they

---

[23] Galen, *De temperamentis* II.6. See *Selected Works*, 258.

[24] Galen, *Methodus Medendi* I.5.1–4, II.1.3, II.3.10. See *On the Therapeutic Method*, trans. Hankinson, 21–22, 40–41, 46.

[25] Galen, *De temperamentis* I.6. See *Selected Works*, trans. Singer, 219.

[26] On the concept of nature in the learned medicine of the Renaissance, see Ian Maclean, *Le monde et les hommes selon les médecins de la Renaissance* (Paris: CNRS éditions, 2006).

[27] As established in the treatise whose title indicates its central argument, the *Quod animi mores corporis temperatura sequantur*, translated in Galen, *Selected Works*, 150–76.

also acknowledged the existence of an immaterial and immortal rational soul, resisting the materialistic reductionism that would explain all psychic functions entirely in terms of the interaction of physical qualities, and so did not disagree—at least not openly—with their natural-philosophical colleagues who frequently defined man as a "rational animal."[28] Only very few—such as the famous Paduan physician Giambattista da Monte—endorsed Galen's heterodox claim that the rational part of the soul simply is the bodily "mixture."[29] Appeals to occult ('hidden') causes and substantial concessions to theological arguments were commonplace.

When it came to understanding the activities of the soul, Renaissance Galenists generally adhered to the sophisticated codifications of Aristotelian faculty psychology formulated by their medieval predecessors and contemporary natural philosophers.[30] There were, admittedly, other important influences: Galen himself had elaborated a subtle, eclectic psychology—recorded principally in the influential *De placitis Hippocratis et Platonis*[31]—and the uses made of Aristotle's *De anima* in learned medicine depended heavily upon late-antique and Arabic interpretations of that work.[32] It was also common for physicians to diverge from Aristotle in a number of important ways, for example by dividing the soul into three parts (nutritive, sensitive, and intellective—the possession of which was routinely said to distinguish men from other animals), or by asserting the primacy of the brain rather than the heart in the governance of the body. But when describing the particular operations of the soul in the body,

---

[28] See R. W. Serjeantson, "The Soul," in *The Oxford Handbook of Philosophy in Early Modern Europe*, ed. Desmond M. Clarke and Catherine Wilson (Oxford: Oxford University Press, 2011), 119–41, at 122–26.

[29] Galen, *Selected Works*, 153, 157; Giambattista da Monte, *Medicina universa*, ed. M. Weindrich (Frankfurt, 1587), 124–25, cited and discussed in Ian Maclean, "Naturalisme et Croyance Personnelle dans le Discours Médical à la fin de la Renaissance," *Journal of the Institute of Romance Studies* 6 (1998): 177–91, at 185–86.

[30] Katherine Park, "The Organic Soul," in *The Cambridge History of Renaissance Philosophy*, Charles B. Schmitt and Quentin Skinner (Cambridge: Cambridge University Press, 1988) 464–84; Dennis des Chene, *Life's Form: Late Aristotelian Theories of the Soul* (Cornell University Press, 2001); Fernando Vidal, *Les sciences de l'ame, XVIe–XVIIIe siècle*. (Paris: Champion, 2006); Serjeantson, "The Soul," at 120–28. On the position of Aristotle in Galenic medicine more generally see Schmitt, "Aristotle among the Physicians," in *The Medical Renaissance of the Sixteenth Century*, ed. Roger French, Ian Lowie, and Andrew Wear (Cambridge: Cambridge University Press, 1985), 1–15; Maclean, *Logic, Signs and Nature*, 83–84, 191–93.

[31] Vivian Nutton, "*De Placitis Hippocratis et Platonis* in the Renaissance," in *Le opere psicologiche di Galeno, Atti del terzo colloquio Galenice Internazionale Pavia, 10–12 settembre 1986*, ed. Mario Vegetti (Naples, 1988), 281–309.

[32] Park, 'The Organic Soul," 467–68.

medical writers inherited and usually adhered rather closely to scholastic faculty psychology. Following the orthodoxy established by Aristotle's *De anima* 1.1, the soul was typically defined as the intelligible 'form' of the living body (or the 'actuality,' ἐντελέχεια, of the body which potentially has life).[33] And following the medieval interpretation, each of the soul's operations, or distinct faculties (δυνάμεις: *vires* or *virtutes* in the Latin tradition), was thought to be directed towards its own object and designated its own function.[34] Although the nature of these faculties—and indeed whether they existed as ontologically separate entities—became increasingly disputed in the course of the sixteenth century,[35] medical works did not often register serious concern with such controversies.[36] These were conventionally deemed to be the territory of the *physicus* rather than the *medicus*,[37] and given that Galen himself had written of the δυνάμεις of the soul as if they were meaningfully distinct, most learned physicians were predisposed to adopt medieval schemes without substantial modification.[38]

Accordingly, when discussing the particular operations of the soul in the body—and they were typically concerned only with its 'organic' (vegetative and sensitive) as opposed to 'intellective' aspects—Renaissance Galenists routinely employed the scholastic terminology of the powers (*vires* or *virtutes*) deemed responsible for perception, cognition, emotions,

[33] See, for instance, Johannes Velcurio, *In philosophiae naturalis partem omnium praestantissimam, hoc est Aristotelis de Anima libros, epitome longe doctissima* (Basel, 1537), I.I, p. 5; Julius Caesar Scaliger, *Exotericarum exercitationum liber quintus decimus, de subtilitate, ad Hieronymum* Cardanum (Paris, 1557), CCCVII.12, fol. 396v ("Anima est forma substantialis perficiens corpus tale, quale deseribit ibi"); Burton, *Anatomy*, 1.1.2.5, vol. 1, p. 147, where the soul is defined as "the perfection or first Act of an Organicall body, having power of life."

[34] Park, "The Organic Soul," 467–68, 470–73, 475–83. As Burton notes, despite the agreement of "most Philosophers" on the definition of the soul in the *De anima*, "many doubts arise about the *Essence, Subject, Seat, Distinction*, and subordinate faculties of [the soul]." *Anatomy*, 1.1.2.5, I, p. 147. For an important earlier discussion in England see Andrew Willet, *De animae natura et viribus quaestiones quaedam, partim ex Aristotelicis scriptis decerptae partim ex vera philosophia, id est, rationis thesauris, depromptae in usum Cantabrigiensis* (Cambridge, 1585).

[35] Park, "The Organic Soul," 477–79.

[36] A notable exception is in Du Laurens, *A Discourse*, 77–80 (*Discours*, 104r–108r).

[37] See, for example, Giambattista da Monte, *Consilia medica* (Nürnberg, 1559), XIX. On the principle that *ubi desinit physicus, ibi medicus incipit*, see Schmitt, "Aristotle among the Physicians," 14–15.

[38] See, for instance: "δύο γὰρ ἔχομεν ἐν ταῖς ψυχαῖς δυνάμεις ἀλόγους." Galen, *Opera Omnia*, ed. Kühn, vol. 5, p. 28. See also the endorsement of Plato's assignation of the three different 'parts' of the soul to the brain, heart and liver in the first book of the *Quod animi mores corporis temperatura sequantur*, in Galen, *Selected Works*, 152ff.

and so on. The most important of these for medical accounts of psychic health and disease were the 'inner senses' of the sensitive soul, usually conceived as imagination (sometimes subdivided into common sense/*sensus communis*, imagination/*virtus imaginativa* and phantasy/*phantasia*), reason (sometimes comprised of the *virtus cogitativa* and *virtus aestimativa*), and memory (*virtus memorativa*), which were often assigned to the anterior, middle, and posterior ventricles of the brain respectively.[39] These powers were thought to operate in conjunction with the bodily organs by means of subtle mediating spirits (animal spirits in the brain, vital spirits in the heart, and natural spirits in the liver), which directed the soul's actions in the body.[40] In turn, the spirits were said to affect the functioning of psychic activities and bodily organs through variations in quantity, quality, and expansion or contraction.[41] The qualities and quantities of the spirits, as with the humours, could be affected or manipulated by internal physical or external environmental factors.[42]

IV

How, then, might these medical-psychological conceptions of body and soul be related to a conception of the self, or a form of subjectivity? On the most basic level, in Galenic medicine every self was composed of these intertwining bodily and psychic elements; and each individual self could be differentiated from other selves—in the first instance idiosyncratically, by its specific humoral mixture (and so its health or sickness), and then by the directly related manner and extent to which the powers of the organic soul operate in the body (or in Aristotelian language, actualize their respective potentialities). As a subject, s/he was thereby constituted as a functional body-soul composite whose primary mode of experience, health or sickness, was radically dependent upon complexionate type, and whose psychic and affective experience—we might say its 'character'—was organized similarly, by the interaction of this complexion

39 Grazia Tonelli Olivieri, "Galen and Francis Bacon: Faculties of the Soul and the Classification of Knowledge," in *The Shapes of Knowledge from the Renaissance to the Enlightenment*, ed. Donald R. Kelley and Richard H. Popkin (Dordrecht: Kluwer, 1991), 61–70.

40 For instance, see Lemnius, *The Touchstone of Complexions*, 7r–8r. See also Walkington, *Optick glasse*, 96–101.

41 For a detailed, orthodox account of the healthy functioning of animal spirits in the brain see Ercole Sassonia, *De melancholia*, in *Opera practica* (Padua, 1639), 18a–b.

42 See L. J. Rather, "The 'Six Things Non-Natural': A Note on the Origins and Fate of a Doctrine and a Phrase," *Clio Medica* 3 (1968): 336–47.

with the animal spirits and the physiological substance of the brain, as well as external events and environmental circumstances. Or, to rephrase this again in Aristotelian psychological terms, the subject was constituted as a ensouled body which engaged in sequences of activities that brought its potentialities into being.

If we relate this conception to some of the most basic and conspicuous figurations of subjectivity and selfhood in Renaissance thought, it is striking in the first instance how different it is from classically modelled views—especially Platonist ones—of the rational 'inner self' as a kind of secret citadel that is the locus of psychic authenticity.[43] Perhaps the most important three *loci* for the latter way of thinking in the Renaissance were, first, the discussion of the Delphic injunction to self-knowledge in the Platonic *First Alcibiades* 128E–133C, where the rational soul, as the part of us that is most perfect and resembles God, is identified as the true self; second, the mention of reason as ὁ ἐντὸς ἄνθρωπος ('the inner man') in *Republic* 589A–B; and finally, Cicero's assertion in *Tusculanae disputationes* I.22.52 that moral self-knowledge concerns soul not body: "Neque nos corpora sumus. Cum igitur *nosce te* dicit, hoc dicit, *nosce animum tuum*."[44] This approach structured Pauline and Augustinian Christian conceptions of the psychic inner self as the location of the divine voice within us,[45] and is ubiquitous in early modern moral and spiritual literature. Its fullest expression, however, can be found in expressly Neoplatonist conceptions of the true self as reason or intellect. According to Marsilio Ficino's summary of the *First Alcibiades*, "the man is the rational soul" because this is the part of us that is capable of self-reflection, that shares in the divine mind in the manner of a stream flowing from its source, and that uses the body as its instrument in order to participate in human affairs.[46] Ficino fleshed out

---

43 Charles Taylor, *Sources of the Self: The Making of the Modern Identity* (Cambridge: Cambridge University Press), 111–207, esp. 115–42.

44 Cicero is here following (ps.-[?])Plato, *First Alcibiades* 129B–131A, 133B–C (in *Plato*, trans. W. R. M. Lamb, 12 vols, vol. 8, pp. 194–205, 210–13).

45 Theo K. Heckel, *Der Innere Mensch: die paulinische Verarbeitung eines platonischen Motivs* (Tübingen, 1993), 11–30, 89–210; Hans Dieter Betz, "The Concept of the 'Inner Human Being' (*ho esô anthrôpos*) in the Anthropology of Paul," *New Testament Studies* 46 (2000): 315–341, at 324ff; Taylor, *Sources of the Self*, 127–42. On this concept before Plato, see Walter Burkert, "Towards Plato and Paul: The 'Inner' Human Being," in *Ancient and Modern Perspectives on the Bible and Culture: Essays in Honor of Hans Dieter Betz*, ed. A. Y. Collins (Atlanta: Scholars Press, 1998), 59–82.

46 "Est autem homo, anima rationalis, mentis particeps; corpore utens. Ex hac definitione illius officium trahitur trifariam distributum. Ut enim rationalis anima est, in seipsam circulo quodam ratiocinationis sese animadvertendo reflectitur. Ut mentis particeps, in divinam mentem velut rivulus in fontem suum refluit. Ut utens corpore, humanis

this Platonic vision at length in the *Theologia Platonica de immortalitate animae* (1469–1474), where, for example, the teaching that "[h]omo est ratio" is glossed with a discussion of the necessity of inner self-cultivation urged in *Republic* 589A–B.[47]

The conception of the true and interior self as rational soul, or mind (*mens* or *animus*), is also readily available in later Renaissance texts of practical ethics that are not squarely in the Neoplatonic tradition. The eclectic philosopher Girolamo Cardano asserted in his *De consolatione libri tres* (1542) that "totus enim homo, animus est."[48] A few decades later, the same assumption about the self underlay the Neostoic Justus Lipsius's separation of "what is not in us but around us" from the 'inner man' of the mind (*animus*) in the *De constantia libri duo* (1584).[49] Notwithstanding the tendency within learned medicine to employ the functionalist conception of soul as a set of capacities, the notion of the inner psychic self was also prevalent in Renaissance Aristotelian moral philosophy. Here the key classical discussion was in *Nicomachean Ethics* X.7, which presents the view that the most perfect happiness for human beings is produced in the activity of contemplation, as the highest virtue of the understanding or theoretical intellect (νοῦς). In one respect, since the theoretical intellect is the "most divine" element in the human being, a contemplative life is superhuman (X.7.8, 1177b26–31); but in another, it is most truly human, since the intellect is the "dominant and better part" and hence the

negocijs gubernandis incumbit.... Philosophiae studio, moralis, mathematicae, theologiae opus est, ut ad seipsum et ad mentem sui causam redeat." *Platonis opera qvae ad nos extant omnia*, trans. Janus Cornarius and comment. Marsilio Ficino (Basel, 1561), 335. See also the discussion of the *First Alcibidades* in Angelo Poliziano, "Letter to Bartolomeo Scala," in Jill Kraye, ed., *Cambridge Translations of Renaissance Philosophical Texts. Vol. 1: Moral Philosophy* (Cambridge: Cambridge University Press, 1997), 194.

47 "Homo est ratio. Post haec iubet Plato, ut interiorem illum hominem nutriamus potius quam bestias illas, ne propter famem, deficiente homine, solae in nobis supersint bestiae [...]." Marsilio Ficino, *Platonic Theology*, trans. Michael J. B. Allen and ed. James Hankins (Cambridge, Mass. and London: Harvard University Press, 2001–2006), 6 vols, XVII.4.7–14, esp. 8–9, vol. 6, p. 56.

48 Girolamo Cardano, *De consolatione*, I, in *Opera omnia* (Lyon, 1660), 592b. As Cardano's English translator puts it: "[a] man is nothinge but his mynd." *Cardanus comforte*, trans. Thomas Bedingfield (London, 1576), 8.

49 "Duo sunt, quæ arcem hanc in nobis Constantiæ oppugnant, Falsa bona, Falsa mala. Utraque sic appello, QUAE NON IN NOBIS SED CIRCA NOS, QUAEQUE INTERIOREM HUNC HOMINEM, ID EST ANIMUM, PROPRIE NON IUVANT AUT LAEDUNT." Justus Lipsius, *De constantia libri duo* (Frankfurt, 1591), I.7, p. 27 (*Two Bookes of Constancie*, trans. Sir John Stradling (London, 1595), 15). See also the (seemingly Platonizing) reference to Anaxagoras in *De constantia* I.11, pp. 36–7 (*Two Bookes*, 28).

"true self," and in this sense, "the intellect more than anything else is man" (X.7.9, 1178a2–8).[50]

In the frequently rehearsed discussions about the relative merits of the contemplative and active lives, Renaissance commentators often saw no fundamental incompatibility between Platonic and Aristotelian ethics,[51] the latter being similarly premised upon a conception of the true self as intellect, whose virtue is manifested in theoretical wisdom, and which is realized most fully in contemplation.[52] Sometimes, as in the *Expositio libri Ethicorum Aristotelis* (1478) by the Florentine humanist Donato Acciaiuoli, this position was glossed with the argument that the speculative operations of the intellect bring us closest to God and spiritual (or 'separate') substances, because this faculty distinguishes us from irrational animals, which have only vegetative and sensitive souls. For Aristotle, as Acciaiuoli pointed out, the human self was to be identified with its most valuable part, and therefore,

> we must strive to lead a life which is similar to that of immortal beings and separate substances, pursuing that life which is based on the best element in us, that is, the mind, reason and intellect. Although the mind is small in mass, because it is indivisible, absolutely unmixed and consequently lacks quantity or magnitude, nevertheless it greatly excels [other faculties] in power, because it rules, in the natural order of things, all the inferior faculties that exist within us. It is also of superior worth because it is unmixed and immaterial. Hence Aristotle says that each of us consist of this, that is, a mind and reason, because it is the principal thing in us. The first conclusion is therefore that each creature seems to be, in some sense, that which

[50] Aristotle, *Nicomachean Ethics*, trans. H. Rackham (London: William Heinemann, 1934), 618–19; see also IX.4.4 (1166a22–3), 534–5 and IX.8.6 (1168b34–1169a2), 552–53. At IX.4.3, 1166a16–17, pp. 534–5, the self is identified in slightly different terms as the reasoning or thinking (διανοητικός) part.

[51] Jill Kraye, "Moral Philosophy," in *The Cambridge History of Renaissance Philosophy*, ed. Schmitt and Skinner, 334–46.

[52] Renaissance interpretations of Aristotle were sometimes influenced by the fourth-century commentator Themistius, according to whom Aristotle's position is that "we are the productive (ποιητικός) intellect." *Themistius on Aristotle on the Soul* (London: Duckworth, 1996), 100, 16–102, 24, pp. 124–27. See, in general, H. P. F. Mercken, "The Greek Commentators on Aristotle's *Ethics*," in *Aristotle Transformed: The Ancient Commentators and their Influence*, ed. Richard Sorabji (London: Duckworth, 1990), 407–43; and E. P. Mahoney, "Neoplatonism, the Greek Commentators, and Renaissance Aristotelianism," in *Neoplatonism and Christian Thought*, ed. D. J. O'Meara (Albany, NY: State University of New York Press, 1982), 169–77, 264–82.

> is most outstanding in it; the mind is that which is most oustanding in man; therefore, each of us seems, in some sense, to consist of a mind.[53]

This form of Aristotelianism was therefore fully in line with the Platonic (and Ciceronian) understanding of the divine character of contemplative activity. The intellect, and so the 'true self' of each individual, has a divine aspect.[54]

However, if the Galenic medical conception of the human subject jars strikingly with such notions of the intellective 'inner self,' a slightly different picture emerges when we turn to ethical considerations of the relationship between the individual and the human community. Here the ambiguity of the tenth book of the *Nicomachean Ethics* was of fundamental importance. Having identified the 'true self' with the intellect, Aristotle proceeds (at X.8.1–3, 1178a8–23) by proposing a contrasting view of the distinctively human subject as an embodied social being with a series of physical and social needs, expressing its nature through the exercise of moral virtues. Here he identifies 'moral activities' that we perform in social interaction, such as justice and courage, and also in our passions, as 'purely human' matters, and these are related not just to our psychological condition but also to our bodily constitution. Since the human subject is by nature a body-soul composite, it is the virtues expressing this composite nature that constitute its experience *qua* human subject. From this point of view, the moral virtues, the standards of which are established by the special intellectual virtue of prudence, and which involve the habits of

[53] "Dicit igitur inprimis post habere oportet eorum sententiam qui monent nos ut sequamur mortalia & humana & eniti debemus vivere ea vita que est similis immortalibus et essentiis separatis et secundum eam vitam que est optima omnium que sunt innobis, id est ipsa mens et ratio et intelllectus qui et si sit parvum mole quia est indivisibile et simplicissimum et perconsequens caret quantitate vel magnitudine molis: tamen vi multum excellit quia imperat ordine nature cunctis potentiis inferioribus que sunt innobis & prestabilitate quoque excedit cum sit simplex & immaterialis. Quare quisque dicit philosophus videtur esse hac idest mens & ratio quia est principalissimum in homine & ideo affert primam conclusionem talem. Id quo quomodo videtur esse unusquisque quod est ideo prestabilissimum. Sed mens est prestabilissimum in homine ergo unusquisque videtur quoquomodo esse mens." Donato Acciaiuoli, *Expositio libri Ethicorum Aristotelis* (Florence, 1478), X.7, fol. 250r. Translation by Jill Kraye, in *Cambridge Translations*, vol. I, p. 55.

[54] "Addit enim quod is qui sic vivit scilicet vita contemplativa non vivit secundum conditionem humanam sed secundum quod aliquid divinum in ipso consistit pro ut videlicet per intellectum habet similitudinem cum substantiis separatis." "Due igitur his insumma videntur esse precipue rationes ad ostendendum speculativam esse supremam felicitatem & esse prestantiorem activa. Unia quia contemplatio est similis operationi divine. Alia quia per contemplationem valde distamus a brutis." Acciaiuoli, *Expositio*, X.7, fols 249r and 253r.

acting in relation to others in accordance with reason and of experiencing emotions in a moderate and rational way, encapsulate the specifically human aspects of subjectivity. This interpretation of the subject can be buttressed by Aristotle's assertion about deliberate choice (προαίρεσις) in VI.2.5, that it involves a union of desire and intellect, and that man is "such an origin of action."[55]

The ambiguity of the *Nicomachean Ethics* in this regard received close attention from Renaissance commentators. Although Acciaiuoli had argued that in some sense the human individual consists principally of "mind and reason," he conceded that "there are two types of rational life: leading one type, he is said to live like a man; leading the other, he is said to transcend the human condition." Since man is distinguished from other animals in the first place by his practical rational faculty, Acciaiuoli concluded from Aristotle's text that "active happiness belongs to the man who is living in a human and political condition, not to the one leading a more excellent and superior life, that is, an intellective life." Properly defined, man is "an intermediate being between other animals and separate essences." His intellective capabilities are divine and constitute his 'principal' essence, but insofar as he has a composite nature, his specifically human capabilities are manifested through the moral virtues, and the rational manner in which he manages his psychic and somatic activities.[56]

Thus, as the German natural philosopher Rudolph Goclenius observed in his *Lexicon philosophicum* (1613), Aristotelians typically diverged from Platonists when it came to understanding the constituent parts of the human being and their relationship. Whereas the latter believed that the

[55] "Hence choice is either desiderative reason or ratiocinative desire, and such an origin of action is a man." Aristotle, *Nicomachean Ethics* VI.2, 1139b4–5, trans. Ross, Ackrill and Urmson (Oxford: Oxford World's Classics, 1998), 139. See also VI.12.6, 1144a6–7, where prudence and moral virtue are said to determine "the complete performance of man's proper function." *Nicomachean Ethics*, trans. Rackham, 366–67.

[56] "Ea [*sc.* vita rationalis] autem est duplex & alia vivere dicitur ut homo: alia vero supra conditionem humanam: est enim ratio in homine ut principium rerum agendarum. Est etiam ratio principium rerum speculandarum, id est mens activa & speculativa & altera agit humana agibilia: alia speculatur ea que sunt.... Ex his colligitur quod activa felicitas competere videtur homini viventi conditione quadam human & civili non viventi praestantiore et potiore in intellectiva quadam vita.... Homo autem videtur esse medius inter alia animalia & essentias separatas [...]." Acciaiuoli, *Expositio*, X.7, fol. 249r–v. The translation is by Jill Kraye, from *Cambridge Translations*, vol. I, p. 53. See also the discussion of προαίρεσις: "Concluditur ergo quod homo est principium intellectus & appetitus & ista electionis & electio rerum agendarum." *Ethics* VI.2 in Acciaiuoli, *Expositio*, 131v–132r, at 132r.

definitive characteristic of man was soul, and regarded the body as merely its instrument, Aristotelians saw the human as both soul and body, bound together a relationship of entelechy.[57] Accordingly, much of the Aristotelian moral philosophy taught in the universities of the Renaissance, and propagated in works of late scholastic moral and political thought, was premised upon a view of the human being as an embodied rational being living in society. As the Bavarian humanist Joachim Camerarius noted in his discussion of *Ethics* VI.2.5 in his 1578 commentary, a socialized conception of the subject clearly accords with the Aristotelian definition of the human being as by nature a political animal in *Politics* I.2, 1253a2–18: "id est ζῶον πολιτικὸν, non νοερόν."[58] And according to the Paduan professor Francesco Piccolomini in his *Universa philosophia de moribus* (1583), ethical inquiry must address itself to the human being who lives "in a community and in the company of other men" not in solitude, and must be concerned with the *summum bonum* not only of his soul, "but of the totality of his composite being." Even the life of moral virtue actualized in the human community, Piccolomini argued, is insufficient to the supreme good of the human being, which has physical as well as psychic needs. "Therefore Theages was right," he concluded, in saying that

---

57 "Platonicis homo proprie est anima. Corpus enim eis nihil hominis est, nisi tanquam possessoris, velut equus aut malleus militis aut fabri. Sed Aristotelicis homo est animi per synecdochen: quia anima est eis homnis pars.... Aristoteli anima corpus informat, ut ἐντελέχεια, non tantum assistit corpori." Rudolph Goclenius, *Lexicon philosophicum quo tanquam clave philosophiae fores aperiuntur* (Frankfurt am Main, 1613), 105b, s.v. "Anima." I owe this reference to Serjeantson, "The Soul," 124.

58 "Et harum consilium porpositumque & voluntas, caussa est: Consilij autem, appetitus, & finis ipsius consideratio. Caussam autem nunc intelligemus ipsius motus principium: quae caussa originis est & efficiens dicitur. Et hoc ipsum principium est hominis. Id est, ista constitutio est humanae naturae, secreta iam ab alijs naturis universis, id quod Cicero splendide & copiose pronuntiavit lib. De Legg. I. Animal hoc provisum, sagax, multiplex, acutum, memor, plenum rationis & consilij, quem vocamus hominem, praeclara quadam conditions generatum esse a supremo Deo. Solum est enim ex tot animantium generibus atque naturis particeps rationis & cogitationis, cum caetera sint omnia expertia. Itaque haec est notio propria hominis, Esse animal rationis particeps: id est ζῶον πολιτικὸν, non νοερόν. Etsi mens & intelligentia rationem quoque complectitur. Nam in vitae huius communitate, quae civilis est congregatio, prudentia consiliorum & in deliberando sagacitas, in primis spectari, & laudem celebritatemque praestantiae & dignitatis conciliare solet. Deliberationes autem suscipiuntur de rebus ijs de quibus consolutationes solent proponi: quae sunt προαιρετά." Joachim Camerarius, *Ethicorum Aristotelis Nicomachiorum explicatio acuratissima* (Frankfurt am Main, 1578), 262–3. Camerarius translates the passage in question thus: "Quam ob rem Consilium ac propositum, vel est mens cum appetitu, vel est appetitus cum cogitatione. Et huiusmodi principium quoddam hominem constituit." *Ethicorum*, 261.

> the supreme good must be suited to the entire man, not just to parts of him. Man is composed of a body and a soul; therefore, his supreme good must arise from a harmonious combination of all those things which are conducive to the perfection of his composite being.[59]

Here there is a closer fit with the Galenic medical conception of the subject as a functional body-soul composite.

The same can be said for the emphasis in mainstream humanistic moral and political thought on virtuous activity as centrally constitutive of human subjectivity. As is well known, humanist moralists and political theorists drew heavily upon Stoic ethics, especially the practical ethics of Cicero and Seneca, to propagate a thoroughly social vision of human flourishing.[60] In the typical accounts, the human being is said to be naturally suited to living with others in a community, the bonds of which are grounded upon a common participation in reason, and manifested in the moral virtues derived from the duties required of us by (rational) nature. This vision was integral to the justifications of political participation produced in the quattrocento by Leonardo Bruni and other Florentines identified by Hans Baron as "civic humanists," whose influence on later generations of European humanists has been much discussed by subsequent scholars of Renaissance political thought.[61]

But it is also possible to detect here a more flexible conception of individualized selfhood. Whilst being grounded upon a concept of universal nature, the Ciceronian identification of the human subject with the morally virtuous character also took account of the different capabilities of specific individuals, permitting the presentation of a diversity of *exempla* of ethical rectitude beyond the model of the ideally wise sage, and what appears to be a conception of individual moral selfhood.[62] According to

[59] Francesco Piccolomini, *Universa philosophia de moribus* (2nd edn, 1594), IX.12, trans. Jill Kraye, in *Cambridge Translations*, vol. I, p. 73.

[60] See Quentin Skinner, *The Foundations of Modern Political Thought* (Cambridge; Cambridge University Press, 1978), vol. I, pp. 88–109, 118–28, 236–62.

[61] Hans Baron, *The Crisis of the Early Italian Renaissance: Civic Humanism and Republican Liberty in an Age of Classicism and Tyranny* (rev. ed., Princeton: Princeton University Press, 1966); J. G. A. Pocock, *The Machiavellian Moment: Florentine Political Thought and the Atlantic Republican Tradition: With a new afterword by the author* (Princeton and Oxford: Princeton University Press, 2003); Skinner, *Foundations of Modern Political Thought* vol. I; *Renaissance Civic Humanism: Reappraisals and Reflections*, ed. James Hankins (Cambridge: Cambridge University Press, 2000).

[62] Cicero, *On Duties*, trans. Walter Miller (London: William Heinemann, 1913), I.46, pp. 50–51. See Sorabji, *Self*, 163–65, and David Sedley, "The Stoic-Platonist Debate on *kathêkonta*," in *Topics in Stoic Philosophy*, ed. Katerina Ierodiakonou (Oxford: Oxford University Press, 1999), 151–52.

Cicero in the *De officiis*—a key text for humanist ethics—nature also gives us a second, specific *persona*: each human being is endowed with a particular talent or set of talents, and so an individual *natura*.[63] Acting well in this life can then be seen not just as conforming to a universal rational standard, but more flexibly as akin to an actor being given a part that is well-suited to his capabilities and then choosing the best way of living up to that part. There is a moral *decorum* of character, which resembles the modern idea of being 'true to yourself.'[64] This conception of a self that is determined by its adherence to moral norms of nature which are grounded both in universal reason and the particular *persona* of the individual is also found in Seneca, who refers the stock question of whether to participate in public affairs to the question of whether such activity accords with the nature of the individual in question.[65]

Accordingly, the principle that different individuals have different needs and capabilities, and so may manifest different forms of moral virtue, became virtually a humanistic commonplace. Renaissance discussions of the relative merits of the active and contemplative lives, as Kristeller observed some time ago, were often concluded with the non-dogmatic acknowledgement that different individuals were suited to different forms of life.[66] As the Neoplatonist Cristoforo Landino suggested in his *Disputationes Camaldulenses* (1472), since both *otium* and *negotium* afforded humans the opportunity to exercise different varieties of excellence, the very best life—as the examples of prince Federico of Urbino, Lorenzo de'Medici and above all, Cicero illustrated—would be a combination of both.[67] With similar implications, in Juan Luis Vives's *Fabula de homine* (1518), Jupiter gives man a variety of parts in different plays in the

---

63 Cicero, *On Duties*, 1.107, 109–10, pp. 108–9, 112–13.

64 Cicero, *On Duties* 1.109–114, pp. 110–17; Sorabji, *Self*, 167.

65 Seneca, *De tranquillitate animi*, 6.1–7.2, in *Moral Essays*, trans. John W. Basore (Cambridge, Mass. and London: Harvard University Press, 1932), 234–37.

66 P. O. Kristeller, "The Active and the Contemplative Life in Renaissance Humanism," in *Studies in Renaissance Thought and Letters*, 4 vols (Rome: Edizioni di storia e letteratura, 1956–96), vol. 4, ch. 12, pp. 197–213, at 207, 210–11.

67 Cristoforo Landino, *Disputationes Camaldulenses*, ed. Peter Lohe (Florence, 1980), 7–8 (on Federico), 11 (on Lorenzo), 42–46 (on Cicero), and the conclusion as stated at p. 13: "Et quoniam id quaeris, ita de utroque vitae genere [*sc.* otium et negotium] disputandum censeo, ut primo singula seorsum prosequar, deinde ea ita inter se conferam, ut, quanvis in hac qua vivimus vita eum tum demum absolutissimum credamus, qui utrunque coniunxerit, tamen, utrum excellentius sit, in primis appareat." For discussion see Bruce G. McNair, "Cristoforo Landino and Coluccio Salutati on the Best Life," *Renaissance Quarterly* 47:4 (1994): 747–69.

theatrum mundi.[68] And according to Montaigne in his essay "De la solitude," the traditional discussion of the respective merits of contemplation and civic activity could only be resolved by taking the natural "complexions" of individuals (their humorally based psychological idiosyncrasies) into account. Some are more suited to activity, others—like Montaigne himself, a mixture of "le jovial et le melancholique, moyennement sanguine et chaude"[69]—to retirement.[70] As Montaigne's comment suggests, by differentiating the ethically appropriate social roles of individuals on the basis of their physiological temperaments and the activities of which they are thereby most capable, the visions of selfhood found in humanist moral writings could sometimes mesh quite closely with Galenic medical conceptions of the human subject.

Despite their substantial debts to pagan sources, it should go without saying that all of these figurations of human nature were Christianized to some extent. It is beyond the scope of this essay to address the complexity of the relationship between the classical and Christian traditions in this territory, and its transformation in the course of the Reformation and counter-Reformation; instead, I shall briefly indicate some of the distinctively Christian theological themes and concepts that are relevant to Renaissance medical psychology and particularly theories of melancholy.

If we are to follow the account of Charles Taylor, probably the most influential vision of selfhood in the Christian tradition was given by Augustine.[71] His elaboration of the interior spiritual domain as the locus both of the 'true self' and the voice of God within us, as we noted above, was built upon the Platonic conception of the psychic 'inner man,' and

[68] Juan Luis Vives, "A Fable about Man," trans. Nancy Lenkeith in *The Renaissance Philosophy of Man*, Ernst Cassirer et al. (Chicago: University of Chicago Press, 1948), 387–93, at 387–88.

[69] Montaigne, *Les Essais*, "De la presumption," 679. See M. A. Screech, *Montaigne and Melancholy: The Wisdom of the 'Essais'* (London: Duckworth, 1983).

[70] "Laissons à part cette longue comparison de la vie solitaire à l'active... Il y a des complexions plus propres à ces precepts de la retraite les unes que les autres. Celles qui ont l'apprehension molle et lasche, et un'affection et volonté delicate, et qui ne s'asservit et ne s'employe pas aysément, desquels je suis, et par naturelle condition et par discours, ils se plieront mieux à ce conseil, que les par tout, qui se passionnent de toutes choses: qui s'offrent, qui se presentent, et qui se donnent à toutes occasions." Montaigne, *Les Essais*, ed. Jean Balsamo, Michel Magnien, and Catherine Magnien-Simonin (Paris: Éditions Gallimard, 2007), I.38, pp. 241, 246–47.

[71] Taylor, *Sources of the Self*, 127–42. See also Brian Stock, *Augustine the Reader: Meditation, Self-Knowledge and the Ethics of Interpretation* (Cambridge, MA, and London: Harvard University Press/Belknap, 1996).

provided, according to Taylor, an account of psychic self-awareness and a "language of inwardness" that represented a "radically new doctrine of moral resources, one where the route to the higher passes within."[72] A language of this kind structures a large proportion of the moral theology and devotional literature of the middle ages and Renaissance, and in important strands of both the Catholic and Reformed traditions spiritual self-examination and self-knowledge were central goals of practical divinity. Here it is enough, perhaps, to recall such familiar and influential figures as Ignatius and William Perkins.[73]

There are numerous complications involved in the process of tracing the influence of Augustinian ideas about inwardness and their reconfiguration in later Christian notions of selfhood—not least those created by the doctrine of the resurrection of the body, which seems to require that the 'true' self should be understood as some kind of body-soul composite that persists in the afterlife.[74] But here I can simply note two of the more conspicuously Christian elements that penetrated Renaissance psychology and medicine via their medieval predecessors. The first is the tendency to ascribe a central role in the passage from cognition to action to the faculty of the will, that for Augustine is the power which after the Fall had become perverted, enslaved by sin, in need of fortification by divine grace, and so the crucial determinant of one's moral and spiritual character. The will had become fully integrated into the Aristotelian faculty psychology of the middle ages and Renaissance, as a rational appetite of the intellective soul working alongside intellect and memory. There had been long-running debates about its freedom, but also, and more pertinently here, about the respective primacy of the will or the intellect in the attainment of beatitude. For those in the Scotist tradition who held that the will was the rational power of the soul ultimately responsible for moving it towards or away from its highest good, it was therefore the central psychic component of moral and spiritual selfhood.[75]

---

72 Taylor, *Sources of the Self*, 139.

73 See, in general, Jean Delumeau, *Le catholicisme entre Luther et Voltaire* (Paris: PUF, 1971); id., *Le péché et la peur: la culpabilisation en Occident* (*XIII*^e^*–XVIII*^e^ *siècles*); and Daniel Andersson, *Closer to God: Practical Divinity and the Struggle for Mind, Body and Soul in Early Modern England* (forthcoming).

74 See Caroline W. Bynum, *The Resurrection of the Body in Western Christianity, 200–1336* (New York: Columbia University Press, 1995); Fernando Vidal, "Brains, Bodies, Selves, and Science: Anthropologies of Identity and the Resurrection of the Body," *Critical Inquiry* 28:4 (2002): 930–74, at 939–50.

75 For two opposed views, representing Thomist intellectualism and Scotist voluntarism respectively, see Coimbra Commentators, *In Libros Ethicorum Aristotelis Ad Nicomachum, Aliquot Conimbricensis cursus disputatione* (Lisbon, 1593), Disp. III, quaest. 3, art. 2,

The second (mostly) Christian concept that infiltrated Renaissance psychology is that of the conscience. This had frequently been bifurcated in medieval accounts into *synderesis*—the innate natural disposition to grasp the ethical premisses of natural and divine law—and *conscientia*—the process of reasoning on the basis of those premisses. Recent work has emphasized the subtle complexity of the early modern reception and transformation of this concept, not least in response to the confessionalization of religious politics in the sixteenth century,[76] but here it suffices to note the position of *synderesis* and *conscientia* within the orthodox Aristotelian psychology of this period. Typically, these powers were not identified as part of an ontologically separate faculty, but were designated as 'innate habits' of the rational power of the intellect. They are sometimes said to work in the manner of a 'practical syllogism' with three parts: *synderesis* proposes, the *dictamen rationis* applies, and the conscience concludes.[77] Together with the will, which they informed, the intellectual powers of *synderesis* and conscience therefore constituted the most important, distinctively spiritual components of moral selfhood.

V

Turning now to melancholy, with a view to arriving at the features of the 'melancholic subject': how did the Renaissance understanding of this condition relate to these schemes of selfhood and forms of subjectivity—medical and non-medical? As has been the case throughout this essay,

and John Case, *Speculum questionum moralium in universam Aristotelis philosophi summi Ethicen* (Frankfurt am Main, 1594), X.7; both are translated in Kraye, ed., *Cambridge Translations*, vol. I, pp. 62, 83. On the importance of the will in Italian humanist views of human nature, see Trinkaus, *In Our Image and Likeness*, vol. 1, pp. 51ff.

[76] Brian Cummings, "Conscience and the Law in Thomas More," *Renaissance Studies* 23:4 (2009), 465–85; Lawrence Witchel, *Casuistry in Seventeenth-Century England: English Protestant Casuistry, Conscience, and Oath-Taking* (Saarbrücken: VDM Verlag, 2009); and, more generally, Douglas C. Langston, *Conscience and Other Virtues, from Bonaventure to MacIntyre* (University Park, PA: Pennsylvania State University Press, 2001).

[77] On the practical syllogism, see Aristotle, *Nicomachean Ethics* VII.3.6–14, 1146b35–1147b19, pp. 388–95, where it is discussed in relation to failures of self-restraint in conditions of madness, drunkenness, and sleep. For a useful summary of its position in Renaissance psychology see Burton, *Anatomy of Melancholy*, 1.1.2.10, vol. 1, pp. 158–59. See also William Perkins, *A Discourse of Conscience, wherein is set downe the Nature, Properties, and Differences Thereof: as also the way to get and keepe good conscience* (Cambridge, 1596), I, pp. 1–5, and 83–86.

I shall offer a general outline and downplay variations across time and space, though it is a well-known feature of the orthodox learned theory of melancholy from the middle ages until the late Renaissance that it was static in many of its fundamental aspects. Well into the seventeenth century, this theory was continually being refined, rather than transformed, by engagements with a number of key ancient texts—mainly the Hippocratic *Aphorisms* and *Epidemics*, and Galen's *De locis affectis* and *De symptomatum causis*.[78] Here I shall be referring mainly to works on melancholy from the later decades of the sixteenth and early decades of the seventeenth centuries, a period when the Galenic medical theory of the condition was being elaborated with a degree of detail that was unprecedented; but the conceptual continuities with earlier medical writings mean that most of my suggestions also hold for the earlier Renaissance.

In the first place, locating the melancholic subject within the functional model of Galenic physiology depends on the fundamental characterization of the condition as one of pathological 'depravation.' In the disease of melancholy, we are told by a host of Renaissance Galenists, some of the somatic and (more importantly) psychological functions of the organism are characterized by a condition of *depravatio*, corruption or perversion from their healthy or naturally functioning state. The material cause of this *depravatio* was typically identified as an excess or corruption of the humour black bile, which as well as upsetting the mixture of particular bodily parts, was thought to affect the spirits and thereby the psychic faculties in the brain. From this process follows the set of familiar melancholic symptoms: apparently groundless emotions of fear and sadness, as well as anxiety, delusions, and hallucinations. This is the basic structure of accounts of the melancholic disease as well as those of the technically healthy melancholic complexion.

Although in the Galenic account black bile was thought to accumulate pathogenically in one of three places—the head, the whole body, or the hypochondrium, giving rise to three distinct subspecies of the disease—it is crucial to emphasize that in each case the part primarily affected, whose functions are 'depraved,' was the brain. The vast majority of learned

[78] For a summary of Renaissance medical teachings on melancholy, viewed through the prism of Burton's *Anatomy of Melancholy*, see Gowland, *Worlds of Renaissance Melancholy*, 33–97.

physicians in the Renaissance followed Galen in this respect.[79] As Girolamo Capo di Vacca, professor of medicine at Padua, put it in his *Practica medicina* (1594), melancholy is defined as "the principal dysfunction of the anterior [ventricle of the] brain, accompanied by fear and sadness, and deriving from a gloomy disposition."[80] Others, such as the Portuguese Jewish physician Eliau Montalto, argued that the heart was affected, as it was the physiological seat of the passionate symptoms of melancholy—but this was in addition to the principal affection of the brain.[81] Bodily symptoms such as sleeplessness, lethargy, and the darkening of the skin were of course also significant, but the psychology of these medical accounts was ultimately more important in determining contemporary conceptions of melancholic experience.[82]

If melancholy was theorized as principally a cerebral condition, albeit one with a host of somatic symptoms, which faculty or faculties of soul in the brain were considered to be dysfunctional? Here again Galen's authority was cited, particularly his explanation in *De symptomatum causis* II. 7. 2 that the conspicuously irrational fear and despondency of melancholics is caused by the darkness of black bile, which by "taking possession of the power of the rational soul," generates fear in the same manner as external darkness.[83] Also important was the discussion of melancholy in the *De locis affectis*, where the emotional symptoms of the condition are said to be caused by the ascent of humoral evaporations through the body to the brain ("the colour of the black bile, casting shadow over the seat of the

[79] Galen, *Omnia tum quae antehac extabant, tum quae nunc primum inventa sunt, Opera in Latinam conversa*, ed. Conrad Gessner, 4 vols (Lyon, 1550), II, cols. 232, 886). See *De locis affectis*, III. 6. 10, *De symptomatum causis*, II. 7. 1.

[80] "delirium melancholicum est functio corrupta principalis, cum timore & moerore, cerebri anterioris, dependens ab affectione tenebricosa." Girolamo Capo di Vacca, *Practica medicina* (Frankfurt, 1594), I. 10, p. 94. See, similarly, Du Laurens, *A Discourse*, 91 (*Discours*, 123r).

[81] Eliau Montalto, *Archipathologia in qua internarum capitis affectionum essentia, causae, signa, praesagia, & curatio accuratissima indagine edisseruntur* (Lyon, 1614), IV. 3, pp. 228–29. Ercole Sassonia was unusual in refraining from identifying the brain as the primarily affected part, implying this question depended on the somatic location of the preponderance of black bile (brain, whole body, or hypochondrium); see *De melancholia*, in *Opera practica* (Padua, 1639), 26a.

[82] Cf., for example, the relative lengths of the accounts of general somatic and mental symptoms given in Burton, *Anatomy*, 1.3.1.1–2, vol. 1, pp. 381–96.

[83] Galen, *De symptomatum causis*, II. 7. 2, in *Galen: On Diseases and Symptoms*, trans. Ian Johnston (Cambridge: Cambridge University Press, 2008), 264 (translation slightly modified).

mind, creates fear").[84] In both works, however, Galen argued further that whilst inducing groundless passions, the dark humour and its vapours in the brain also induce "false imaginings" and hallucinatory derangements, as well as suicidal impulses.[85] Renaissance physicians commonly inferred from these arguments that melancholy involved the depravation of the soul's rational faculties, specifically the imagination (hence the hallucinations), and sometimes also the intellect (hence the extreme passions and suicides).[86] Capo di Vacca, who as we have seen identified the anterior ventricle of the brain as the affected part, also states that rational intellect in the middle ventricle can be simultaneously (if temporarily) affected.[87] For Montalto, the emotional and hallucinatory symptoms of melancholy originated in faulty cognition—melancholics were irrationally fearful and sad about things, because their rational faculty did not overrule their crazed fantasies—which meant for him that reason and imagination were both depraved in the disease.[88] This position was reiterated at greater length with reference to Aristotle's *De anima* in the early seventeenth century by the Paduan professor Ercole Sassonia, in his *De melancholia* of 1620.[89]

To summarize the description of the melancholic in these texts, then: the melancholic is primarily constituted in psychological terms as a person whose rational faculties of imagination and intellect are dysfunctional, on account of the effects of black bile or its vapours upon the brain, with the result that he or she suffers extreme emotional perturbations. Indeed, one of the distinctive features of the later Renaissance theory of the disease can be found in the detailed elaboration of the relationships between the melancholic humour and its vapours, the animal spirits, and the deranged phantasms of the imagination.[90] All the authors

---

84 "atrae bilis color, mentis sedem tenebris similem reddens, timorem efficit." Galen, *Opera*, ed. Gessner, col. 890. He is referring here to those suffering from the inflammation of melancholic humours in the hypochondrium.

85 Galen, *Opera*, ed. Gessner, cols 889–90.

86 See, for instance, Galen, *Aliquot opera ... De Inaequali intemperie Liber I. De Differentiis & causis morborum, symptomatumque Libri VI. De Iudiciis Libri III. De Curatione per sanguinis missionem Liber I*, trans. and comm. Leonhart Fuchs (Paris, 1549[?]–1555), 138–39; Giambattista Da Monte, *Consilia medica* (Nürnberg, 1559), consil. XVI, XIX, XVIII.

87 Capo di Vacca, *Practica medicina*, I. 10, p. 94.

88 Montalto, *Archipathologia*, IV. 3, pp. 224–30.

89 Ercole Sassonia, *De melancholia*, pp. 5a–7b.

90 I discuss this in more detail in "Melancholy, Imagination, and Dreaming in Renaissance Learning," in *Diseases of the Imagination in Early Modern Europe*, ed. Yasmin Haskell (Turnhout: Brepols, 2011), 53–102. For a discussion of the effects of melancholy on the power of memory, see Markus Bauer, "Melancholie und Memoria: Zur Theorie von

mentioned above concerned themselves with the effects of corrupted spirits in the brain—which generate what Capo di Vacca identified as "shadowy phantasms"[91]—and theorized a direct relationship between the qualities of these spirits and the resultant psychological derangement. Most obviously, as Montalto noted, dark and murky spirits generated terrifying sense-images, which was "the most powerful reason why melancholics are never without fear or despondency, because the black humor, the cause of the disease, infuses the seat of the rational soul with perpetual night."[92] Ercole gave an extensive account of the diverse effects of corrupted spirits upon the melancholic imagination, explaining the means by which the qualities of coldness, heat, gloominess, dilation, contraction, disordered motion, motion "against nature," and the imprinting of humoral sense-species upon the spirits, create particular imaginative derangements. If the cold and moist phlegm is involved, for example, a melancholic might suffer the delusion that he is made out of snow; if the animal spirits are gloomy, he is fearful and sad, but also habitually loves solitude and obscure places, imagines death, the dead, devils, and other dark objects.[93] Perhaps most suggestive for the concerns of this essay are imaginative depravations that were self-delusions about one's physical qualities and characteristics. "One thinkes himselfe a giant," wrote Burton, "another a dwarfe; one is heavy as lead, another is as light as a feather... Another thinkes himselfe so little, that he can creepe into a mousehole: one feares heaven will fall on his head: a second is a cock.... A Baker in *Ferrara*... thought he was composed of butter, and durst not sit in the sunne, or come neere the fire for feare of being melted." Such examples were frequently recycled in Renaissance medical texts.[94]

Gedächtnisschwund und fixer Idee im 17. Jahrhundert," in *Ars memorativa: zur kulturgeschichtlichen Bedeutung der Gedächtniskunst, 1400–1750*, ed. Jörg Jochen Berns and Wolfgang Neuber (Tübingen: Niemeyer, 1993), 313–30.

91 Capo di Vacca, *Practica medicina*, I. 10, pp. 94–95.

92 "Haec potissima causa est, quare melancholicos timor, ac moeror nunquam deserant, quia nempe ater humor, passionis materia, animae rationalis domicilio perpetuam offundit noctem." Montalto, *Archipathologia*, IV. 7, pp. 242–3, quote at p. 243.

93 Ercole Sassonia, *De melancholia*, 12b, 17a–20a, 28b–29a.

94 Burton, *Anatomy*, 1.3.1.4, p. 402. For a discussion of the common melancholic delusion of being made of glass, see Gill Speak, "An Odd Kind of Melancholy: Reflections on the Glass Delusion in Europe (1440–1680)," *History of Psychiatry* 1 (1990): 191–206.

VI

We can now address some of the ways in which this medical psychology of melancholy relates to non-medical conceptions of selfhood. To recap: if the subject, in the terms of Galenic medicine, is a functional body-soul composite, whose activities and experience of health or sickness are dependent upon the humoral mixture, then the specifically melancholic subject is one that is functionally corrupt—more particularly, it is a subject with powers that are radically vitiated. Or in Aristotelian terms, the melancholic subject is one whose natural human potentialities, particularly his or her capacities as a 'rational animal,' are imperfectly actualized. What are the implications of this for the melancholic's moral selfhood? To the extent that the melancholic is afflicted by extreme and irrational passions, his or her experience is constituted as a vicious one in which the capacity to actualize one's potential excellence as a human being is seriously hindered; remedying this is sometimes said to be a matter for ethics or divinity rather than medicine,[95] but beyond this there is little discussion of melancholy in the higher echelons of Renaissance moral philosophy.

What little there is, however, occurs principally within the Aristotelian or Stoic traditions.[96] In the first, which clusters around Aristotle's discussion of ἀκρασία ('bad mixture') in the seventh book of the *Ethics*, temperamental melancholics are described as impulsive people who do not rationally deliberate, but follow their imaginations and are subject to intense desires (VII.7.8, 10.3–4, 14.5–6). These passages were related to the Galenic understanding of melancholy by Renaissance commentators such as Acciaiuoli, Pietro Vettori, and Jacques Lefevre D'Étaples. Whilst Aristotle had specified that melancholics were only partially vicious, and not unjust—they did not deliberately harm others, and were easily corrected (V.10.3–4)—they were nevertheless seen to be morally impaired in that they were indisciplined, and prone to imaginative derangement and excessive passions.[97] Given that on one reading at least (following VI.2.5) the exercise of deliberate choice is what defines the human for Aristotle,[98]

[95] As in Du Laurens, *A Discourse*, 81 (*Discours*, 109r).

[96] For an outline, see Gowland, "The Ethics of Renaissance Melancholy," *Intellectual History Review* 18 (2008): 103–17.

[97] Gowland, "The Ethics of Renaissance Melancholy," 104–106.

[98] Cf. Aristotle, *Nicomachean Ethics* VII.10, 1152a17–19, where it is made clear that the ongoing discussion of ἀκρασία pertains to those who do not properly engage in deliberate choice (προαίρεσις).

its pathological absence in the melancholic subject, which is noted by Du Laurens,[99] would imply that in this Aristotelian view the moral selfhood of the melancholic was vitiated in a radical sense.

A similar picture emerges when we consider Stoically influenced moral writing. From this perspective, the solitary sadness of the melancholic could represent either a vicious deviation from the natural duty of the self to participate in public affairs, or a threat to the moral *persona* of the philosopher, in which the pursuit of wisdom required the soul's movements to be in accordance with right reason. For Burton, human beings "are all brethren in Christ, or at least should be, members of one body," bound together in a community by natural virtue and charity; but the melancholic man is typically "unwilling to undertake any office" and unsociable, loving solitude and exhibiting a host of misanthropic vices.[100] Even if (following the Neoplatonic theory of Ficino) solitary melancholics can be "of a deepe reach" and "excellent apprehension" in philosophy, their judgement is unreliable, "profound ... in some things, although in others, *non recte judicant inquieti*.... They count honesty, dishonesty, friends as enimies," and "many of them" are "desperate harebraines, rash, carelesse, fit to be Assasinates."[101] For Du Laurens, the dysfunctioning of the melancholic's depraved imagination and reason represents the degradation of faculties "which extol and advance man, above all other living creatures," representing his divine excellence, justifying his governance of the world, and "which give him the title of a sociable and politike living creature."[102] But this corruption is also mirrored in the manner in which the melancholic lives, as a "savadge creature, haunting the shadowed places, suspicious, solitarie, enemie to the Sunne, and one whom nothing can please, but onely discontentment." Du Laurens makes the implications for the moral selfhood of the melancholic clear, inviting his readers to "iudge and weigh if the titles which I have heretofore given to man, calling him a divine and politique creature, can any way agree with the melancholike person."[103] The melancholic subject here is less than human.

[99] "I will adde also that one thing which *Aristotle* mentioneth in his Ethickes, as that they love change of things, and for this cause are not so fit for consulations of great importance." Du Laurens, *A Discourse*, 85 (*Discours*, 115r).

[100] Burton, *Anatomy*, 1.1.1.1., vol. 1, p. 126; 1.3.1.2, vol. 1, pp. 394–95; 3.1.3.1, vol. 3, pp. 29–33. On Burton's Stoicism see 11–15, 166–69, 227–30, 271–75, 281–85.

[101] Burton, *Anatomy*, 1.3.1.2, vol. 1, pp. 391–92.

[102] Du Laurens, *A Discourse*, 73, 80 (*Discours*, 99v–100r, 107v–108r).

[103] Du Laurens, *A Discourse*, 82 (*Discours*, 110v).

What of the melancholic's spiritual experience? Here we can point first to the high degree of interchangeability between moral vice and spiritual sinfulness in many moral-theological works, but also to a number of spiritual concepts that were absorbed into the symptomatology in Renaissance medical accounts—for example, the physical symptom of lethargy, which represents the absorption of the patristic concept of *acedia*, sloth, into Galenic medical doctrine.[104] But in terms of the psychological account I have been focusing on here, insofar as the melancholic is chronically sad, fearful, and generally unable to govern his passions, in the final, moral-spiritual, analysis it is the rational intellectual faculty of the will that is most at fault. Learned medical authors are generally uninterested in this, but it is clearly expressed more popular works, such as Burton's *Anatomy*, where melancholy, like every disease, is said to originate in the sin of Adam,[105] and where it is explained in detail that "once," before the Fall, our sensitive appetites—our emotions—were "well agreeing with reason," but "now," after the Fall, we have a "depraved will," so that "*Reason* is over borne by *Passion*.... And thence come all those head-strong Passions, violent perturbations of the Minde."[106] The novel account of the specifically religious form of the disease in the third Partition of the *Anatomy* also fleshes out the spiritual dimension of particular kinds of melancholic experience. Here, the *synderesis* and the conscience, acting by means of the 'practical syllogism' prominent in Calvinist casuistry, are identified as the "greatest cause" of spiritual despair, and depicted as "a thousand witnesses to accuse us" that effects a "deepe apprehension" of our "unworthinesse."[107] In the last Subsection of the work, Burton explores the manner in which the "cauterized consciences" of religious melancholics express faulty reasoning,[108] as a result of their "distempered phantasies," or perhaps demonic interference. Despairing thoughts may well, he says,

104 The classic account is Siegfried Wenzel, *The Sin of Sloth: Acedia in Medieval Thought and Literature* (Chapel Hill: University of North Carolina Press, 1967). See also Noel Brann, "Is Acedia Melancholy? A Re-examination of this question in the light of Fra Battista da Crema's *Della cognitione et vittoria di se stesso* (1531)," *Journal of the History of Medicine and Allied Sciences* 34 (1979): 180–99.

105 Burton, *Anatomy*, 1.1.1.1, vol. 1, pp. 121–28.

106 Burton, *Anatomy*, 1.1.2.11, vol. 1, pp. 160–61.

107 As I have claimed elsewhere, this is developed by Burton into a critique of contemporary Calvinism, and it represents the striking manner in which religious concerns not only came progressively to infiltrate medical orthodoxy after the Reformation, but also, in the hands of some authors, to effect its politicization. Gowland, *Worlds of Renaissance Melancholy*, 139–204.

108 Burton, *Anatomy*, III, p. 429.

"proceed [...] from a crazed phantasie, distempered humours, [or] blacke fumes which offend [the] braine [...]."[109] Here we can see the meshing of the Galenic medical and spiritual discourse; the melancholic experience is simultaneously one of psychic dysfunction and spiritual malaise. The melancholic appears to be, spiritually speaking, 'all too human.'

Finally, we can return briefly to the widely shared idea that the 'true' core of the self, or the 'inner' self, is the reason or intellect. As I noted above, to the extent that melancholics are said to have a damaged intellectual faculty, this clearly implies that from a Neoplatonic point of view, their selfhood—what is essentially and individually their own—is seriously impaired. This brings us to a paradox in the Platonic conception of the self, since it was this faculty of the soul, the intellect, that was considered to be divine rather than human, and in this sense represents a self that is to some extent de-individuated, and part of God.[110] And it is this paradox that is most clearly expressed in Marsilio Ficino's influential doctrine of genial melancholy, elaborated first in his *Theologia Platonica* (1482) and later in his *De vita libri tres* (1489), and found reverberating throughout Renaissance medical writing on the disease.[111] For Ficino, when the conjunction of humoral physiology and astral movements produces not melancholic disease but melancholic genius—bringing powers of prophecy, philosophical insight, poetic creativity and so on—this is not presented as a fulfilment of the human self's rational-intellectual capacities, or even an enhancement of these capacities. It is precisely the opposite, a condition of divine fury, an inspired state of self-alienation. It is, in Ficino's terms, a form of *vacatio*, an 'emptying' out of the self, when the rational soul loses its attachment to the body and is "seized by the divinity"[112]—and so a 'release' of the ensouled self from its human bodily prison so that it is free to reunite itself with God. In those moments of rapture, the melancholic does not have a human self, and in that sense, is no longer human.

---

109 Burton, *Anatomy*, 3.4.2.6, vol. 3, p. 433.

110 Sorabji, *Self*, 115–36. This is also the case for certain interpretations of Aristotelian ethics, e.g. by John Case (Kraye, *Cambridge Translations*, vol. I, pp. 60–66) and the Coimbra Commentators (*ibid.*, 81–5). Obviously I cannot discuss the topic of the immortality of the soul, and Averroist controversies concerning the shared intellect here.

111 On Ficino's legacy in the Italian Renaissance, see Noel L. Brann, *The Debate over the Origin of Genius During the Italian Renaissance* (Leiden and Boston: Brill, 2002).

112 Marisilio Ficino, *Platonic Theology*, trans. M. J. B. Allen, ed. James Hankins (Cambridge, Mass. and London: Harvard University Press, 2001–6), 6 vols, XIII.2, at vol. 4, pp. 162–63.

VII

As we have seen, the relationships charted here between philosophical conceptions of the self and Galenic medical theory are in some respects implicit and speculative. It is rare to find learned physicians theorizing such relationships explicitly, and the division between the learned cultures of medicine, moral philosophy and theology in this era—rooted in the separate organization of university faculties—tended to discourage sustained or detailed inquiries of this nature. However, we have also seen that in certain cases it is possible to discern awareness of significant connections between philosophical conceptions of the self, Galenic constructions of subjectivity, and theories of melancholy, and to draw out some of the implications of such connections for an understanding of the melancholic subject.

Before ending with a suggestion about how such implications can be brought together, we can make a number of general observations about the nature of the subjectivity on display here. First, there is virtually nothing in the medical writing that resembles a language of interiority. It is true that melancholics are often said to have a complex inner life, being described as anxious, consumed with self-hatred, subject to peculiar emotional experiences such as the bittersweet *voluptas dolendi*,[113] and with their gaze habitually turned inwards (Burton calls this distinctive form of painful self-relation "melancholizing").[114] But in medical texts such characteristics are simply identified and classified as pathological symptoms that are caused by dysfunctions or corruptions of specific psychic powers. Beyond that, except in one or two unusual cases that incorporate poetic quotations, learned medical discourse just does not go. Unsurprisingly, physicians eschew the exploration of emotional interiority as a matter of course, ceding that ground to contemporary spiritual and literary-poetic discourse.[115]

---

[113] See Petrarch, *De remediis utriusque fortunae libri II* (Lyon, 1577), II.xciii, p. 732; Burton, *Anatomy*, I, lxix–lxxi. For a Foucauldian reading of Petrarchan interiority see Strozier, *Foucault, Subjectivity, and Identity*, 175–208.

[114] Burton, *Anatomy*, 2.2.6.2, II, p. 107.

[115] A partial exception to this judgment is Jacques Ferrand, *De la maladie d'amour eou melancholie erotique* (Paris, 1623), the second, expanded, and more humanistic edition of the same author's *Traicté de l'essence et guérison de l'amour ou melancholie erotique* (Toulouse, 1610)—a work by a professional physician that contains an unusual quantity of literary quotations and allusions.

Second, and for closely related reasons, there is no clearly individuated figuration of melancholic selfhood in this medical discourse. Although Galenic physicians routinely acknowledge the importance of tailoring their knowledge to the individual patient, and frequently discuss the case-histories of melancholic individuals—as in Pieter van Foreest's *Observationes et curationes* (first edition 1588)[116]—there is no properly individualized melancholic 'self' in these texts. Melancholics have their own biographies, but *qua* melancholics they are subjects, constituted by reference to general symptomatological schemes, and the narratives of their case-histories (again, hardly surprisingly) are conducted in order to extract diagnostic or therapeutic knowledge that will be either universalizable, or applicable to other patients. In Renaissance medical works—and here there is a notable contrast with the Calvinist autobiographies that were common in seventeenth-century England[117]—biographical information that would be intrinsic to the selfhood of the individual patient in the case history is by definition extrinsic to the concern of the physician, who has to treat many patients. What occurs in these texts is the discursive construction of a more or less generalizable melancholic subjectivity, constituted primarily in terms of patterns of related causes and symptoms. These are considered, by implication, to structure the pathological experience of each individual sufferer.

Nevertheless, as the medical works quoted at the beginning of this essay suggest, Renaissance authors did perceive in melancholy, particularly in its symptoms and their causes, a condition that affected the sufferer's sense of him- or herself, in ways that went to the core of what it was to be a human being. The diseased melancholic subject, as we have seen, was constituted in Galenic terms as one whose rational faculties were radically dysfunctional. That melancholic subjectivity, as we have also seen, was elaborated in relation to some of the key vectors of selfhood in the dominant strains of contemporary moral philosophy and spiritual discourse: reason, intellect and will; imagination and passion; contemplation and activity; and, drawing upon all of these, conceptions of the divine or human nature of man and his faculties. These aspects of melancholic subjectivity suggest that from the point of view of Renaissance learning, to experience the disease of melancholy was to experience the duality of the

---

[116] Pieter van Foreest, *Observationum et curationum medicinalium ac chirurgicarum opera omnia quatuor tomis digesta* (Rouen, 1653), bk. X.

[117] See Katherine Hodgkin, *Madness in Seventeenth-Century Autobiography* (Houndmills and New York: Palgrave Macmillan, 2007).

human condition: to be psychically, morally, and spiritually impeded or corrupt, and encapsulate the fallen nature of man—to have a self that is radically imperfect; but also still to be a divine creation, capable of receiving grace, and in certain conditions perhaps—to be able to transcend that radically imperfect human self and reunite, as pure soul, with God.[118]

[118] On the duality of Renaissance theories of human nature see Trinkaus, *In Our Image and Likeness*, and id., *Adversity's Noblemen: The Italian Humanists on Happiness* (New York: Columbia University Press, 1940). It is nicely expressed in relation to the melancholic complexion by Walkington: 'The melancholick man is said of the wise to be *aut Deus aut Daemon*, either angel of heaven or a fiend of hell: for in whomsoever this humour hath dominion, the soule is either wrapt up into an *Elysium* and paradise of blesse by a heavenly contemplation, or into a direfull hellish purgatory by a cynicall meditation." *Optick glasse*, 64.

MUSIC AND SPIRIT IN EARLY MODERN THOUGHT

Penelope Gouk

The relationship between music and spirit in the early modern period is essentially to do with health and well-being. For as Henry Peacham observed in his *Compleat Gentleman* (1622): "The Physitians will tell you, that the exercise of Musicke is a great lengthener of the life, by stirring and reviving of the spirits, holding a secret sympathy with them..."[1] As I will show in this essay, the belief that music's sympathetic action on the spirit could restore and maintain well-being was remarkably enduring, my examples of this belief spanning the fifteenth to the eighteenth centuries. It was also held throughout this period that music was particularly useful as a cure for melancholy, a disease to which scholars were especially prone.[2]

Both these ideas were embedded within a conceptual framework where health was regarded as a proper balance between the bodily humours as well as a harmony between the body and soul, either of which could be disturbed by a variety of external factors that resulted in disease. The physician's role was to diagnose the imbalances that his patient suffered from (for example, melancholy was due to an excess of black bile or choler in the blood) and to prescribe appropriate changes in diet and exercise to counteract their ill effects.[3] Although it might seem surprising, we have very little documentary evidence of physicians suggesting that their patients should listen to music.[4] However there are indications that even without

[1] Henry Peacham, *The Compleat Gentleman* (London, 1622), 97. I owe this reference to Tom Dixon.

[2] Music is briefly noted as a remedy on pp. 40–41 of Timothy Bright's *Treatise of Melancholie* (London, 1586), the earliest English text on this affliction. Robert Burton's *Anatomy of Melancholy* (Oxford, 1621) also contains a section on "Music a Remedy," in which he details its effects.

[3] For further discussion of the physiological mechanisms underpinning melancholy and its cure see Penelope Gouk, "Music, Melancholy and Medical Spirits in Early Modern Thought," in *Music as Medicine: The History of Music Therapy since Antiquity*, ed. Peregrine Horden (Guilford: Ashgate, 2000), 173–94.

[4] The examples most often cited date from the early eighteenth century and involved two patients suffering with fevers finding relief through music. These cases were discussed in "Observation sur un musicien guéri d'une fièvre avec délire par la musique," *Histoire de l'Académie Royale des Sciences, anneé 1707* (Paris, 1730), 7–8 and "Observation sur une

the recommendation of a physician early modern individuals consciously used music as a remedy for melancholy, especially lovesickness.[5]

My reason for exploring the links between music and spirit stems from an interest in early modern understandings of what we would now call music's emotional effects and their relevance to health. Chiefly following Aristotle, the nature of sound and music were topics traditionally treated in the context of the soul, which unlike today was identified as an important subject of natural philosophical and also medical enquiry, as well as being central to moral philosophy and theology.[6] This was because the soul was thought to play an essential role in all physical and mental actions including sense perception and motor activity, motions that were mediated by the spirit or what was often called the sensitive soul.[7] It is also important to realize that during this period the emotions were generally called the passions or affections, and were thought of as actions of the soul that lie midway between acts of reason and acts of the senses. It was a subject which seemed to receive renewed attention from the early seventeenth century, the most influential work on this topic probably being Descartes's *Les passions de l'âme,* first published in 1649 and translated into English a year later. An earlier English example of this genre is the Jesuit Thomas Wright's *The Passions of the Minde* (1604), in which he explains that "those actions then which are common with us, and beastes, wee call Passions, and Affections, or perturbations of the mind."[8] If the passions are not moderated according to reason the soul is afflicted with some

fièvre violente et délire guéris par la musique," *Histoire de l'Académie Royale des Sciences, anneé 1708* (Paris, 1730), 22–23. For Brocklesby's discussion of a musical cure for grief, see below.

[5] In the early seventeenth century a servant from Somerset wrote to one of his master's friends about a visit, asking him to bring a particular musician with him "to drive off Melancholly." See Christopher Marsh, *Music and Society in Early Modern England* (Cambridge: Cambridge University Press, 2010), 66. On self-help in the case of lovesickness see Linda Phyllis Austern, "Musical Treatments for Lovesickness: The Early Modern Heritage," in *Music as Medicine*, ed. Horden, 213–45.

[6] On the medieval background, see Charles Burnett, "Sound and its Perception in the Middle Ages," in *The Second Sense: Studies in Hearing and Musical Judgement from Antiquity to the Seventeenth Century*, ed. Charles Burnett, Michael Fend and Penelope Gouk (London: The Warburg Institute, 1991), 43–69.

[7] A fuller discussion of the sensitive soul and its faculties is found in Katherine S. Park, "The Organic Soul," in *The Cambridge History of Renaissance Philosophy*, ed. C. B. Schmitt and Quentin Skinner (Cambridge: Cambridge University Press, 1988), 464–84.

[8] Thomas Wright, *The Passions of the Minde in Generall* (2nd ed. n.p., 1604), 7. For an introduction to the passions, see Thomas Dixon, *From Passions to Emotions: The Creation of a Secular Psychological Category* (Cambridge: Cambridge University Press, 2003).

malady. But these stirrings in the mind also alter the humours, hence it is not only physicians of the soul who need to understand their effects but also physicians of the body.

So far I have been using the word spirit (and spirits) as though its meaning is self-evident. But what does 'spirit' actually signify, derived as it is from the Latin *spiritus*? Just like today, in early modern times the term was used in a variety of contexts and with a range of different and even conflicting meanings. For example, at one extreme it could denote an alcoholic liquid which had gone through the process of distillation. At the other end of the spectrum it could signify a wholly incorporeal entity such as the Holy Spirit, an invisible demon, the animating principle in man and animals (*spiritus* or *pneuma*, the breath of life), or the soul at the moment of death.[9] But spirit also referred to various vaporous substances that mediated between matter and non-matter, and this mediating role is especially clear for the kind of spirit that I propose to concentrate on here. This, or rather these, were the subtle, highly refined substances or fluids (distinguished as natural, vital, and animal) which permeated the blood and bodily organs and linked body and soul, and which were known as the medical spirits.[10] However, it is significant that the medical spirits were often associated with some of the other kinds of spirit I have already mentioned. For example, there was always the implication that the universal manifestation of spirit—the spirit of the Lord or the Holy Spirit—acted on individuals via the medical spirits to cultivate the 'spirit within.' Also, as we will see, there tended to be 'contamination' between the medical spirits and the spirit of nature or world soul which was a feature of Stoic and then Neoplatonic philosophy, an essentially magical doctrine within which both music and spirit had an important role to play.[11]

Despite the implied promise that I will deal generally with the early modern period, in fact this paper will concentrate on the work of four authors, three of them English, of whom two were writing in the early

[9] See for example the entries for 'spirit' in the *Oxford English Dictionary Online*, http://dictionary.oed.com/.

[10] Although most physicians followed Galenic tradition in adopting this tripartite division it is notable that Timothy Bright, for example, insisted that it was a distinction of "diverse offices of one spirit," rather than a real diversity in nature. See his *Treatise of Melancholie*, 43.

[11] D. P. Walker, "Medical Spirits in Philosophy and Theology from Ficino to Newton," *Arts du Spectacle et Histoire des Idées* (Tours: Centre d'Etudes Supérieures de la Renaissance, 1984), 287–300.

seventeenth century. The rationale behind my selection is a desire to highlight some striking similarities, if not continuities, in thinking about music and spirit that can be traced across nearly three centuries, and which also have their precedents in antiquity.[12] As I have just suggested, one source for some similarities that I have found is their roots in Platonic or Neoplatonic philosophy, elements of which can be found for example in the writings of Richard Brocklesby, an eighteenth-century London physician who published a short philosophical treatise on the application of music to disease in 1749.[13] Including Brocklesby allows me to reject the conventional idea that 1700 is a natural cut-off point for the early modern period. At the same time he conveniently harks back to the earliest author whose work I am considering here, the late-fifteenth-century Florentine philosopher and priest Marsilio Ficino. Thus for example Brocklesby explicitly cites Ficino's *Commentary on Plato* to support a discussion of mental disorders and his claim that music composes the motion of both the animal spirits and the mind.[14] Ficino's extensive editions of and commentaries on Plato and his followers were chiefly responsible for the dissemination of Neoplatonic philosophy across Europe, especially after the publication of his *Opera omnia* in 1576. However, the text to which I shall pay most attention is Ficino's *De vita libri tres* or *Three Books on Life* (1489), a work which proved to be a starting point for many later discussions of melancholy, including how to use music as a therapeutic tool.[15]

This leads us to my next two authors who come after Ficino chronologically, the Jesuit priest Thomas Wright whose *Passions of the Minde* (at least the expanded 2nd edition of 1604) contains a chapter on music's effects, and Francis Bacon, his importance here being that he envisaged a new kind of experimental philosophy in which the nature of music's

---

[12] I make a similar claim in my essay "Raising Spirits and Restoring Souls: Early Modern Explanations for Music's Effects," in *Hearing Cultures: Essays on Sound, Listening and Modernity*, ed. Veit Erlmann (Oxford and New York: Berg, 2004), 87–105.

[13] Richard Brocklesby, *Reflections on antient and modern musick, with the application to the cure of diseases. To which is subjoined, an essay to solve the question wherein consisted the difference of antient musick, from that of modern times* (London, 1749). In fact the first English text devoted to music's medicinal effects was the apothecary Richard Browne's *Medicina Musica: Or, A Mechanical Essay on the Effects of Singing, Musick, and Dancing.* [*Containing their uses and abuses, and demonstrating by clear and evident reasons, the alterations they produce in a human body*] (London, 1729).

[14] Brocklesby, *Reflections*, 26.

[15] For the discussion in this essay I have used *Marsilio Ficino Three Books on Life. A Critical Edition and Translation with Introduction and Notes*, ed. Carol V. Kaske and John R. Clark (Binghampton, NY: The Renaissance Society of America, 1989).

effects constituted a significant topic for investigation. Indeed I propose to start this paper by focusing on Bacon's treatment of music and spirit in his *Sylva Sylvarum* (1626), with a view to showing how on the one hand he drew on an intellectual tradition effectively started by Ficino and on the other he was to influence later generations of natural philosophers, including Brocklesby.

Francis Bacon's understanding of music's operation on spirits was intended to form part of his new, experimentally grounded method of discovering truths about the world. Specifically, the investigation of music's effects, including its effects on human nature, was to form part of a new subject of acoustics, a branch of physics which Bacon identified as a higher kind of natural magic.[16] The association between experiment and magic was not coincidental, since the practice of *natural* magic (in contrast to the demonic kind) concentrated on the manipulation of hidden, that is 'occult,' forces that operated throughout nature that could not easily be conceptualized in scholastic terms.[17] By contrast, the idea of practising *science* was incomprehensible before Bacon incorporated magic into his new kind of experimental philosophy, which was enthusiastically taken up by natural philosophers in the later seventeenth century and beyond.

This process of incorporation is evident in the way Bacon writes about the study of what he calls "audibles" in the *Sylva*, a subject which he had already identified as "acoustica" in his *De dignitate et augmentis scientiarum* of 1623.[18] On the one hand this discipline was to investigate the nature and causes of sounds (and note that Bacon identified music as proportional and ordered sound) and on the other it was to have an operational side, the deliberate manipulation of sounds to produce specific effects at a distance, especially through the action of sympathy, what we today call resonance. Because music in particular could dramatically alter "manners" (i.e. outward behaviour) and move the passions this empirical

---

[16] For further details see Penelope Gouk, *Music, Science and Natural Magic in Seventeenth-Century England* (New Haven and London: Yale University Press, 1999), esp. ch. 5. On the wider context of music in Bacon's writings, see Andrea Luppi and Elizabeth Roche, "The Role of Music in Francis Bacon's Thought: A Survey," *International Review of the Aesthetics and Sociology of Music* 24:2 (1993): 99–111.

[17] The linkage between natural magic and experimental science explored in Gouk, *Music, Science and Natural Magic* is also discussed in John Henry, *The Scientific Revolution and the Origins of Modern Science*, 2nd edn (Houndsmills and London: Palgrave, 2002), ch. 4.

[18] See *The Works of Francis Bacon*, ed. J. R. Spedding, L. Ellis, and D. D. Heath, 14 vols (London, 1857–74), I, 542. This term was translated as "Acoustique art" in *Of the Advancement and Proficiencie of Learning... Interpreted by Gilbert Watts* (Oxford, 1640), 135.

investigation into "audibles" came within the framework of the doctrine of man, as a form of medicine. Indeed, in Bacon's classification of knowledge, music and medicine were both arts connected to the body because of their potentially beneficial effects on the human spirit, especially the capacity to promote health and long life. Both Ficino in the fifteenth century and Brocklesby in the eighteenth also regarded music as a form of medicine partly because of its benefits as a means of prolonging life.

Before looking into music's properties in more detail it will be helpful to discuss Bacon's conception of spirit (*pneuma, spiritus*) in general and how he saw spirits operating in the universe as a whole, not just within the human body.[19] As D. P. Walker and Graham Rees have explained, Bacon's pneumatology owed a significant debt not only to Ficino and Paracelsus but also to two more recent Italian scholars, Bernardino Telesio and Agostino Donio.[20] In brief, Bacon believed that the cosmos was made up of tangible matter and two kinds of pneumatic substance. The first of these were lifeless spirits or "pneumaticals" present in both inanimate and animate bodies, being principally air and having a natural tendency to multiply and escape to the ambient air. The second kind were animate, vital spirits, a category in Bacon's system that subsumed the normal Galenic medical spirits of the natural, vital and animal kinds. These vital spirits governed growth and decay and were also the efficient cause of all animal and human activity, including all mental processing.[21]

Another name for these vital spirits was the sensible soul, which served as the instrument of the rational soul. In *De augmentis scientiarum* (1623) Bacon describes the lower, sensitive soul as an invisible, vapour-like corporeal substance "endowed with the softness of air for receiving impressions, and with the vigour of fire for launching actions" which in "perfect" animals is located chiefly in the head, runs through the nerves, and is replenished by the spiritous blood of the arteries. It was responsible for

[19] The principal sources on Bacon's cosmological theories are Graham Rees, "Francis Bacon's Semi-Paracelsian Cosmology and the Great Instauration," *Ambix* 22 (1975): 81–101, 61–73; idem, "Matter Theory: A Unifying Factor in Bacon's Natural Philosophy?" *Ambix* 24 (1977): 110–25; and idem, "Atomism and 'subtlety' in Francis Bacon's Natural Philosophy," *Annals of Science* 37 (1980): 549–71. For the operations of spirits within the body, see K. R. Wallace, *Francis Bacon on the Nature of Man* (Urbana, Ill., 1967).

[20] Rees, "Francis Bacon's Semi-Paracelsian Cosmology;" D. P. Walker, "Francis Bacon and *Spiritus*," in *Science, Medicine and Society in the Renaissance: Essays to Honor Walter Pagel*, ed. A. G. Debus (New York: Science History Publications, 1972), II, 121–30 (This is reprinted in D. P. Walker, *Music, Spirit and Language in the Renaissance* (London: Variorum, 1985)).

[21] For the Renaissance background on *spiritus* see Park, "The Organic Soul."

motor activity, sense perception and the lower mental functions including the imagination. In short, "as Bernardino Telesio, and his disciple Agostino Donio have in some measure not quite uselessly asserted... This soul might better be called by the name *Spiritus*."[22] In the *Historia vitae et mortis* (1623) Bacon explains how a knowledge of the *spiritus* has an immediately practical use: under ideal conditions, it is condensed and glows with a gentle heat, a state conducive to the prolongation of life. Without care, however, the *spiritus* becomes attenuated and/or overheated, which eventually leads to senility and death. Like Ficino in *De vita*, Bacon suggests a number of ways to maintain the integrity of the *spiritus*, including the avoidance of strong passions. Gentle passions, by contrast, are good because they strengthen and condense the *spiritus*.[23] Music is an important means of moderating passions, although it is also capable of arousing them.

So how does music affect the *spiritus*, and why can its effects be so strong on the listener? In his discussion of "audibles" in the *Sylva* Bacon observes that the sense of hearing strikes the spirits "more immediately" and "more incorporeally" than the other senses, including vision. And, although he does not say so explicitly, Bacon seems to follow Avicenna's view that sounding bodies, like visible objects, give off images, remarking that "the species of audibles seem to participate more with local motion, like percussions or impressions made upon the air."[24] Some bodies, because of an equality in their "parts" or "pores," produce musical sounds. In the case of hearing, these audible species enter the ear directly and cause either pleasure or pain as they mingle with the *spiritus* (he says nothing about the ear's anatomy), a phenomenon which is particularly clear in the case of concords and discords of music. Bacon observes that musical sounds can also produce a sympathetic response in inanimate bodies such as musical instruments. This sympathy occurs as a result of the audible species mingling with their pneumatic parts, in the same way that they mingle with the human *spiritus*. For Bacon the phenomenon of sympathy, or sympathethic vibration, was a distinctive part of the natural

22 Quotation taken from the translation in Walker, "Francis Bacon and *Spiritus*," 121–22, who took the Latin from *Works of Francis Bacon*, ed. Spedding et al., I, 606.

23 Walker, "Francis Bacon and *Spiritus*," 122.

24 *Sylva Sylvarum*, § 268. For further discussion of Bacon's theory of hearing see Penelope Gouk, "Some English Theories of Hearing in the Seventeenth Century: Before and After Descartes," in *Second Sense*, ed. Burnett et al., 95–113. On the medieval background see Charles Burnett, "Sound and its Perception in the Middle Ages," in *Second Sense*, 43–69.

world that lent itself to his new experimental method. While the causes of sympathy were 'occult' in scholastic terms (that is they were not manifest to the senses and so were not susceptible to physical explanation), in the context of natural magic and Bacon's experimentalism they were regarded as a fundamental explanation for many phenomena.[25]

As well as having an affinity with air, its medium, and the airy substance of *spiritus* there is something special about organized musical sound that communicates itself to the *spiritus* which then takes on its patterned movement. As Bacon observes, the idea that music imitates the characters and affections of the soul by virtue of its movement was held in antiquity, the different Greek modes (or *harmoniai*) reputedly having the power to make men warlike or effeminate, to make them feel solemn or to incline them to pity, and so forth.[26] Bacon appears to agree that music can do this, the cause being that

> the sense of hearing striketh the spirits more immediately than the other senses, and more incorporeally than the smelling... harmony, entering easily, and mingling not at all, and coming with a manifest motion, doth by custom of often affecting the spirits and putting them into one kind of posture, alter not a little the nature of the spirits, even when the object is removed.[27]

It is important to note that Bacon does not seem to be thinking of "harmony" in the abstract here, but has specific musical forms in mind to which the spirits have their analogue:

> And therefore we see that tunes and airs, even in their own nature, have in themselves some affinity with the affections: as there be merry tunes, doleful tunes, solemn tunes; inclining men's minds to pity; warlike tunes, &c. So it is no marvel if they alter the spirits, considering that tunes have a predisposition to the motion of the spirits in themselves. But yet it hath been noted, that though this variety of tunes doth dispose the spirits to variety of passions conform unto them, yet generally music feedeth that disposition of the spirits which it findeth.[28]

---

[25] John Henry, "Occult Qualities in the Experimental Philosophy: Active Principles in Pre-Newtonian Matter Theory," *History of Science* 24 (1986): 335–81.

[26] For Plato and Aristotle's views on the modes or *harmoniai*, and a discussion of the *harmoniai* more generally, see Andrew Barker, *Greek Musical Writings Volume I: The Musician and His Art* (Cambridge: Cambridge University Press, 1984), ch. 10 and 11.

[27] Bacon, *Sylva*, § 114.

[28] Bacon, *Sylva*, § 114.

Bacon himself did not speculate further on the relationship between music and the passions, although he devoted several sections of the *Sylva* to identifying the outward, physical signs of these inner perturbations.[29]

By contrast, Wright was more expansive in his treatment of music, which as a Jesuit he believed could be used to elevate the mind to devotion, although regrettably it might also be used for dissolute levity and lead to debauchery. (This ambiguous power of music was at the core of the Reformation debate about the appropriate place of music in worship and everyday life.)[30] Following Aristotle, Wright classified the passions as either pleasurable or painful.[31] These could be recognized by outward motions of the body, in behaviour, dress, gesture, speech and manners.[32] He also had a clear idea of why passions affect the body as well as the soul. When an object is perceived by the imagination (by means of the animal spirits) the sensitive faculty signifies to the soul whether or not the appetite should be followed. If it is pleasurable (concupiscible) it will result in animal spirits moving from the brain, the seat of the sensitive soul, via the nerves, which he calls "secret channels," to the heart, the seat of the passions, which thereby becomes dilated. By contrast, a painful (irascible) appetite leads to the heart contracting and the gathering of melancholy blood around it, resulting in an imbalance of the humours and mental disquiet.[33]

Wright acknowledges four competing explanations for the power of music.[34] The first argues for a "certain sympathy" between the soul and music, while the second invokes God's general providence for producing a spiritual quality in the soul which then stirs up a passion. For his third explanation Wright suggests that the sound itself passes through the ears and goes to the heart, which it then "beateth and tickleth" to produce "semblable passions." However, it is the fourth explanation that Wright thinks most likely, namely

[29] Bacon, *Sylva*, §§ 714–22.

[30] On the debate as it developed in England and its consequences, see Marsh, *Music and Society*, ch. 8.

[31] Wright, *Passions*, 24.

[32] Wright, *Passions*, 104–38.

[33] Wright, *Passions*, 45.

[34] Wright, *Passions*, 159–72, "How passions are moved with music and instruments." See also Gouk, "English Theories of Hearing," esp. 101–102.

> that as all other sences have an admirable multiplicitie of objects which delight them, so hath the ear… so in musicke, divers consorts stirre up the heart, divers sorts of joyes, and divers sorts of sadness or pain…[35]

Surprisingly, Wright's guarded opinion is quite similar to that of Richard Brocklesby, who also took the view that the mind has an "inexplicable faculty" to be pleased or displeased with certain airs in the same way it is delighted or dissatisfied with perceptions of the other senses.[36]

Brocklesby published his *Reflections on Ancient and Modern Music, with the Application to the Cure of Diseases* in 1749 with a view to promoting the experimental use of music in the cure of mental diseases such as madness and melancholy. Although Brocklesby himself never wrote systematically on natural philosophy, we know that he regarded Bacon as "the prime and chief philosopher of all ages" and used the latter's *Sylva Sylvarum* as a model for his own experimental method.[37] In brief, Brocklesby identified the animal spirits in the nerves (i.e. equivalent to the rarest form of Bacon's *spiritus*) as the essential link between body and mind, and argued that the temperament and complexion of the body is a 'true index' to the moral habits of the mind, while at the same time the habits of the mind influence the animal spirits and grosser parts of the body:

> For as hath been observed, nature herself has assigned to every emotion of the soul, its particular cast of the countenance, tone of voice, and manner of gesture. And the whole person, all the features of the face and tones of the voice answer, like strings upon musical instruments, to the impressions made on them by the mind.[38]

Brocklesby's main purpose was to persuade his readers of music's powers on both the body and mind, which can be shown experimentally. As part of his argument, he observes that the operation of all medicines depends almost entirely on the motion they appease or excite, and that music is no different in that it is a kind of universal incentive to motion or rest.

Of most relevance to us here is Brocklesby's discussion "on the powers of musick in disorders of the mind," the context in which he uses Ficino's

---

35 Wright, *Passions*, 168–171.

36 Brocklesby, *Reflections*, 14.

37 Brocklesby, *Reflections*, 33.

38 Brocklesby, *Reflections*, 17–18. On the use of the word 'emotion' in its modern sense rather than the more common language of the 'passions' in use in the eighteenth century see Graham Richards, "Emotions into words—or words into emotions?," in *Representing Emotions: New Connections in the Histories of Art, Music and Medicine*, ed. Penelope Gouk and Helen Hills (Aldershot: Ashgate, 2005), 49–65, esp. 53 and n. 12.

commentary on Plato to argue that music composes the motion of the animal spirits as well as the mind, which has to be well-balanced so that particular affections or passions do not disrupt the body unduly.[39] Having noted that the passions that produce the most alterations on the body are "anger, grief, excessive joy, enthusiasm in religion or love, the panick of fear and such-like," he goes on to point out that both ancient and modern evidence proves these to be the passions that have been allayed by music. In sum, if we allow that the mind is a powerful agent in particular diseases, there is a good reason to use music to allay the extreme passion of grief and sorrow, in other words, melancholy.[40]

Now I propose to look at the fifth chapter of Brocklesby's *Reflections* because it treats in detail of "the retardation of old age by the application of music," the process of prolonging life also being one of Bacon's guiding philosophical aims. Brocklesby observes that one of the principal causes of decay and premature death is the waste of animal spirits which the mind uses in producing innumerable alterations on the body. This process of depletion should make our chief goal the production of a fresh supply of spirits, or failing this the conservation of such spirits through the control of strong passions, both strategies having being recognized by Bacon as fundamental to longevity. Brocklesby is clear that the right steps for the prolongation of life will never be undertaken by the "vulgar herd of mankind," partly because most people gratify each "passing fancy" which uses up the spirits, and also partly because the required steps for delaying death are so complex they can only be practised by a few.[41]

These rare beings prove to be philosophers, the evidence being that "philosophic and abstemious men" have been notable among those who have achieved a very long life. In antiquity these included men like Democritus and Plato, in modern times they include "mathematical philosophers in particular" (although he does not mention whom he has in mind). Again we find Brocklesby citing Francis Bacon as a source of inspiration, whom he says asserted in his *Historia vitae et mortis* (1623) that "temperance and a Pythagoric life" is most conducive to longevity. By way of amplifying this claim Brocklesby notes that Plato and Pythagoras were both masters of music and geometry, suggesting that the use of music, and frequent attention to it, might promote long life. Given that he has already

39 Brocklesby, *Reflections*, 29, cited again on p. 60, where Brocklesby indicates that he is using a Leiden edition of Ficino which I have not yet been able to locate.

40 Brocklesby, *Reflections*, 33–34.

41 Brocklesby, *Reflections*, 72.

demonstrated music's power to divert and maintain the spirits, and that Bacon says that an invigoration of the spirits is the best way to prolong life, Brocklesby proposes that it might be a good idea for people pursuing this goal to put music to trial and to "recreate their spirits every day with a piece of good music."[42]

This discussion of music's integration into a "Pythagoric life" by Brocklesby gives me the opportunity now to turn my attention towards the earliest and possibly most influential Western text on this subject, namely *De triplici vita* or *Three Books on Life* by the Florentine Neoplatonist Marsilio Ficino.[43] It was first published in 1489 but like most of Ficino's other works, especially those on Platonism, *De vita* went through a number of later editions.[44] The significance of this work is that it was the first medical text intended to help philosophers maintain their spiritual health, which is impaired by too much study. For just like Brocklesby, Ficino is mindful of the bad effects of intense mental activity on the spirits. In fact (anticipating Bacon here) he also uses the word *spiritus*, and says that this hot substance is "defined by the physicians as an airy vapour of the blood used by the soul for the exercise of the exterior and interior senses," a definition which would not have looked amiss to Brocklesby.[45] Above all it is the faculty of imagination that the scholar exercises in his daily contemplations.

In fact the illness to which scholars are constitutionally prone proves to be melancholy, which according to Galenic doctrine was simply an unpleasant disease involving an imbalance of the humours, notably an excess of black bile in the blood, which dries up with too much heat. Indeed much of *De vita* is taken up with perfectly conventional methods for countering the effects of melancholy, including recommendations for diet and daily regimen. What is new in Ficino, however, is the connection he makes between melancholy, music and the spiritual life of the Platonic (but hopefully also Christian) philosopher ultimately seeking union with

---

42 Brocklesby, *Reflections*, 74.

43 On the legacy of this work see the editors' "Introduction" to *Three Books on Life*. The earliest modern discussion of Ficino's treatment of music is found in the first two chapters of D. P. Walker, *Spiritual and Demonic Magic from Ficino to Campanella* (London: The Warburg Institute, 1958). Another valuable source on Ficino's musical magic is Gary Tomlinson, *Music in Renaissance Magic: Toward a Historiography of Others* (Chicago and London: Chicago University Press, 1993).

44 Almost thirty editions of *De vita* were published between 1489 and 1647; see Tomlinson, *Music in Renaissance Magic*, 143–44.

45 Quotation from *Three Books on Life*, Bk 1, ch. 2, 110–11.

the divine, a context in which music serves as a vehicle for spiritual purification.[46] I should mention here that Ficino was not only a skilled musician and a priest but also identified himself as a follower of Pythagoras and Plato, dedicated to both religion and philosophy.[47] Thus in addition to two books appropriately entitled "On a healthy life" and "On a long life" the third book of *De vita* is entitled "On fitting one's life to the heavens" and holds out the promise of immortality, through practising a form of spiritual medicine designed more for the soul's salvation than the body's health. As Ficino wrote to his friend Francesco Musano,

> The body is indeed healed by the remedies of medicine; but spirit, which is the airy vapour of our blood and the link between body and soul, is tempered and nourished by airy smells, by sounds, and by song. Finally, the soul, as it is divine, is purified by the divine mysteries of theology.[48]

This third book, which not coincidentally is where music appears as part of the treatment for melancholy, is concerned with attracting heavenly influences, the virtues and powers of the planets, which can be used to enhance one's own *spiritus*. Early modern physicians routinely used planetary positions to understand their patients' constitutions and temperament, but in Ficino's hands astrology became a powerful means of spiritual purification, that went far beyond prevailing notions of its proper limits. And as we have just learned, he thought that one of the most effective means of tempering the *spiritus* was through the use of sounds and song.[49] Here we can see a distinct similarity with Bacon's ideas, on nurturing the spirit, although it is not clear whether Bacon drew directly on Ficino or not.

At the simplest level, Ficino thought that music has a stronger effect on man than anything transmitted through the other senses, because its medium, air, is of the same kind as the *spiritus*. Sounds combine directly with the spirits in the inner ear and are conveyed to the soul (which itself is similar to musical consonance) and also affect the whole spirit dispersed

46 Peter Serracino-Inglott, "Ficino the Priest," in *Marsilio Ficino: His Theology, His Philosophy, His Legacy*, ed. Michael J. B. Allen and Valery Rees (Leiden, Boston & Köln: Brill, 2002), 1–14. See also Angela Voss, "The Musical Magic of Marsilio Ficino" in the same volume, 227–42.

47 Christopher S. Celenza, "Pythagoras in the Renaissance: The Case of Marsilio Ficino," *Renaissance Quarterly* 52:3 (1999): 667–711.

48 Marsilio Ficino, *The Letters of Marsilio Ficino* (London: Shepheard-Walwyn, 1975), I, 40.

49 On Ficino's astrological music see Walker, *Spiritual and Demonic Magic*, 12–24; Tomlinson, *Music in Renaissance Magic*, 101–44; Voss, "Musical Magic."

throughout the body. The second reason why music has this power is because it transmits movement and is itself moving, song being "the most powerful imitator of all things." It imitates the affections of the soul, and also reproduces bodily gestures, human movements and moral characters, so that it provokes "both the singer and hearer to imitate and perform the same things." This explanation seems to have been based on Ficino's reading of the pseudo-Aristotelian *Problems*, which include two on music that ask why hearing alone affects the moral character, the answer being that sound has movements which are of the same nature as actions, and actions have a moral character.[50] As Walker points out, Ficino seems to be the first Renaissance author to take seriously the ancient Greek belief that music affects character and behaviour, and also the first to suggest practical ways of recreating the effects of ancient music.[51]

The practical techniques Ficino offers in *De vita* are for a kind of magical music that draws down planetary influences into the performer's *spiritus*, a practice which he believed used to be carried out by Pythagoras and his disciples in antiquity, who were particularly interested in the sun's (Apollo's) influence. What Ficino's Pythagorean music was like is quite hard to ascertain, and in fact, despite some modern attempts to recreate its sounds, it is impossible to reconstruct with any authenticity, just as it was impossible for Ficino himself to reconstruct the music of Pythagoras.[52] However, leaving this caveat to one side, a few conjectures about Ficino's musical experiments can still be made. According to Walker, Ficino's cryptic remarks on the subject suggest that words taken from the *Orphic Hymns* (believed at the time to be by Orpheus himself and newly edited by Ficino) were to be sung to the accompaniment of the *lira*, a word used at the time in Italy for various kinds of stringed instruments, as well as for those used in ancient Greece. The kind of *lira* that Ficino probably had in mind was the *lira da braccio*, a bowed stringed instrument actually used by Italian court improvisers to accompany their lyric poetry in a manner which was thought to resemble that of the ancient poets and orators. In essence, Ficino says that you have to make the meaning of the words, the melody to which you sing those words, and the gestures and movements

50 Walker, *Spiritual and Demonic Magic*, 8–9.
51 Walker, *Spiritual and Demonic Magic*, 25–26.
52 *The Secrets of the Heavens*, a CD recording of the Hymns of Orpheus set to music by the Marini Consort (RVRCD53), invites the listener to experience the music of the spheres in a form which follows Ficino's description of his astrological music.

with which you accompany them, 'fit' with the character and song of the planet whose gifts you want to receive.

What I want to emphasize is that whatever form they actually took, these musical techniques already presume that music is by itself capable of nourishing the *spiritus* and altering a person's disposition by occult means. However, the benefits of music can be enhanced by astrology. In particular, Ficino recommends creating songs to the sun god Apollo, to counter the malignant effects of Saturn, the planet associated with a melancholic temperament. Underlying his suggestions for aligning one's *spiritus* to a planet's character are a series of related, and essentially musical, principles. The first Ficino took from the Neoplatonic philosopher Plotinus, whose writings he was editing at the time.[53] This originally Stoic principle was the *spiritus mundi*, an extremely fine substance akin to the human *spiritus* that permeates the cosmos and is the medium of occult actions that can take place over great distances. The affinity between parts of the universe are maintained by tension or *tonos* in the way that the strings on one lyre can vibrate with those on another at a distance. The second principle derives from Plato's *Timaeus*, that both the universe and man are constructed on the same harmonic proportions, so the use of anything having the same proportions as a certain heavenly body will make your spirit similarly proportioned. Last is the principle already mentioned, that music imitates affections and moral attitudes, and therefore a planet's character can be imitated in music which can then draw its influence into the *spiritus*.[54]

Ficino's music-spirit theory had mixed fortunes after his death, but we can still trace elements of it in Bacon and Brocklesby's thought. Thus it turns out that although Bacon does not have anything to say about astrological music, and basically disapproved of magic, he nevertheless believed that music's affective power was magical since it was a phenomenon that relied on sympathy between music and spirit and had a particularly strong effect on the imagination. As such, it could be investigated experimentally with a view to controlling the passions, a goal which Brocklesby also thought worthwhile (as did Wright). But we should note that Bacon's cosmology also assumed an identity between the substance and actions of the human *spiritus* and an aetherial substance that distinctly resembles

---

53 Tomlinson, *Music in Renaissance Magic*, 85–88; Brian Copenhaver, "Astrology and Magic," in *Cambridge History of Renaissance Philosophy*, 264–300.

54 Walker, *Spiritual and Demonic Magic*, 14–18.

the *spiritus mundi*, an affinity which he thought could explain the power of fascination, for example.[55]

What is surprising is that this elision between these two substances was still being made well into the eighteenth century, most notably by the architect of a new cosmology. Thus the 1713 edition of Isaac Newton's *Principia mathematica* ends with the conjecture that all bodies contain a "very subtle spirit" by which particles of bodies attract each other, and all sensation and motion in animals take place. In the second English edition of his *Opticks* (1717), Newton again suggests that animal motion (including sensation and perception, especially hearing and sight) might be performed by the vibrations of a subtle spirit. He also suggests that the harmonic vibrations of this substance might explain why light is divided into seven principal colours in the same way that there are seven degrees in the musical scale. He further suggests that this vibrating spirit also fills the whole universe and is the medium for attractive forces such as magnetism, electricity and gravity.[56] Indeed, Newton envisaged the universe as God's sensorium, and the universal aether or *spiritus*, the vehicle through which He exercises His divine will, just as the human *spiritus* in the form of the animal spirits in the brain and nervous system serve as the vehicle for the human will. It was important to Newton that God was able to intervene in the workings of the world, actions which were carried out through operations of the spirit. This was an explicitly anti-Cartesian position because Newton rejected Descartes's idea that all motion in the universe was endowed at the time of its creation and simply followed mechanical laws.[57]

Although he does not say so directly, Brocklesby also seems to have a Newtonian concept of an active principle in nature, a view which he uses to refute the idea that Descartes's mechanical philosophy is sufficient to explain music's operation on the bodily organs. Those who reduce its effects to the "mechanical undulatory pulsation of the air, on the extremities of the nerves" are clearly wrong, not least he says because music excites commotion in the mind first, rather than the body.[58] By contrast, Brocklesby thinks that the vital functions of all animals, including man, can only be accounted for with reference to a vital principle that needs reinforcing from time to time by the active cause which initially created

[55] See Walker, "Medical Spirits."
[56] Isaac Newton, *Opticks* 2nd edn (London, 1717), 328.
[57] For the intellectual background to this position see Henry, "Occult Qualities."
[58] Brocklesby, *Reflections*, 17.

them—a belief that he says was held by the "Platonists of old": "A spirit feeds [the world] within, and, infused throughout its limbs, a mind stirs the mass and mingles itself with the great body."[59]

This emphasis on an active principle in nature distinctly recalls Newton's belief in the constant intervention of God in the world system. In fact, Brocklesby's attack on the validity of mechanical explanations was part of a broader trend in English physiology from the mid-eighteenth century onwards.[60]

In this paper I have used the relationship between music and spirit as a pathway for exploring similarities in thinking, especially about emotions or passions, between several authors whose ideas have not previously been seen as connected.[61] In my view, I think it is particularly striking to find certain patterns of thought, best described as magical, continuing well beyond the conventional cut-off point of 1700 as the end of the early modern period.[62] However, although my goal is to trace continuities or similarities over a long period of time, I am aware that these authors were writing in rather different contexts from each other, which have to be kept in mind. Ficino was a philosopher and priest whose primary aim was to offer an esoteric form of spiritual or soul medicine to a small group of scholars, a practice that drew influences from the heavens into the sensitive soul. For Wright, who was also a man of the church, music was just one of the means through which the passions could be controlled and harnessed for good rather than evil ends. Both Bacon and Brocklesby regarded music's effects as a phenomenon to be investigated experimentally, with a view to improving the practice of medicine.

However, although they expressed themselves differently, all four men concurred that music can alter the passions through its motion and that this process is effected through a spirit or spirits which connect the body to the soul. Ficino and Bacon called this medium *spiritus*, which Wright and Brocklesby identified as the animal spirits. They all seem to have

59 Brocklesby, *Reflections*, 25. This comes from the sixth book of the *Aeneid* and is Anchises' philosophizing rather than a philosophical account of the world. I owe this attribution to Leofranc Holford-Strevens.

60 See Theodore M. Brown, "From Mechanism to Vitalism in Eighteenth-Century English Physiology," *Journal of the History of Biology* 7 (1974): 179–216.

61 In this regard I have extended the time frame used by D. P. Walker in "Medical Spirits from Ficino to Newton" to argue for a continuity of ideas about *spiritus*.

62 Here I follow, but also extend, the time frame used in my own *Music, Science and Natural Magic* as well as that found in Charles Webster, *From Paracelsus to Newton: Magic and the Making of Modern Science* (Cambridge: Cambridge University Press, 1982).

followed Galenic medical theory in thinking of this entity as an airy, vital substance distilled from the blood that flows through the nerves and is responsible for sense perception, motor activity and lower mental functioning. Ficino, Bacon and Brocklesby thought that, because the use of the mind and its faculties involves the motion of this vital substance, it gradually becomes depleted, an effect which can lead to illness and even eventually death. As well as replenishing spirit, music can also "compose" its motion when it is disordered because of its own harmonically organized nature. Indeed, music can imitate particular passions by impressing the spirits with their motion and thereby may counter the effects of other passions. To sum up, my authors implicitly agreed with each other that music can have therapeutic or medicinal effects because of its similarity to spirit, and that these effects should be taken seriously (Brocklesby in particular hoped to encourage the use of music in the treatment of mentally afflicted patients).

It would seem appropriate at this point to ask what kinds of music are associated with particular passions, since they are evidently connected. Disappointingly, there is very little said about actual music in these texts, except in Brocklesby's case. In the first place Brockelsby offers his readers a fascinating case study of a Scottish gentleman whose deep melancholy was eventually overcome when his doctor arranged for a harpist to play "soft and solemn sounds" on a daily basis.[63] His second example is an anecdote of a small child who was observed by his musical parents to be full of good humour after hearing some "sprightly airs" of music. By way of experiment his father played some "chromatic and graver strains" at which the child became melancholy and sad, "which temper was remov'd as soon as pleasanter music was played."[64] In addition to these cases Brocklesby actually identifies two works by Handel which he thinks do move the passions, a quality which is apparently not shared by most modern compositions because they disregard the "laws of the rhythmus or variation of time, which is the very soul of harmony," in other words, they do not observe the proper metre in setting poetry to music.[65]

The works Brocklesby mentions approvingly are Handel's music for *Milton's L'Allegro, il Penseroso ed il Moderato* and also that for *Acis and Galatea*, works that of all his music keep "truest to the rythmus and there-

---

[63] Brocklesby, *Reflections*, 34–36.
[64] Brocklesby, *Reflections*, 36–37.
[65] Brocklesby, *Reflections*, 76.

fore afford more delight in general, than anything else of the kind."[66] Here Brocklesby seems to be speaking from direct experience of Handel's music: the first of these works was premiered on 27 February 1740 at the Royal Theatre of Lincoln's Inn Fields, while *Acis* (composed during 1718–19) was performed regularly in London up through 1741. With Brocklesby's interest in the passions in mind, the crucial feature of *L'Allegro*, for example, is that it has two main protagonists, each being the personification of a mood, the "joyful" man and the "contemplative" or "melancholic" man, passions which are conveyed both through the dialogue and the music used to accompany these verses.[67]

While much of this essay has been focused on the spirits that mediate between body and soul, I have also addressed the nature of other kinds of spirit that were thought to be similar if not identical to animal spirits, a connection that links music's effects to other forces at work in man and nature. I have shown that both Ficino and Bacon believed in a very rare substance or substances that acted as the medium for planetary influences and other hidden forces in nature just as *spiritus* acted within the body. But instead of showing that this essentially magical way of thinking about the universe just died away, as is generally thought to have happened in the Enlightenment, I have argued that some of its characteristics are discernable in Newton's cosmology. His was a dynamic universe in which the deity was presumed to intervene by means of the *spiritus mundi* or world spirit just as other vibrating substances served as media for gravity, light and sound. A similar spirit seems to have operated in Brocklesby's cosmos, which he describes in Platonic terms as a "great body" in which a mind mingles and "stirs the mass" or, in other words, infuses life into matter. In conclusion, we have seen music conceptualized in the early modern period as an animating principle which shares its characteristics with the life force, a relationship which can explain why it can have such an immediate effect on body, soul and spirit.

---

66 Brocklesby, *Reflections*, 77.

67 For example one might contrast the opening song by L'Allegro, "Hence loathed melancholy" with his next air, "Haste thee nymph," in George Frideric Handel, *L'Allegro, il Penseroso ed il Moderato*, Christine Brandes, Lynne Dawson, David Daniels, Ian Bostridge, Alastair Miles, Bach Choir, Ensemble Orchestral de Paris, cond. John Nelson, 2 CDs (Virgin Classics 7243 5 45417 2 8, 2000), CD 1, tracks 1 and 5.

INDEX